HOLISTIC NURSING

Barbara Blattner, R.N., M.P.H.

Prentice-Hall, Inc., Englewood Cliffs, N.J. 07632

Library of Congress Cataloging in Publication Data

BLATTNER, BARBARA.
   Holistic nursing.

   Includes bibliographical references and index.
   1. Nursing.   2. Holistic medicine.   3. Nursing—Psy-
chological aspects.   I. Title.   [DNLM: 1. Philosophy,
Nursing.   2. Nursing care.   3. Holistic health.   WY 86
B644h]
RT42.B53   610.73   80-39521
ISBN 0-13-392571-4
ISBN 0-13-392563-3 (pbk.)

Editorial/production supervision by Fred Bernardi and Ros Herion
Interior design by Fred Bernardi
Cover design by Jerry Pfeifer
Manufacturing buyer: John Hall

Printed in the United States of America

10 9 8 7 6 5 4 3 2 1

Prentice-Hall International, Inc., *London*
Prentice-Hall of Australia Pty. Limited, *Sydney*
Prentice-Hall of Canada, Ltd., *Toronto*
Prentice-Hall of India Private Limited, *New Delhi*
Prentice-Hall of Japan, Inc., *Tokyo*
Prentice-Hall of Southeast Asia Pte. Ltd., *Singapore*
Whitehall Books Limited, *Wellington, New Zealand*

contents

7018834

iii

foreword

Holistic living can assist you in upgrading your health, performance, and well-being; it is healing for the whole person—body, mind, and spirit. Today, holism is assuming phenomenal popularity and importance even among the lay public. This holistic approach aims at enhancing our total well-being, in part through self-awareness. By learning to gauge our own innate energy, potential weaknesses, and strengths, we can all benefit from this approach. True, it requires a great deal of self-discipline and willpower, but we must not lose sight of the vital awareness that in the final analysis each of us is responsible for his or her own health and well-being. Otherwise, no matter what new treatments are developed, we will continue to be plagued by stress-induced diseases.

Holistic Nursing presents an integrated view of health and health care services. We all know that an overload of stress depletes the body, mind, and spirit. Therefore the book places its emphasis on self-assessment, self-care, and self-direction so that students will better be able to relate to themselves, their families, and their community. By paying attention to the body's internal needs, one can recognize the need for a balance in one's lifestyle and activity. In addition, reducing stress by coping with stress-causing situations at work and at home is discussed as an integral part of the framework of this book. To health care providers, the influence of occupational stress, both upon themselves and upon their patients, is of utmost concern.

Yet I believe we can adjust our personal reactions to enjoy fully the eustress of success and accomplishment without suffering the distress commonly generated by frustrating friction and purposeless, aggressive behavior against our surroundings. In order to arrive at this stage, we must strive to practice a code of ethics based not on blind superstition, inspiration, or societal traditions, but on scientifically verifiable laws that govern the body's maintenance of homeostasis.

My own work reflects my view that holistic health can create personal fulfillment. From what the laboratory and the clinical study of somatic diseases has taught me concerning stress, I have developed three general principles readily applicable to everyday living. I have summarized these precepts as follows:

1. *Find your own natural predilections and stress level.* People differ with regard to the amount and kind of work they consider worth doing to meet the exigencies of daily

life and to assure their future security and happiness. In this respect, all of us are influenced by hereditary predispositions and the expectations of our society. Only through planned self-analysis can we establish what we really want. Many people suffer all their lives because they are too conservative to risk a radical change and break with traditions.

2. *Altruistic egoism.* The selfish hoarding of the good will, respect, esteem, support, and love of our neighbor is the most efficient way to give vent to our pent-up energy and create enjoyable, beautiful, or useful things.

3. *"Earn thy neighbor's love."* This motto, unlike "Love thy neighbor as thyself," is compatible with our biological structure; and although it is based on altruistic egoism, it could hardly be attacked as unethical. Who could blame a person who wants to assure homeostasis and happiness by accumulating the treasure of other people's benevolence? Yet this makes one virtually unassailable, for people would not attack and destroy those upon whom they depend.

Holistic Nursing shows the practicing nurse how to apply the notions of humanistic caring so that everyone can achieve their maximum potential. Every individual can effectively change his or her lifestyle, and react in his or her own way, to reach toward the goal of high-level wellness. What it comes down to is: *Fight for your highest attainable aim, but do not put up resistance in vain.*

Hans Selyé
International Institute of Stress
Montreal, Quebec

preface

Holistic Nursing proposes a conceptual model for nursing education and practice. It defines holistic nursing as the conscious application of the life processes of self-responsibility, caring, human development, stress, lifestyling, communication, problem solving, teaching/learning, and leadership and change in the intrapersonal, interpersonal, and community systems through preventive, nurturative, and generative nursing activities to help clients help themselves move toward high-level wellness. Essentially, *Holistic Nursing* is an integrated process-oriented approach to promoting health in a variety of settings and populations. It uses innovative theories and methodologies applicable to nursing and consistent with holistic health philosophies as well as orthodox medical content.

This book does not attempt to catalogue the infinite variety of holistic health options now available to health care consumers and practitioners. It does offer some criteria for evaluating and selecting quality health services with clients. The conceptual framework of the book helps sort our differing health practices and perspectives and encourages critical appraisal as a responsibility of both nurse and client.

This book grew out of a course the author designed as part of a total curriculum revision by the students and faculty of San Francisco State University, Department of Nursing. "Introduction to Holistic Nursing" was developed, taught, and evaluated for four semesters and contributed much to this textbook. The overwhelming enthusiasm and contributions students and faculty brought to the course left no doubt that a book bringing the concepts, wealth of reading material, and self-exercises together into a cohesive whole was a necessity. Nursing service colleagues echoed the plea for more information and application of holistic nursing concepts to everyday practice. The result is a trimmed, tightened, and tested piece of work that reflects the birth pangs of a new approach to nursing.

Original features distinguish *Holistic Nursing* from its predecessors and contemporaries. First and foremost, the book encourages self-assessment, self-care, and self-direction on the part of the student. With guidance and continuous "feedback," the student can self-experience and analyze responses to each of the exercises contained in the chapters and appendices. The hypothesis has been proposed and tested that a nurse who can look at and critique her own self-responsibility, caring, human development, stress, lifestyling, communication, problem solving, teaching/learning, and leadership and change processes, is a nurse who can learn to assess these processes in clients. A nurse who is engaged in the ongoing task of self-development, lifestyle modification, learning, and change is one who can nurture that striving in a client. Likewise, most of the self-assessment material has been evaluated and modified by students.

Second, *Holistic Nursing* presents a unified conceptual framework revolving around nine central life processes, each of which encompasses one or more current theories or positions with substantiating data. Each process could in itself become a book, but time and space constraints dictated choice of only a few major theories that apply directly to nursing. Certainly, the use of holistic theories and practices in nursing is only beginning.

Third, although the idea of a process approach to nursing education is not new, three of the life processes mentioned in this text are, to my knowledge, original to nursing education, that is, self-responsibility, caring, and lifestyling. Nursing has traditionally inferred this content indirectly. Chapters 2, 3, and 6 are devoted strictly to these essential processes.

Fourth, the emphasis of this book is on high-level wellness, although all the concepts also apply to illness settings and problems. The text begins where students usually find themselves—somewhere on the health, or at least asymptomatic, end of the health–illness continuum. The connection is quickly drawn between lifestyle, health, and illness. Preventive, self-nurturative, and generative lifestyle modifications are suggested specifically in the areas of self-responsibility, nutrition, fitness and conditioning, stress reduction and management, and environmental awareness. Clinical examples, self-tests, and current research all emphasize the importance of lifestyling to attain optimal health.

Fifth, the client is viewed as the chief agent of health maintenance and illness prevention. The nurse role is discussed as that of a caring colleague with major teaching and health counseling functions. The ultimate goal of health care is self-care. The nurse generates whatever alternatives necessary to assist the client in attaining that level within the scope of the situation and individual capabilities.

Sixth, examples of life processes in action are taken from alternative health modalities and settings when possible. Holistic approaches are advocated and defined, although exhaustive descriptions were not feasible. Holistic nurses are encouraged to become familiar with alternative as well as orthodox healing philosophies and methods. Various cultural healing methods are described in the hope that holistic nurses will see not only the rituals but the underlying common belief structures.

The book is organized in a sequential manner with each chapter, or life process, building on the preceding material. Occasionally, the student is asked to turn to the appendices for examples of health assessments, questionnaires, or inventories. The first chapter attempts to give an overview of holism, health, holistic health and medicine, and holistic nursing. Key concepts and life processes are pinpointed and trends identified. Subsequent chapters explore in more detail the ideas presented in Chapter 1.

The objectives for each chapter may be turned into general study questions for the student to answer while reading. Referring to the objectives frequently is recommended as a way to stay on track while covering an enormous amount of material. Chapter 6, Lifestyling, is broken into five parts to facilitate comprehension of a large amount of content, much of it new.

Including both masculine and feminine pronouns throughout the text caused tedious reading. Therefore, the feminine pronoun denotes the nurse, and the masculine most often describes the client. No sexist slur is intended.

The hope of the author is that this exciting positive approach to health and wholeness will be grasped by students and faculty and shared with clients and colleagues. The nurses who assimilate this framework and use it in their practices are the researchers who will bring forth data that will revolutionize nursing and health care as we now know it.

ACKNOWLEDGMENTS

Appreciation is extended to the faculty and students at San Francisco State University who experienced, evaluated, and expanded the life process concepts and activities with me. I am especially grateful to Sarah LaBrier, the tireless creative co-coordinator of the first holistic nursing course, who helped me develop and test many of the innovative ideas and teaching strategies contained in this book.

Acknowledgments also go to the nurse reviewers whose fine comments and works in the field of nursing education and holistic nursing encouraged and guided me: Fay L. Bower, Sylvia E. Hart, Elizabeth O. Bridston, Pat Hess, Gloria R. Burgess, Marjorie Buck, and Patricia E. Moeller.

Thanks to all the technical experts who made the coalescence of this book possible:

1. To Jim Donahue, my typist, who believed in the ideas behind the words and made them readable.
2. To Fred Bernardi, my precise and persevering copy editor, who combined wit with his perceptive questions and suggestions.
3. To Ros Herion, my book production editor, who was able to take both the smaller and the larger view in bringing hundreds of last-minute details together harmoniously.
4. To Fred Henry, my editor, who had faith in me and the concept of holistic nursing and helped me to make it a reality.

Finally, I am ever grateful to my family and friends for their unfailing support and belief in me. To my parents, John and Natalie Thorpe, who have modeled humanistic health caring for as long as I can remember. Most of all, my heartfelt thanks go to my husband, Simon Blattner, who taught me how to fight for an idea I believed in and whose time had come.

Barbara Blattner

Chapter 1
introduction to holistic nursing concepts

CHAPTER OUTLINE

CHAPTER OBJECTIVES

1. Contrast the World Health Organization's definition of health with current ideas about high-level wellness and optimal health, citing at least two prominent authorities.
2. Trace the development of Eastern and Western concepts of health and illness.
3. List the four components of holistic health as outlined by one authority in the chapter.
4. Define terminology relating to theory development in nursing and briefly describe this evolution citing major nursing theorists.
5. Differentiate preventive, nurturative, and generative nursing activities and intrapersonal, interpersonal, and community systems.
6. Describe the nine life processes used by holistic nurses in their preventive, nurturative, and generative activities with clients.

As society changes, so do nursing education and practice. Information, research, and theory are being generated and disseminated at a rate with which even the most conscientious of practitioners cannot keep pace. As more professionals become subspecialized technocrats, the need to bring together basic theories and philosophies about nursing into a comprehensive whole becomes imperative.

Competition and astronomical costs characterize our medical care system. Health care suffers, and consumers respond with anger, distrust, and legal action. The caring and cooperation between health professional and client, which are needed to facilitate health and healing, have become outdated virtues. A return to *caring* in health care is mandated.

The American people, once known as fiercely independent and proud of their diverse cultural backgrounds, have given up their rights to their bodies, their health, and their cultural healing practices. As the health care system medicalizes our lives and national budget, people are feeling the need to return to simpler, more self-sufficient lifestyles and healing methods congruent with their value systems.

Holistic Nursing proposes a conceptual framework from which to view a group of concepts, theories, and processes applicable to nursing and complex health-care problems. Many of these ideas have been tested; others are being practiced and researched. The task of this book is to weave them into a coherent whole to form the basis for a holistic nursing practice sensitive to the needs of society.

AN OVERVIEW OF HOLISM AND HEALTH

One of the most confusing issues that surrounds holistic health, medicine, and nursing is that of clearly defining terminology. The words "holistic" and "health" are both derived from the same Anglo-Saxon root, *hal*, which can mean "whole," "to heal," "sound," or "happy." The word may also be spelled with a *w* added to the base *ho* (from the later Middle English), which accounts for the word "wholistic," which is often used interchangeably with "holistic."

The Greek work *holos* means "whole," from which Arthur Koestler in 1967 coined the word "holon," to mean a "self-contained whole" when seen from below in any hierarchical system and a "dependent part" when seen from above in that system. [17] (The popular laser technique—holography—is also derived from this word.)

Development of Holistic Thought

Specific references to the development of holistic thought are difficult to pinpoint, although literature that pertains to holism generally is enormous. In 1926, Jan Christian Smuts specifically addressed *Holism and Evolution,* basing his ideas on the views of Hegel, Darwin, and others. Smuts had two intense interests—philosophy and biology. He disagreed with the analytical method employed by the life sciences to study organisms. He thought there was more to learn about the human body than could be gained from taking each part (cell, system, etc.) and studying it in isolation. He felt there was something more that pulled everything together in harmony and caused the organism to maintain itself in a fluctuating environment. He termed this organizing process "holism."

The notion of holons incorporates the idea that, depending on the position of the observer, parts can be wholes *or* the whole parts. This heretical proposition has been labeled by modern physicists as the "uncertainty principle" and is reflected by David Bohm's classic statement:

> We have reversed the usual classical notion that the independent "elementary parts" of the world are the fundamental reality, and that the various systems are merely particular contingent forms and arrangements of these parts. Rather we say that inseparable quantum interconnectedness of the whole universe is the fundamental reality, and that relatively independent parts are merely particular and contingent forms within this whole. [7, p. 138]

The position which this quote represents poses an obscure riddle not unlike those of the Eastern mystics:

> Things derive their being and nature by mutual dependence and are nothing in themselves. [7, p. 138]

The important concept contained in "holos" and "holism" is the idea of systems fluctuating to adapt to changing environments. Analyzing a system—a mathematical or biological system, for example—can be performed in various ways by various observers at various times to yield various results—each different but equally valid. Modern physicists are saying that uncertainty and variability are in themselves principles on which we must base our thinking.

More recently, D.C. Phillips has taken the works of Smuts and others and identified a holistic thesis which includes the following five points:

1. The analytic approach as typified by the physicochemical sciences proves inadequate when applied to certain cases, for example, to a biological organism, to society, or even to reality as a whole.
2. The whole is more than the sum of its parts.
3. The whole determines the nature of its parts.
4. The parts cannot be understood if considered in isolation from the whole.
5. The parts are dynamically interrelated or interdependent. [33, p. 6]

Strictly speaking, then, holism is a philosophical and biological concept which implies wholeness, relationships, processes, interactions, freedom, and creativity in viewing living and even nonliving entities. This holistic philosophy will form the basis for a holistic nursing model to be proposed later in this chapter.

Changing Definitions of Health

Holism is beginning to encompass an even broader definition when it is applied to the health sciences. Definitions of health are often matters of preference that depend on educational and cultural backgrounds and frames of reference.

In 1947, the World Health Organization made an attempt at a biopsychosocial definition of health:

> Health is a state of complete physical, mental, and social well-being and not merely the absence of disease or infirmity. [47, 1: pp. 1–2]

Current trends show health defined in a positive sense rather than by contrasting it to what it is not.

In 1958, Halpert Dunn coined his now classic definition of health as:

> . . .an integrated method of functioning which is oriented toward maximizing the potential of which the individual is capable, within the environment where he is functioning. [15, pp. 5–6]

Dunn emphasized that health or wellness was not a fixed, standardized goal to be strived for, but an ongoing process toward an ever higher potential of functioning. He saw this directional concept, which he termed "high-level wellness," as a preventive idea involving not only the individual, but also his family and community.

Seven years later, René Dubos, the public health microbiologist and philosopher, described health as an expression of fitness to the environment, as a state of adaptedness. [14] He quoted Katherine Mansfield, who died of tuberculosis, as writing, "By health I mean the power to live a full, adult, living, breathing life in close contact with what I love—the earth and the wonders thereof . . . .I want to be all that I am capable of becoming." [14, p. 351]

Don Ardell, a health planner, takes the concepts of wellness, prevention, and adaptation and arrives at the following:

> . . .high level wellness is a lifestyle-focused approach which you design for the purpose of pursuing the highest level of health within your capability. A wellness lifestyle is dynamic or ever-changing as you evolve throughout life. It is an integrated lifestyle in that you incorporate some approach or aspect of each wellness dimension (self-responsibility, nutritional awareness, stress management, physical fitness, and environmental sensitivity). [1, p. 65]

Dr. George Sheehan, sports physician, cardiologist, and marathoner, also views health from an adaptive standpoint, but laces his definition with strong implications for self-responsibility and determinism:

> Health is man adapting, man striving, man living the present and thrusting himself into the future. [40, p.91]

Ivan Illich, one of the more well-documented social critics of our time, describes health as "the intensity with which individuals cope with their internal states and their environmental conditions."

Illich goes on to say in his essay titled "Health as a Virtue" in his book, *Medical Nemesis,* that:

> Health designates a process of adaptation. It designates the ability to adapt to changing environments, to growing up and to aging, to healing when damaged, to suffering, and to the peaceful expectation of death.
>
> Health designates a process by which each person is responsible . . .responsible for what he has done, and responsible to another person or group.
>
> . . .The greater the potential for autonomous adaptation to self, to others, and to the environment, the less management of adaptation will be needed or tolerated [from professionals].

Illich concludes the book with the statement:

> Healthy people are those who live in healthy homes on a healthy diet in an environment equally fit for birth, growth, healing, and dying; they are sustained by a culture that enhances the conscious acceptance of limits to population, of aging, of incomplete recovery and ever-imminent death. Healthy people need minimal bureaucratic interference to mate, give birth, share the human condition, and die. [22, pp. 271–72]

Our definitions of health have begun to change, as have our beliefs and theories about wellness and illness.

PHILOSOPHIES AND BELIEF SYSTEMS ABOUT HEALTH AND ILLNESS

Although many cultural perspectives on health and illness exist, only two of the major forces that currently influence holistic health will be mentioned here. The term "paradigm" is chosen to describe some of these positions. Paradigm, as first described by Thomas Kuhn and applied in Figure 1–6, is a set of concepts held by a group of people with similar interests or backgrounds. [23] A paradigm is a useful conceptual framework because it holds certain assumptions that everyone concerned believes in and operates from. A paradigm usually has a special language which facilitates communication among members, and thus saves time and energy. The problem with paradigms is that any knowledge outside a specified realm is greeted with distrust and skepticism.

Throughout this text several sets of seemingly opposing paradigms will be examined, beginning with those of the Taoists and Confucianists and continuing with those of the holists and reductionists, Behaviorists and Humanists, and those who espouse Western and Eastern Perspectives on health. My position is that different paradigms share more than is realized, and that by listening to another point of view and agreeing on a common terminology some of the differences might be solved. The narrow view and the larger view both have something to offer.

Western Perspective

Western scientific knowledge began in the sixth century B.C. with the Greeks, who sought to discover the essential nature of things. In the fourth century B.C., Aristotle organized this knowledge into spirit and matter. Thus began the dualism which has shaped Western thought for 2,000 years. In the fifth century B.C., Hippocrates focused on matter and hypothesized the relationship between disease and the physical environment. This "miasma" theory was supported for years until Henle (in 1874) formulated the conditions to prove "germ theory."

It was Pasteur who actually demonstrated the existence of these microorganisms. Both theories worked well in contributing to the prevention of certain diseases, such as malaria and dysentery, and Pasteur's germ theory had two valuable aspects—one being the idea that specific microorganisms had specific effects, and the other being the belief that the resistance of a host to a specific disease was important.

The concept that specific agents (microorganisms) cause certain diseases (effects) was a great step in medical research because it aided the development of causal thinking in analyzing disease. The unfortunate point of medicine's gearing its research in this direction was that it implied only one way of looking at a health problem—from either the agent's or the host's point of view. Even our present disease classification system is based on the microbe or its effects (symptoms) on the host—for example, as in tuberculosis or cystitis. The host's own ability to reshape the disorder or its symptoms was not considered in this medical approach.

During the second half of the nineteenth century, epidemiologists* found that the agent-host diad was not sufficient to analyze all disease processes. The broader triad of agent-host-environment was synthesized, and this theory has dominated medicine ever since. Western medicine has drastically improved its knowledge of each of the components of this triad. We have witnessed the exponen-

---

*Epidemiologists study the distributions and determinants of states of health in the human population. [42, p. 3]

tial growth of such related fields as microbiology, immunology, recombinant genetics, biomedical engineering, ecology, and others. But the analysis of the unique relationship of the agent-host-environment variables to each other and to the resulting states of health or illness in individuals and populations was overlooked and/or ignored.

Medicine was not alone in its struggle out of the dark ages. Quantum physics fought its own battle to overcome the classical Newtonian paradigm that governed the collective scientific mind of the world from the seventeenth through the nineteenth centuries. Classical physics was and still is an appropriate method of conducting empirical research and analysis. It is based on several philosophies about how truth or knowledge is obtained, as outlined in the following list:

1. All complex ideas are built from a basic group of simple ideas or principles, and all knowledge can be reduced to these elements. *(Reductionism)*
2. All matter is made up of basic building blocks, the smallest of which is the atom. These can be separated and studied in their most minute form. Matter and spirit are separate entities. *(Atomism)*
3. The mind is like a machine with simple components which can be analyzed and demystified. *(Mechanism)*

Another school of thought, whose proponents called themselves the Rationalists, was led by René Descartes. To Descartes, mind and matter were separate realities. Anything material, such as the body, could be analyzed and categorized. Mind and body were in no way connected. This philosophy is known as Cartesian Dualism.

The aforementioned assumptions held sway in the scientific community until the end of the nineteenth century. It is no wonder that the science of medicine should model itself on such powerful and persuasive philosophies. The biomedical model has formulated its own assumptions which have worked remarkably well for purely physical pathologies.

Some of the assumptions of the biomedical paradigm are:

1. All aspects of human health can be understood in physical and chemical terms.
2. The aim of medical science is to analyze the structure and function of the human body in more and more detail.
3. The prerequisite basic sciences in the study of medicine are anatomy, physiology, biochemistry, molecular biology, and microbiology.
4. Study of the mind and its pathology is a separate medical specialty known as psychiatry.
5. Therapy consists of physiochemical interventions on the body machine. [42, p. 9]

The biomedical model will be mentioned throughout this text as a valid but limited paradigm upon which nursing has been based. Medicine and nursing need a broader model to encompass psychosocial, cultural, spiritual, nutritional, and environmental factors. Nursing is in the process of building that model.

Eastern Perspective

Thousands of years before the Greeks were developing their Western view of the world, the roots of Eastern mysticism were beginning in India with Hinduism. The Eastern philosophies of India, China, and Japan would not fall prey to the separate realities of mind and matter. All of life was seen as a whole from a religious perspective.

Hindus considered the body to be an integral part of the human being, unseparated from the spirit. If Hinduism was somewhat mythological, Buddhism was concerned with the mundane human condition and methods of coping with it. Buddha preached the Four Noble Truths, two of which bear repeating here:

> First, the human situation is fraught with frustration. This difficulty arises from the fact that everything around us is impermanent and transitory. Suffering results from resisting the natural ebb and flow of nature. Second, humans suffer when they cling or grasp onto a fixed view of life. This quality of separating and trying to confine the fluid forms of reality was considered ignorance by Buddha. As mankind continues to cling to its firm reality, it becomes trapped in a vicious circle called "samsara" in which every action generates further actions and each question poses new questions. This never ending chain of cause and effect is called "karma." [7, p. 95]

By the sixth century B.C., just as the Greeks were separating body and mind, the Chinese were developing two distinct philosophical schools of thought—Confucianism and Taoism. Confucius transmitted culture, social organization, common sense, and practical knowledge to his disciples. Taoism was concerned with nature and the discovery of its Way (or Tao). Taoists advocated following the natural order of things, acting spontaneously, and trusting intuition.

These two schools would seem to polarize Chinese thinking in the same way that dualism would divide Western thinkers. This did not occur, however, because opposite poles, opinions, and points of view were considered complementary and were respected as different aspects of the same question by the Chinese.

The best depiction of the Tao—the Way, process, or order of nature—is the "T'ai-chi T'u" symbol (Figure 1-1) or "Diagram of the Supreme Ultimate."

> The diagram is a symmetric arrangement of the dark yin and the bright yang, but the symmetry is not static. It is a rotational symmetry suggesting, very forcefully, a continuous cyclic movement. [7, p. 107]

The yin and yang pair have become the fundamental concept of Chinese thought. Inherent in the concept are the male and female stereotypical characteristics attributed to each sex. Figures 1-2 and 1-3 graphically depict and enumerate the characteristics of the yin-feminine and yang-masculine principle of Chinese thought and medicine.

The Institute for the Study of Humanistic Medicine (now called Synthesis

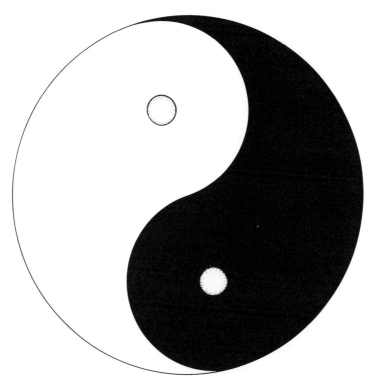

The circle represents the 'Tao' or 'T'ai Chi'
(Supreme Ultimate)

The white is the 'Yang' force
(heat, expansion, the creative, male, positive)

The black is the 'Yin' force
(cold, contraction, the receptive, female,
negative)

FIGURE 1-1 The "T'ai-chi T'u" Symbol

Graduate School) has chosen the masculine and feminine principle as the point from which to view current medical practice in Western medicine:

> The diagram suggests the equality of power and mutual interdependence of these two vast human principles. It is based on the philosophy that the power of the masculine principle is materialized by the power of the feminine principle, which makes potential energy into concrete reality. It summons up the possibility that the knowledge and will of the masculine principle require the compassion and harmony of the feminine principle and vice versa in order to be nondistinctive and to be whole. [4, p. 12]

Traditional Chinese medicine is based on the balance of the yin and yang in the human body, and any illness is seen as a disruption of this balance. The inside

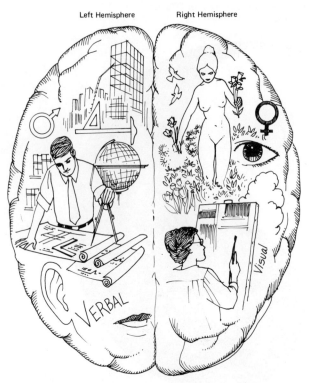

FIGURE 1–2 Left and Right Hemispheres of the Brain and Their Specialized Functions

of the body is yang, the body surface is yin; the back of the body is yang, the front is yin. Some of the organs of the body are yin, some yang. The balance among all these parts is maintained by a continuous flow of "chi," or vital energy, along a system of "meridians" which contain acupuncture points. Each organ has a meridian associated with it. Yang organs have yin meridians and vice versa. Whenever the flow between yin and yang is blocked, illness occurs and can be cured by sticking needles into accupuncture points along the meridians to stimulate and restore the flow of chi.

Another important concept in Chinese medicine is the Relationship of the Five Elements of Wood, Fire, Earth, Metal, and Water. It is believed that the mutual breeding and controlling of these elements can transform disease, change the relationship of the internal organs to each other, balance emotional and physical health, as well as balance man and his environment. Despite other philosophical differences, the thought from the *I-Ching* that in order for disease to occur there must be a "stealthy" evil and a weakened body, suggests strong parallels to Western ideas about health.

Western psychiatry has theorized related archetypal patterns of male and female in human consciousness (see Chapter 4). Studies in the area of the psychol-

Who Proposed It?		
Many sources	Day	Night
Blackburn	Intellectual	Sensuous
Oppenheimer	Time, History	Eternity, Timelessness
Deikman	Active	Receptive
Polanyi	Explicit	Tacit
Levy, Sperry	Analytic	Gestalt
Domhoff	Right (side of body)	Left (side of body)
Many sources	Left hemisphere	Right hemisphere
Bogen	Propositional	Appositional
Lee	Lineal	Nonlineal
Luria	Sequential	Simultaneous
Semmes	Focal	Diffuse
I Ching	The Creative: heaven masculine, Yang	The Receptive: earth feminine, Yin
I Ching	Light	Dark
I Ching	Time	Space
Many sources	Verbal	Spatial
Many sources	Intellectual	Intuitive
Vedanta	Buddhi	Manas
Jung	Causal	Acausal
Bacon	Argument	Experience

FIGURE 1-3 The Two Modes of Consciousness: A Tentative Dichotomy

From *The Psychology of Consciousness* by Robert Ornstein. Copyright © 1972 by W. H. Freeman and Co. Reprinted by permission of Viking-Penguin, Inc.

ogy of consciousness find physical support for both dimensions of consciousness. The split-brain phenomenon was reported in *Scientific American* in 1967 and has been an area of study for Dr. Robert Ornstein in San Francisco. It is believed that the left hemisphere is predominantly concerned with what the Chinese would call the yang mode of consciousness, while the right hemisphere appears to account for the yin or feminine mode which is involved with visualization and dreaming.

There is an increasing body of evidence to support the split-brain phenomenon, that is, that there are two modes of consciousness corresponding to each half of the brain which is specialized according to certain predictable functions (see Figure 1-2). Early research was performed on animals and then on severe epileptics in which the *corpus callosum*—the communication channel between the left and right cerebral hemispheres—was severed. Figure 1-3 summarizes the findings of over fifteen researchers and writers who have studied the analytic and intuitive aspects of the split-brain.

From anatomy and physiology, it is known that the left side of the body is primarily controlled by the right side of the cortex. Conversely, the right side of the body is controlled by the left side of the cortex. Each hemisphere shares some functions and both sides participate in most activities. The majority of people have predictable functions for which a particular hemisphere has responsibility. Most people in contemporary Western society are left-hemisphere-dominated. The challenge to holistic nurses is to nurture, enhance, and bring into balance the historically suppressed right hemisphere mode of consciousness for health and wholeness.

Two major points of view about health and illness have been presented. They are by no means all-inclusive. Native American healers, curanderos of South America, and Filipino healers represent a few more of the many exciting healing philosophies and practices not mentioned. Each has its own approach, ritual, and contribution to make. Some cultural healing philosophies have commonalities, which are mentioned in Chapter 8.

Belief in the healer and/or the healing method, currently termed "placebo effect" is one such common thread and has received a great amount of attention recently. In Latin, the word *placebo* means "I shall please." In medicine it is considered "an inactive substance or preparation given to satisfy the patient's symbolic need for drug therapy, and used in controlled studies to determine the efficacy of medicinal substances." [26]

Dr. Jerome Frank, of Johns Hopkins Medical School, theorizes that the symbol (placebo) triggers a healing visualization in the client. [18] The implications for further mind over body research are countless. The important factor is the expectation or belief of the person being healed or healing himself.

Scientists have long recognized that about one third of all patients get relief from pain when they are given placebos. It has only recently been found that the endogenous pain killer, endorphin, is produced when a placebo is administered for pain. The literature contains numerous references to many kinds of antibiotic, antihypertensive, antihistimine-like effects produced by placebos. What specific chemicals are responsible for the varied effects is still unknown.

Scientific investigations are being conducted to define the placebo's effects and limitations. Pharmacologically active drugs always effect more than the designated target organ or system and often produce undesirable side effects. Perhaps channeling the powerful placebo could decrease these untoward effects. Why some people respond to placebos and others do not is another topic for research and discussion.

In addition to the placebo effect, a whole realm of brain sciences as they relate to health and healing is opening up. A recent symposium sponsored by the University of California, San Francisco Continuing Education in Health Sciences, and The Institute for the Study of Human Knowledge, explored the healing brain, the benefits of laughter, the effect of stress on the immune system, and the specialization of the two halves of the brain.

Over fifty years ago, Smuts summarized the mind-body connection more ably than he may have realized:

> Mind in "volition" is an inner self-direction of the structure of Body. Body, giving rise to mental "sensation," is simply performing that mutation or creative leap, which we have found at every other state of evolution . . .

Mind and Body as elements in the Human Personality influence each other because of their co-presence in this creative whole of personality . . .It is the Holism in which they both "live, move, and have their being" that is the real explanation of whatever happens or appears to happen between them. It is the third which is greater than both of them, that really counts. To me this is the last word in the relations of mind and body, of the spiritual and the physical. It may sound strange and mystic; but it is the simple fact that the whole in this case, personality, makes all the difference. [41, pp. 270–71]

HOLISTIC HEALTH

Holistic health, although a seeming restatement of terms, has only come into popular usage in the past ten years. It is difficult to get a universally accepted definition of the phrase and many practitioners have given up trying.

Dr. Don Fink, professor at the University of California, San Francisco School of Medicine, defines holistic health as:

A term being used currently to describe concepts and practices of health care that transcend or radically alter current health care practices. Included under this rubric are concepts of humanistic medicine, alternative health care, pre-primary care, and altered provider-patient relationships. [17, p. 23]

Each of these concepts will be addressed throughout the text within the framework of holistic nursing.

Humanistic Medicine

Each of the subconcepts of holistic health warrants explanation. The first—*humanistic medicine*—encompasses all the medical specialties and espouses some of the ideas contained in humanistic psychology. Although humanistic medicine deals with illness, it focuses on the presence of health in the person who happens to be ill. All illness has a meaning for the individual and part of the role of the helper is to help the person discover the message and the positive value of the illness. For example, some illnesses force people to stop, take stock of their lives, and perhaps, embark on new life courses. In other words, clients can be helped to grow through a seeming tragic loss of role, self-esteem, body-image, and so on.

Clients cannot be seen only as diseases or diagnoses. The role of the professional is more than that of technical specialist. Clients and helpers cooperate and collaborate to devise new approaches to health. The client is encouraged to assume increasing responsibility for choices.

Every client is viewed as a unique, feeling individual with potentials for strength, wisdom, and untapped resources. Health is the maintenance of the dynamic relationship of body, mind, and spirit in a constantly fluctuating society and environment. Humanistic medicine is attempting to work within the present health care system, helping it move toward the holistic approach. The basic tenets of humanistic medicine are held by most of those who support the holistic philosophy.

Alternative Health Care

The second concept included in holistic health—*alternative health care*—is defined as a choice between two exclusive possibilities for a situation presenting a choice. Alternative usually means, when applied to alternative health care, a choice or the opportunity to choose among several possibilities. Alternative health care can be seen in four different ways.

Accepted Medical Techniques Applied in a New Way

The first way refers to the more extensive use of American medical techniques applied to problems for which they have been either insufficiently or ineptly utilized. An example would be applying hypnosis to an obesity problem rather than prescribing a diet pill. Hypnosis has long been accepted by the medical community but has not been applied specifically to obesity until recent years.

New Techniques for Old Problems

Another use of the term alternative health care is in reference to the utilization of newer techniques. Included in this category are techniques such as autogenic training and biofeedback. The research on these newer techniques is still being conducted and reported but it is certainly increasing in scientific community acceptance.

Nonmedical Techniques for Health Problems

The third use of alternative health care is in reference to nonmedical techniques to treat health problems. This would mean using approaches like polarity, massage, rolfing, and tai-chi in an effort to optimize health. An example of this meaning of alternative in the area of pathology and healing would be the use of "Therapeutic Touch" or the use of visualization and imagery in the treatment of cancer.*

Non-Western "Unscientific" Techniques

Finally, alternative health care is often used to describe certain highly organized health systems, concepts, and practices that are apart from Western scientific medicine. Examples of these would be Chinese acupuncture, acupressure, American Indian healing systems, and shaman healing practices to relieve pain. Chapter 8 will describe a few of these systems in more detail.

*A glossary of some holistic terms currently in use can be found in Figure 1-4.

FIGURE 1-4 Glossary of Holistic Terms

Reprinted with permission of M. Lawrence Podolsky and Modern Medicine Publications, from "Wholistic Medicine: What Is It, Who Practices It, Who Needs It?" *Modern Medicine,* 44, no. 13 (July 1977), 76–93.

Acupuncture: Insertion of fine needles or wires along established "meridians" in the body.

Bates method or Bates eye system: Philosophy and exercises that enable user to see without glasses.

Bioenergetic and Reichian therapy: Explores the relationship between love, depression, anxiety, and transcendental experience and the body's energy flow.

Bioenergetic workshop: Relates energy flow to body tension and emotional release.

Biofeedback: Electroencephalographic, electromyographic, galvanic skin response, and temperature recordings are used to ascertain focuses of general anxiety and tension; once these are recognized, through proper training individuals can learn to abort the onset of such symptoms as bruxism, hypertension, torticollis, tension and migraine headaches, Raynaud's phenomenon, stuttering, insomnia, and phobic reactions.

Biorhythms: A method of finding natural, cyclical human rhythms and discovering how artificial environment masks and interferes with them.

Birth without violence: Stems from the work of Frederick LeBoyer. Upon delivery, babies are immersed in warm water and all traumatic influences such as bright light and loud noises are removed.

Chakra analysis: Measures level of reality, psychologic state, and spiritual state (karma).

Dance therapy: Rhythmic movement, using dancing of all kinds, to encourage grace with exercise in a noncompetitive atmosphere.

Feldenkrais: A method (developed by Dr. Moshe Feldenkrais) of "functional integration": altering habitual movement responses through education of the central nervous system.

F. M. Alexander technique: A discipline of conscious control for self-improvement, stressing the relationships of breathing, speaking, rest, effort and stress, and balance.

Gestalt experience or process: A way of learning to be more fully present, more whole or centered, and more alive.

Graphology: A study of handwriting to reveal ambitions, fantasies, goals, and talents as well as thinking patterns, social habits, physical condition, and state of maturity.

Healing experience: By teaching ourselves to respond to our internal as well as external environment, we can release unwanted emotions, symptoms, and maladaptive habits. As the mind-body becomes attuned, it acts in accord with its changing experience.

Iridology: Looking into the eyes for telltale signs of illness, anxiety, or disturbing influences.

Jin Shin Jyutsu: A type of massage administered by applying finger pressure along the acupuncture meridians.

(continued)

Kinesiology: Use of muscle-testing indicators and muscle-strengthening techniques. Stresses manipulation at origin-insertion, neurovascular and meridian therapy.

Life change index: Measures factors causing anxiety or stress, e.g., "Foreclosure of mortgage = 30 points," "Traffic ticket = 11 points." More points mean more chances of becoming ill.

LiTE program: Life-threatening Illness, Therapy, and Education. Based on the belief that constructive attitudes, emotions, and habits can strengthen the natural immune system of the body against disease.

Natural birth control: Participants learn four methods of calculating fertile and infertile days, using astrology and lunar phases as well as traditional rhythm method.

Nutrition-health-activity profile (includes nutrition evaluation profile): Questions about dietary preferences and symptoms, e.g., Do you drink tap water? Do you use iodized salt? Do you smoke?

Rolfing: A technique of manipulation developed by Dr. Ida P. Rolf, an organic chemist at Rockefeller Institute. Rolfing applies manipulative force to the fascia, thus "lengthening and centering the body along its vertical axis together with an increased engagement of the deep musculature."

Senoi dream work: Application to dreams of techniques derived from the Senoi ("dream people") of the central Malay peninsula. These enable one to remember dreams with vividness and lucidity and to exercise control over the dream state.

Shiatsu: Finger pressure techniques combined with massage, some overlapping with jin shin jyutsu (q.v.), and with meditation and exercise.

Somatic psychology: Aimed at increasing mind-body integration through psychodiagnostics, psychotherapy, hypnosis, and meditation.

Spiritual consultation: Exploring energy fields that surround living matter (energy patterns, thought patterns) with the assistance of a clairvoyant or psychic.

Tai-chi-chuan: A system of exercises, performed slowly in a continuous series of simple and graceful movements, originating in China over a thousand years ago during the T'ang Dynasty.

Transpersonal group: A group experience designed for those struggling to integrate their spiritual and personal aspects. It focuses on individual Dharma or life path together with gestalt and Jungian dream work, fantasy, and meditation.

Unstressing: A combination of meditation, autogenic training, systematic desensitization, relaxation exercises, and biofeedback.

Yoga: Basic asanas (postures), principles of balance, deep breathing, and meditation.

FIGURE 1-4 (continued)

Preprimary Care

The third concept—*preprimary care*—is defined as a health care system which consists of health care problems that are managed by people themselves. Included in this class are the entire self-help and self-care movement. An example is the women's self-help movement in which groups of people get together and pool their cultural healing practices and knowledges to help each other. Self-care will be described in more detail in Chapters 2 and 3.

Altered Provider-"Patient" Relationship

Finally, and perhaps most important in holistic health, is the *altered provider-patient relationship.* The use of the word "patient" is inaccurate, except in the lowest or first level of the activity-passivity model pictured in Figure 1–5, in which the patient is a dependent person. Passive receiving is often what the word "patient" connotes. The health practitioner-patient relationship can be described as a typical parent-child relationship.

For the remainder of this book the word *client* will be used to denote a person seeking optimal health, usually enlisting the support of a health care provider.

According to Drs. Szasz and Hollender, there are two more levels which increase the client's independence. [45] Level two exists when the patient is still ill but is perceived as being aware of what is going on and capable of following directions and of exercising some judgments. Szasz and Hollender compare this to the relationship between an adolescent and a parent. [45]

FIGURE 1-5 Altered Provider-"Patient" Relationship Model

Adapted from Don Fink, "Holistic Health: Implications for Health Planning," *American Journal of Health Planning*, 1 (July 1976), 23–31.

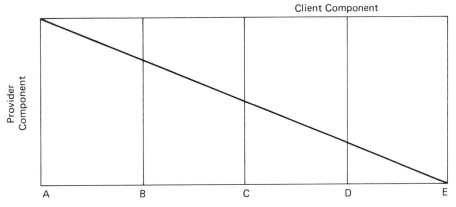

A—Activity/passivity
B—Guidance/cooperation
C—Mutual participation
D—Patient as primary provider
E—Self care

The third level is termed mutual participation, in which the health care person helps the client to help himself. This could be described as a collegial relationship. The health care person has most of the knowledge, but it is shared with the client.

The fourth level, added by Dr. Fink, views the client as the primary provider, who bears responsibility for health or illness, and who is recognized as the primary healer. [17] The health care person, whether physician or nurse, is merely a consultant, providing counsel and assistance whenever called upon.

The fifth, final, and highest level of the grid is that of self-care. We are hearing more and more about this trend as health care costs and health insurance premiums skyrocket. Self-health care is being encouraged by Kaiser Permanente and now by Blue Cross/Blue Shield. This level exists when the individual requires no outside assistance. The individual is able to create his own reality, his own health, and is considered to be the best resource for achieving his own level of optimal wellness. This self-help phenomenon is gathering momentum as the marketplace is flooded with *"Take Care of Yourself"* manuals [46] and such over the counter self-diagnostic technology as early pregnancy testing kits.

One of the fears expressed by proponents of the biomedical approach to health is that self-care and holistic approaches will bring about a barrage of misdiagnoses, unnecessary emergencies, and preventable deaths. Use of any one approach to the exclusion of all others is always dangerous, as is demonstrated by a study which found that 4 percent of psychiatric consultations requested for clients proved to be "obvious organic diseases" which had been erroneously diagnosed by the referring physician as psychiatric, "believing that the patient's symptoms were imaginary." [31; Saraway and Koran as quoted in Pelletier, p. 29]

Holistic Medicine

Dr. Kenneth Pelletier in his book, *Mind As Healer; Mind As Slayer,* describes a set of premises that constitute the basis of what he determines to be a holistic perspective. The premises are familiar:

1. The whole person is treated through an integrated approach.
2. Each individual is unique and represents a complex interaction of body, mind, and spirit.
3. The patient and the health practitioner share the responsibility for the healing process. The patient's responsibility is to become an active participant, exercising his volition in regard to his own health, lifestyle, and further development.
4. Health care is not exclusively the province or responsibility of orthodox medicine. Diagnosis and treatment of pathology is a medical concern. The creation of a lifestyle conducive to health maintenance and personal fulfillment is beyond the limited scope of pathology correction. Included in this idea is a multidisciplinary approach requiring mutual interaction and enrichment among many professions oriented towards helping clients achieve their own level of wellness.
5. Illness is seen as a creative opportunity for the patient to learn more about himself and his fundamental values.
6. The practitioner must come to know himself as a human being. [32, pp. 318–21]

Dr. Pelletier feels that those in the healing professions must become acquainted with their own emotional nature, personality conflicts, and weaknesses, and generally engage in a process of self-exploration. Included in this idea is the exhortation to health professionals to go beyond the constraints of disease and death, to "follow the part of the heart." [32; Don Juan as quoted in Pelletier, p. 322] Throughout this book self-exploration, self-responsibility, and humanistic caring will be emphasized and encouraged.

THE GROWTH OF THE HOLISTIC HEALTH MOVEMENT

Depending on which use of the words alternative health care is chosen, the holistic movement can be considered as either thousands of years old or hundreds of years old. The Chinese medical system has been in existence for thousands of years. Western medicine can trace holistic healing back to Homeopathy, Hippocrates, and the New Testament. Very few methods other than prayer, touch, and word were used in these healing processes.

More recently (in 1958), a center for self-healing exploration and personal development was begun. This center was founded in Meadow Lark, California, by Dr. Evart Loomis. Dr. Loomis subscribes to two beliefs. The first is that mental and emotional tensions, coupled with toxins in the body, lie at the root of illness. [1] The second is that the human body has an innate root wisdom in which it maintains or recovers its own perfection when it is allowed to function unhindered. [1] A typical program at Meadow Lark would involve taking a very complete series of medical and attitude inventories, as well as spending time with a counselor. Two major programs might be prescribed: one might be biofeedback, yoga, polarity, massage therapy, or art and color workshops; the other program would be a nutritional one. This would include large quantities of whole grain foods, many raw vegetables, juices, and fruits. There would be no processed or canned goods, no refined sugar, no foods with any preservatives in them, no coffee, tea, chocolate, or carbonated beverages. The program can guarantee a certain amount of consistency and control because it is a residential one.

The pioneering holistic health and wellness focus of Dr. Loomis has been replicated in Dr. John Travis' Wellness Resource Center in Mill Valley, California. Dr. Travis has developed the directional diagram, as pictured in the appendices at the end of this book.

This model is based on the high-level wellness concept described in 1961 by Halpert L. Dunn. [15] Dunn pictured wellness as the times when a person is alive with glow of good health with wellness, "alive to the tips of his fingers, with energy to burn, tingling with vitality. At times like these the world is a glorious place!" [15, p. 2] Most people, most of the time, are somewhere between this and the other end of the health continuum. The definition of health used by the World Health Organization calls for all wellness states to happen together—wellness of the body, of the mind, of the spirit, and of the environment.

Dunn makes another interesting point that doctors, nurses, and health workers tend to focus on disease, disability, and death to the exclusion of these wellness factors. He hypothesizes that this is because their training is as curers of disease rather than as advocates of positive wellness. Health practitioners are trained to find disease more interesting than wellness. Dunn feels it is easier to fight against sickness than to fight for a condition of greater wellness. The attitude of the health care person often reflects those of patients or clients—that is, when patients are sick they want to get well. But when they are free from sickness, these same people are rarely interested in becoming more well. As long as they have no symptoms, why should clients worry about working toward an even higher plane of wellness?

If a client enrolled in John Travis' Wellness Resource Center program, he would find himself taking a series of nutrition and activity profiles and a medical history. Then he would be given a program which includes the following:

1. Relaxing
2. Experiencing self
3. Removing barriers
4. Improving communications skills
5. Enhancing creativity
6. Envisioning desired outcomes
7. Taking full responsibility for self
8. Loving

The Wellness Resource Center program focuses on four major areas—stress control, self-responsibility, nutrition, and physical fitness. [1, p. 9] These areas will be referred to as *human lifestyling elements* throughout this book. This term was coined in 1975 by John C. McCamy, to express the concept of lifestyle change to achieve optimal health. [25, p. 3]

Lifestyle refers to the beliefs, values, and needs of the total person. Lifestyle is the person's unique way of living. This includes everything from an individual's communication skills to methods of solving financial problems. Dr. Travis has a traditional medical background, but he found a great need for wellness medicine. The Wellness Resource Center is attempting to make an impact not only on preventive health but also on the orthodox illness-oriented medical care system.

Many other holistic health centers are beginning to surface across the country.* (See appendices for a general list of holistic organizations.) They stress humanistic health care, high-level wellness, and unity of body/mind/spirit. The health worker and the client become coworkers toward optimal well-being. Holistic practitioners believe that an illness often enables and motivates an interest in the lifestyle changes required for personal growth and better health. Differences between holistic and orthodox medical care are well demonstrated in Marilyn Ferguson's diagram pictured in Figure 1–6.

---

* Since the focus of this book is optimal and preventive health, the numerous alternative healing centers dealing with specific illnesses and their treatment will not be emphasized.

OLD PARADIGM OF MEDICINE	NEW PARADIGM OF MEDICINE
Treatment of symptoms.	Search for patterns, causes.
Specialized.	Integrated, concerned with the whole patient.
Emphasis on efficiency.	Emphasis on human values.
Professional should be emotionally neutral.	Professional's caring is a component of healing.
Pain and disease are wholly negative.	Pain and disease may be valuable signals of internal conflicts.
Primary intervention with drugs, surgery.	Minimal intervention with Appropriate Technology, complemented with full armamentarium of non-invasive techniques (psychotechnologies, diet, exercise).
Body seen as machine in good or bad repair.	Body seen as dynamic system, a complex energy field within fields (family, workplace, environment, culture, life history).
Disease or disability seen as entity.	Disease or disability seen as process.
Emphasis on eliminating symptoms, disease.	Emphasis on achieving maximum body/mind health.
Patient is dependent.	Patient is (or should be) autonomous.
Professional is authority.	Professional is therapeutic partner.
Body and mind are separate; psychosomatic illnesses seen as mental; may refer to psychiatrist.	Bodymind perspective; psychosomatic illness is the province of all health care professionals.
Mind is secondary factor in organic illness.	Mind is primary or co-equal factor in all illness.
Placebo effect is evidence of power of suggestion.	Placebo effect is evidence of mind's role in disease and healing.
Primary reliance on quantitative information (charts, tests, dates).	Primary reliance on qualitative information, including patient reports and professional's intuition; quantitative data an adjunct.
'Prevention' seen as largely environmental: vitamins, rest, exercise, immunization, not smoking.	'Prevention' synonymous with wholeness: in work, relationships, goals, body-mind-spirit.

FIGURE 1-6 Changing Times, Changing Paradigms

Adapted from *The Aquarian Conspiracy: Personal and Social Transformation in the 1980s,* copyright © 1980 by Marilyn Ferguson. Published by J. P. Tarcher, Inc. Used by permission.

A CONCEPTUAL MODEL FOR HOLISTIC NURSING

Holistic nursing incorporates many of the ideas of holistic health, holistic medicine, and wellness medicine. It differs from them, however, in that it is based on a firm and different set of concepts called the conceptual framework. A *conceptual framework* is usually a theoretical construct which serves as a decision-making guide for building, in this case, a nursing curriculum. [3, p. 6] Do nurses recognize and see value in such a framework?

A small study was conducted at the University of Wisconsin, Milwaukee, in the baccalaureate nursing program to determine the value, if any, of conceptual frameworks to new graduate nurses. [19] Questionnaires were received from sixty-nine graduate nurses who had four to nine months of nursing experience. Seventy percent of the respondents felt that "a concept of nursing provided a basis for a unified approach to their practice of nursing." [19, p. 548] The researchers concluded that the graduates used a conceptual framework in their practice and were able to distinguish their nursing role from those of other professionals. The study also suggested that identification and use of a conceptual framework of nursing while still in a baccalaureate program positively influenced professional practice later on.

The conceptual framework for nursing was originally proposed in 1975 by Shirley Chater as a foundation on which to build a curriculum. [9] It has been used by Fay Bower as a basis for making nursing decisions. [6] Em O. Bevis has elaborated on it and incorporated those processes she feels to be essential in nursing to help clients achieve optimal wellness. [3] The six subprocesses she identified are (1) stress-adaptation, (2) decision making, (3) communication, (4) learning, (5) human development, and (6) change. [3, p. 14] These life processes now form the basis for developing a holistic nursing conceptual model for this book.

Evolving Nursing Models

Nursing practice has undergone several major model changes; current models focus on stress, problem solving, human needs, maturation, interaction, medicine, and/or a synthesis of all these. [5] Recent years have seen nursing theories drawn from the basic behavioral and social sciences and applied uniquely to nursing problems and situations. Continuing nursing research is adding to the *nursing* data base and contributing to theory building.

The holistic nursing model presented in the next section and used throughout this text is derived from several sources. Smuts' original notions about holism, for example, flowing, growing, expanding, and evolving; and Em O. Bevis' definition of process as it relates to systems theory terminology and to nursing. [41; 5] Nursing is defined as a process rather than as a function or as a circumscribed amount of content. *Processes use* theory and facts to achieve a specified goal. For example, holistic nurses use certain processes such as problem solving, human development, and communication in every nurse-client interaction they engage in in order to promote high-level wellness.

Bevis describes processes as having three characteristics: (1) purpose or goal, (2) organization or specific method or structure, and (3) infinite creativity or innovation. [3, p. 14] The holistic nursing model proposed is made up of nine "life processes" that meet Bevis' criteria. Six of them are so-called by Bevis and others. [3, p. 14] Purpose, organization, and innovation also describe the systems approach now used universally to analyze tasks and problems in all spheres of life from business to nursing. Chapter 8 explains the application of the systems view of life and its relationship to holistic nursing.

The nine life processes are used by holistic nurses on themselves and with individuals, families, and communities to prevent illness, to nurture health and wholeness, and to generate creative ways of living and healing. Three of the life processes are new to the process model of nursing and make it particularly holistic. These processes are self-responsibility, caring, and lifestyling. Each element of the holistic nursing model will be briefly described in the next section; an entire chapter of the text will then be devoted to each of the nine life processes defined.

The Holistic Nursing Model

The very nature of holism incorporates the idea of overlapping, interweaving, continuously changing processes. Figure 1–7 gives a graphic representation of this dynamic relationship in the holistic nursing model.

Intrapersonal, Interpersonal, and Community Lifespaces

The goal of nursing is to use preventive, nurturative, and generative activities to assist clients towards achieving their own high-level wellness. This is done by purposefully utilizing the nine life processes of self-responsibility, caring, stress, lifestyling, human development, problem solving, communication, teaching/learning, and leadership and change with self, client, and community. These processes are focused in one, two, and/or three systems, areas, or lifespaces.

The first area is the *intrapersonal* system, environment, or lifespace, that is, the nurse or client with his own unique value system, beliefs, fears, needs, etc. The second, the *interpersonal* system, is defined as groups of two or more people, such as families or the nurse and a client. The third area of holistic health nursing practice is the *community* system, which is comprised of a group of people having a common interest and organization. The three systems are interrelated, interdependent, and are worked in simultaneously. The focus, introductory level, and length of this text dictate a major emphasis on the intrapersonal lifespace. However, some interpersonal and community applications will be included for demonstration purposes. This interconnectedness occurs again in the three kinds of activities nurses engage in—preventive, nurturative, and generative.

Preventive, Nurturative, and Generative Nursing Activities

Preventive nursing activities are those which maintain and promote health and prevent health disruption. Preventive nursing activities comprise the major thrust of this text. Specific terminology and methods as they relate to preventive nursing will

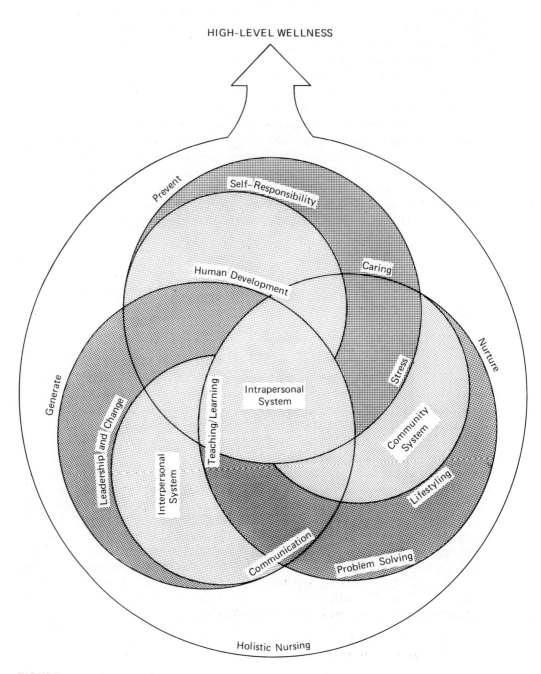

FIGURE 1-7 The Holistic Nursing Model

be described in Chapters 5 and 6. *Nurturative* activities are those involving caring, comforting, supporting, and sustaining. *Generative* activities are those creative nursing actions which foster innovative healing techniques that encourage client, family, and community self-care and self-help. Researching alternatives to orthodox methods of practice in a basic or applied investigation are included in generative nursing.

The practitioner may be plagued with blurring of definitions and need help distinguishing one type of activity from another. There will often be some overlapping of function when devising nursing care. It is important to include *all three types* of nursing measures in a holistic nursing-care plan.

Clinical examples appear in the following diagram:

PREVENTIVE NURSING ACTIVITIES

1. Enforce environmental safety program in clinical setting
2. Carry out isolation procedures
3. Conduct wellness inventory and health hazard appraisal
4. Explain stress-reduction to hypertensive client
5. Teach prenatal nutrition class

NURTURATIVE NURSING ACTIVITIES

1. Encourage angry client to express feelings
2. Support family of dying relative
3. Provide massage to clients
4. Use positive reinforcement and caring in teaching a retarded child activities of daily living
5. Use therapeutic touch or "Laying On Of Hands" with a comatose client

GENERATIVE NURSING ACTIVITIES

1. Help desirous clients to explore alternative healing methods
2. Institute self-care group in senior citizen centers and convalescent homes
3. Teach assertiveness and self-help to third-world groups
4. Gather data on clients willing to experiment with new holistic techniques
5. Teach body therapies/massage to prospective parents and couples

---

The Self-Responsibility Life Process

Self-responsibility is a sense of accountability for one's own well-being. It assumes self-awareness. It is the cornerstone of holistic health nursing. To be self-aware means to know and care for oneself, to recognize one's own limitations as well as one's strengths. It includes a person's ability to create a negative state of being filled with ill health, unhappiness, and accidents. By the same token, a positive state of being can be created.

People are responsible for their own bodies and minds. They can choose sickness or health. They can have control over their lives and minds, their bodies, and their health. Self-responsibility begins first with the nurse. This is self-responsibility at the intrapersonal level. This responsibility can then facilitate the nurse-client relationship in the interpersonal system. Finally, self-responsibility can be extended to include the nursing care of the community system.

The Caring Life Process

Milton Mayeroff is a philosopher who has attempted to define caring and its ingredients in a fashion particularly applicable to holistic nurses. [24] Caring for a person in the most significant sense is helping him to grow and to actualize himself. Caring as helping another grow and actualize himself is a process, a way of relating to someone that involves development in the same way that a friendship can only emerge in time through mutual trust and a deepening and qualitative transformation of that relationship. [24, p. 1]

It is believed by Mayeroff that caring has a way of ordering people's values and activities around it. Caring can then provide a basic stability in a person's life. Through caring a person lives the meaning of his or her own life. Nurses learn first to care for themselves and their significant others and to apply this process to their clients in a mutually growing relationship. The process of caring is examined by looking at and experiencing its ingredients individually and then reordering them into the whole. The previously discussed concept of humanistic medicine is inherent in this process of caring.

Paterson and Zderad have effectively and eloquently described the meaning of humanistic nursing. They view nursing as an experience "lived between human beings." [30] Humanistic nursing is seen as

> more than a benevolent and technically competent subject-object one-way relationship guided by a nurse in behalf of another. Rather it dictates that nursing is a responsible searching, transactional relationship whose meaningfulness demands conceptualization founded on a nurse's existential awareness of self and of the other. [30, p. 3]

Nursing, above and beyond its clinical specialty areas based on the Western medical model, is a human response to a human situation. It supersedes functional and illness-oriented boundaries and concerns itself with the actualizing of the human potential as much as is humanly possible given the client's life situation.

The Human Development Life Process

Human development includes those processes by which a person grows and matures (in the genetic biological sense) in a sequential predictable fashion as well as becomes a unique ever-changing person with increasing capacities for change and achievement towards self-actualization. Nurses should review their own process of growth and development from genetic determinants to psychosocial influences. They trace the emergence of the self and self-esteem. They recognize and apply developmental principles and selected theories to their own growth process. Theories representing intellectual, psychosocial, moral, and motivational development are applied to self and then to clients.

Nurses are able to define and assess normal developmental parameters in others. They are able to identify deviations from normal and to refer for correction. They can counsel and teach preventive and promotive health measures to individuals and families. They can utilize and mobilize community resources to help individuals or communities solve health problems which can maximize conditions for normal development.

Nurses are able to predict high risk populations for developmental problems and crises. They can plan individual and group preventive health programs based on their assessment.

Certain age specific health problems are of particular interest to holistic nurses. One of these is the plight of the senior citizen in our youth-oriented culture. To disengage or self-actualize is the question families and health professionals alike are studying and asking themselves. Selected self-development strategies are proving effective in this burgeoning area of gerontology. The holistic nurse is prepared to implement and teach these innovative ideas and methods in the institutional and community setting.

The Stress Life Process

Stress is viewed as the "nonspecific response of the body to any demand made upon it." [38, p. 472] Terminology surrounding Selyé's stress concept is defined, critiqued, and broadened to encompass newer ideas now being researched (as presented in Chapter 5).

A holistic nurse in an illness setting understands the homeostatic mechanisms effected by the Local and General Adaptation Syndrome. She is aware of current research pertaining to the origin, treatment, and rehabilitation of the "Diseases of Stress."

The holistic nurse in a wellness setting assesses her own level of stress using various personality inventories, lifestyle questionnaires, and physiologic measurements of fitness. The nurse may survey numerous methods of coping with stress, including stress-reduction methods, conditioning the body and mind to better withstand stress, and using crisis anticipation and intervention techniques.

The nurse who practices holistic nursing is able to assist clients to evaluate their own stress responses and their ability to tolerate stressors. Potentially stressful maturational and situational situations can be identified with the client.

The holistic nurse views the intrapersonal and interpersonal systems experiencing stress as continually exchanging energy with the environment in a dynamic relationship. Community implications of stress are recognized and local, national, and worldwide implications and responsibilities are analyzed.

The Lifestyling Life Process

Lifestyling incorporates the holistic nurse's knowledge and skills about health-promotive and disease-preventive behaviors which are consciously applied to manage stress and its related effects, specifically in the areas of self-responsibility, nutrition, fitness and conditioning, stress reduction, and environmental awareness. Following the various inventories evaluating wellness and health risk status, the nurse can make an assessment, pinpoint problem areas, and contract with clients for lifestyle changes that can be managed by the client with nurse support, if needed. Individualized stress-reduction and conditioning programs can be designed for and with the client.

The holistic nurse is aware of and helps the community to become alert to environmental stressors. Community organizations can be encouraged to take responsibility for organizing and sponsoring lifestyle modification and education programs that are indicated.

The Communication Life Process

Communication is all the ways—verbal and nonverbal, conscious or unconscious—that one mind influences and effects another. [37]

Nurses use communication assessments, exercises, and techniques to determine their own communication styles, strengths, and weaknesses and to express their feelings and emotions. Nurses need to evaluate their own communication patterns and styles for effectiveness, efficiency, feedback, and clarity.

Nurses use communication interpersonally with clients in a similar but more purposeful fashion to:

1. obtain information about the client, for example, through interviewing.
2. encourage the client to express feelings, concerns, and questions.
3. give clients feedback they need or request.
4. teach and explain unclear areas about which the client has concerns or questions.

Each of these purposes of communication can be broken down into subpurposes for further study and specific practice. Each type of communication has a series of suggested techniques (verbal and behavioral) which can work effectively to satisfy the goal of that communication with minimal strain and maximal satisfaction for both sender and receiver.

After mastering interpersonal communication, theories, suggestions, and methods, the nurse investigates and applies the principles to facilitate group function. The nurse analyzes groups, their goals, and the effectiveness of their communication. A beginning understanding of community organization and development assists the nurse to help community groups articulate health needs coherently. Appropriate communication channels are explored and utilized in the community lifespace.

The Problem-Solving Life Process

Problem solving is the process of gathering, organizing, classifying, and sorting data into an assessment, formulating a goal and a plan, carrying it out, and evaluating its effectiveness. The overall goal is optimal health, whatever that may be for the particular person.

The holistic nurse looks at her own method of solving problems. She then compares this method to the scientific approach and the nursing problem-solving process. A useable logical method of dealing with client problems is determined. Other more intuitive methods of thinking and reasoning are explored. A criterion for evaluating whatever methods are chosen is decided upon.

The problem-solving method is applied to hypothetical clinical cases and situations with individuals, families, and communities. The client develops his own method of viewing and solving health problems with and eventually independent of nursing support. Preventive, nurturative, and generative holistic nursing actions are examined, evaluated, and modified accordingly.

Research is an essential part of problem solving. It is the base on which the profession of nursing is built and from which it will grow. From the moment the nurse establishes a rationale for a problem or action, she uses the research process. From critique to use of research in clinical practice, the nurse begins to create areas of interest in which to conduct her own studies or participate in the studies of others. New frontiers of holistic nursing theory and practice will emerge from these research projects.

The Teaching/Learning Life Process

Learning is a change in attitude and behavior as a result of practice and experience. Teaching is the process of creating an environment in which learning can occur.

Nurses are constantly modeling and communicating attitudes and practices about health and illness. Three theories of learning are especially useful to holistic nurses attempting to encourage clients to change health practices and lifestyles to promote high-level wellness and prevent illness.

The learning theories described in Chapter 9 are stimulus-response, Gestalt, and humanistic learning theories, and they all play their part in any learning incident.

One of the single most important roles the nurse plays is that of teacher. It is essential for the nurse to become sensitive to her own teaching/learning styles and needs. She needs to recognize what kinds of learning and methods stimulate self-discovery and mastery. Awareness of what motivates learning in self will help the nurse to appreciate the teaching/learning style of clients.

In the holistic approach, the nurse acknowledges that the client is teaching the nurse more about his experience of health or illness. This experience is valued by the nurse who strives to help the client design for himself a teaching/learning package that is stimulating, continuous, expanding, and flexible.

The nurse must acknowledge the validity of self-learning, self-motivation, and self-critique in both her learning and the learning of the client, family, and community. Every nursing action, whether it be protective, nurturative, or generative, involves teaching. The client's attitudes toward health, health care systems, and health care professionals are learned through each nurse-client interaction. Sensitivity, timing, and knowledge are crucial to teaching in the interpersonal and community lifespaces.

The Leadership and Change Life Processes

Change is the planned adaptation to shifts in the environment. It requires premeditated thought and problem solving. The process of executing change to obtain a group goal while encouraging growth is *leadership*. Planned change is a function of good leadership and the two processes should go hand in hand.

The nurse finds herself in a variety of leadership positions and roles. The nurse evaluates her development as a leader. She may not have been the acknowledged leader in a personal or professional situation, but she may have performed part of a leadership function. The nurse assesses her abilities and strengths as a leader and maximizes them in creating an environment in which healing and health can occur. This may mean motivating and mobilizing other members of a group to change.

In order to foster change in an individual, family, community, or institution, the nurse needs a sound knowledge of the principles of change and management. These are elaborated on in Chapter 10. Leadership and change require expertise in every process and skill previously described and more. Leadership and change demand continuous learning and development on the part of the nurse.

The nurse must be flexible and able to project and predict needs of clients and trends in health care. The nurse should be conversant with current professional and political issues which may effect the client, the health worker, and herself. The leader understands the channels of power and how to use them to effect changes.

The Holistic Nursing Model and the Components of Holistic Health

A graphic summary of the holistic nursing conceptual framework is shown in Figure 1–7. In this holistic nursing model all the life processes are pictured as they are used with and by the nurse and the client toward their mutual goal of high-level wellness.

A conceptual framework for holistic nursing has been proposed. The three major areas that have been summarized are:

1. the arenas that holistic nurses simultaneously operate in; that is, the intrapersonal, interpersonal, and community lifespaces.
2. the kinds of activities holistic nurses perform with clients; that is, preventive, nurturative and generative.
3. the life processes all holistic nurses have an in-depth knowledge, understanding, and beginning application of; that is, self-responsibility, caring, human development, stress, lifestyling, communication, problem solving, teaching/learning, leadership and change.

High-level wellness has been defined as a general goal within the context of individual sociocultural and situational variables. The dynamic nature of the life processes in nurses and clients as well as in health and illness is projected on a perpetually changing continuum. The nurse who believes in and utilizes this conceptual framework is said to be practicing holistic nursing.

The four components of holistic health, that is, humanistic medicine, alternative health care, preprimary care, and altered provider-"patient" relationship are appropriately woven into each of the life processes. The holistic philosophy and systems approach to health and health-care problems is likewise included throughout the text. Whenever possible, an Eastern perspective is utilized to balance our predominantly Western view of the world. The intent is to help nursing expand and broaden its knowledge and practice base and to stimulate innovative ways of viewing health and healing. The future of holistic nursing lies in the hearts, minds, and hands of its creative and critically thinking practitioners.

REFERENCES FOR CHAPTER 1

[1] Don B. Ardell, *High Level Wellness* (Emmaus, Pa.: Rodale Press, 1977).

[2] Herbert Benson and Mark D. Epstein, "The Placebo Effect, A Neglected Asset in the Care of Patients," *JAMA,* 232, no. 12 (June 23, 1975), 1225–27.

[3] Em Olivia Bevis, *Curriculum Building in Nursing* (St. Louis: C. V. Mosby Company, 1973).

[4] Anita Blau, Laura Hively, and Naomi Remen, *The Masculine Principle, The Feminine Principle, and Humanistic Medicine* (San Francisco: The Institute for the Study of Humanistic Medicine, 1975).

[5] Fay L. Bower and Em O. Bevis, *Fundamentals of Nursing Practice* (St. Louis: C. V. Mosby Company, 1977).

[6] Fay L. Bower, *The Process of Planning Nursing Care* (St. Louis: C. V. Mosby Company, 1977).

[7] Fritjof Capra, *The Tao of Physics* (Boulder, Colo.: Shambhala Publications, 1975).

[8] Rick Carlson, *The End of Medicine* (New York: John Wiley & Sons, 1975).

[9] Shirley Chater, "A Conceptual Framework for Curriculum Development," *Nursing Outlook,* 23, no. 7 (July 1975), 428–33.

[10] Gretchen Crawford and others, "Evolving Issues in Theory Development," *Nursing Outlook,* 27 (May 1979), 346–51.

[11] Norman Cousins, *Anatomy of an Illness, as Perceived by the Patient* (New York: W. W. Norton & Co., 1979).

[12] Norman Cousins, "The Holistic Health Explosion," *Saturday Review,* March 31, 1979, pp. 17–20.

[13] Norman Cousins, "The Mysterious Placebo, How Mind Helps Medicine Work," *Saturday Review,* October 1, 1977, pp. 9–16.

[14] René Dubos, *Man Adapting* (New Haven, Conn.: Yale University Press, 1965).

[15] Halpert L. Dunn, *High-Level Wellness* (Arlington, Va.: R. W. Beatty Company, 1961).

[16] The Faculty, San Francisco State Department of Nursing, *A Conceptual Framework* (unpublished document, 1977).

[17] Don Fink, "Holistic Health: Implications for Health Planning," *AJHP,* no. 1 (July 1976), 23–31.

[18] Jerome Frank, "The Faith That Heals," *The Johns Hopkins Medical Journal,* 137 (August 1975), 127–31.

[19] Dorothy Hagemeier and Carol Hunt, "Do New Graduates Use Conceptual Frameworks?" *Nursing Outlook,* 27, no. 8 (August 1979), 545–48.

[20] Ernest R. Hilgard and Gordon H. Bower, *Theories of Learning,* 4th ed. (Englewood Cliffs, N.J.: Prentice-Hall, Inc., 1975).

[21] "How Placebos Work—New U.C. Findings," *San Francisco Chronicle*, August (n.d.) 1978.

[22] Ivan Illich, *Medical Nemesis* (New York: Bantam Books, 1977).

[23] Thomas Kuhn, *The Structure of Scientific Revolutions,* Foundations of the Unity of Science, vol. II, no. 2 (The University of Chicago Press, 1958).

[24] Milton Mayeroff, *On Caring* (New York: Barnes & Noble Books, 1971).

[25] John C. McCamy and James Presley,

Human Life Styling (New York: Harper & Row, 1975).

[26] Benjamin F. Miller and Claire B. Keane, *Encyclopedia and Dictionary of Medicine, Nursing, and Allied Health* (Philadelphia: W. B. Sanders Co., 1978).

[27] Harry Nelson, "New Holistic Medicine: The Spirit Grows," *Los Angeles Times,* May (n.d.) 1977, pp. 1 and 32.

[28] Dorothea Orem, *Concepts of Nursing Practice* (New York: McGraw-Hill Book Company, 1971).

[29] Robert Ornstein, *The Psychology of Consciousness* (New York: Penguin Books, 1977).

[30] Josephine G. Paterson and Loretta T. Zderad, *Humanistic Nursing* (New York: John Wiley & Sons, 1976).

[31] Kenneth R. Pelletier, *Holistic Medicine* (New York: Delacorte Press, 1980).

[32] Kenneth R. Pelletier, *Mind as Healer, Mind as Slayer* (New York: Dell Publishing Co., 1977).

[33] D. C. Phillips, *Holistic Thought in Social Science* (Stanford, Ca.: Stanford University Press, 1976).

[34] Martha Rogers, *An Introduction to the Theoretical Basis of Nursing* (Philadelphia: F. A. Davis Company, 1970).

[35] Sister Callista Roy and Sharon Roberts, *Theory Construction in Nursing and an Adaptation Model* (Englewood Cliffs, N.J.: Prentice-Hall, Inc., 1980).

[36] Sister Callista Roy, "Relating Nursing Theory to Education: A New Era," *Nurse Educator,* IV, no. 2 (March/April 1979), 16–21.

[37] Jurgen Ruesch and Gregory Bateson, *Communication* (New York: W. W. Norton & Co., 1951).

[38] Hans Selyé, *The Stress of Life,* 2nd ed. (New York: McGraw-Hill Book Company, 1978).

[39] Sherry L. Shamansky and Cherie L. Clausen, "Levels of Prevention: Examination of the Concept," *Nursing Outlook,* 28, no. 2 (February 1980), 104–08.

[40] George Sheehan, *On Running* (Mountain View, Ca.: World Publications, 1975).

[41] Jan Christian Smuts, *Holism and Evolution* (New York: Macmillan, 1926).

[42] David Sobel, ed., *Ways of Health* (New York: Harcourt, Brace Jovanovich, 1979).

[43] Justin F. Stone, *Tai Chi Chih!* (Albuquerque, N.M.: Sun Publishing Co., 1974).

[44] Mervyn Susser, *Causal Thinking in the Health Sciences* (New York: Oxford University Press, 1973).

[45] Thomas S. Szasz and Marc H. Hollender, "A Contribution to the Philosophy of Medicine," *Archives of Internal Medicine,* 94 (1956), 585–92.

[46] Donald M. Vickery and James F. Fries, *Take Care of Yourself* (Reading, Mass.: Addison-Wesley Publishing Co., 1977).

[47] World Health Organization, "Constitution of the World Health Organization," *Chronicles of WHO,* 1 (1947), 1–2.

Chapter 2
self-responsibility

CHAPTER OUTLINE

CHAPTER OBJECTIVES
1. Define self-responsibility as it relates to holistic nursing.
2. Describe five steps involved in moving toward an altered state of self-awareness.

3. Describe two exercises for increasing self-responsibility in both nurse and client.
4. List four advantages and two disadvantages of keeping a journal.
5. Discuss the two types of role relationships and one example of a potential problem in these relationships.
6. List some of the characteristics of the "sick role" and the "good patient." What expectations do these stereotypes encourage on the part of the health practitioner and client?
7. Explain the major idea underlying locus of control. Differentiate an internally versus an externally controlled individual.
8. Describe contracts and share care and explain how they both encourage client self-responsibility.
9. Explain one way in which the federal government is encouraging self-responsibility through legislation.

If any concept comes close to describing the essence of holistic health, it is that of self-responsibility. Holistic nursing believes that every human being, no matter how defenseless or dependent, has a natural desire and tendency for self-direction and determinism. Holistic nurses recognize self-responsibility as a basic developmental task. Holistic nurses first assess themselves and then their clients in terms of self-responsibility. Second, holistic nurses nurture, support, and generate the individual's goal of total responsibility for self.

The definition of self-responsibility will be broadened to mean the reflective response of the self to freely choose from a variety of alternatives. This definition assumes the development of a set of personal and professional values consistent with holistic nursing. The more narrow interpretation of self-responsibility merely as those professional obligations incurred in and through the practice of nursing is thus magnified significantly.

The nurse is encouraged to evaluate the concepts and methods outlined in this chapter intrapersonally, as if the nurse were the client. Any knowledge gained from this experience can then be applied to colleagues, friends, and clients.

More orthodox content, such as development of self-concept, body image, and self-esteem will be alluded to briefly, but will be explored more fully in Chapter 4.

New findings encompassing self-awareness and selected holistic techniques; self-responsibility for states of health, disease, and accidents; and nurse, client, and "patient" roles in various states of health will be examined in this section. The concept of locus of control as a determinant in bio-psycho-social adaptive processes will be introduced and will serve as a link to Chapters 5 and 6. Self-control of states of consciousness, autonomic processes, and states of health will be applied to the interpersonal, group, and larger community setting.

SELF-AWARENESS

The study of self-responsibility begins with a prerequisite process—awareness or consciousness of self. This developmental experience begins at birth and produces thinking, feeling, acting persons, who recognize themselves as playing different roles and consciously displaying different aspects of themselves. The development of the sense of self is initially unconscious, but at some point the person consciously or out of habit chooses the person he/she will become. Illness occurs when people don't grow and develop their potentials or when they become blocked by a crisis or a series of events which stunt and twist their growing images of themselves.

Awareness is the first step to autonomy or responsibility. Berne defines awareness as the capacity to "see a coffee pot and hear the birds sing in one's own way, and not the way one was taught." [6] Awareness means living here and now, knowing how we feel, and where we are relative to time and space.

Inherent in becoming self-aware is an almost removed passive acceptance of the situation as it is, not as how it should be or ought to be. Fritz Perls, the Gestalt therapist, feels that awareness can be nurturative and a serious step toward healing. [40] Awareness is unpredictable in that we can't figure out where it will lead since it involves a new way of looking at ourselves and others. Eastern mysticism demonstrates the lack of clarity in "knowing and seeing" that occurs in meditative states of consciousness, which fosters self-awareness.

Mind and Spirit Awareness

Pelletier summarized Shapiro and Zifferblatt's research on the five steps involved in moving toward a deep meditative state—an altered state of self-awareness.

1. The individual sits in a physically centered posture and breathes in a calm, effortless way.
2. The person focuses attention on breathing, for example, and does so in a relaxed, deliberate way.
3. The person learns to self-observe without a reactive effect and without becoming habituated to the task.
4. The person is able to desensitize himself to whatever is on his mind—thoughts, fears, or worries.
5. The meditator is able to eventually remove all covert thoughts and images, thereby allowing him to "let go" of cognitive labels, "reopen" the senses, and be more receptive to internal and external stimuli. [39, pp. 205–6]

When this state is achieved, it can be utilized to view any intrapsychic and environmental situation the client and/or helper chooses.

The self-awareness described is a type of consciousness that permits the mind to introspect upon itself without the use of external physical methods. Achieving this level of consciousness characterized by alpha rhythm electroencephalograph patterns is easily attainable and increasingly easy to document through scientific instrumentation. [39, p. 242] The difficulty with meditative states or the intuitive insights gained during these experiences is describing them. The problem is not unlike that expressed by some artists asked to explain their work. The language we use is designed to communicate logical, linear ideas, not, for example, the great "Aha's" of clarifying insights often associated with great scientific discoveries.

The type of knowledge gained in these nonintellectual states is termed absolute as opposed to the rational type which is a product of reasoning or experiment. The words often used to describe rational thought and processes include name, categorize, compare, discriminate, measure, quantify, etc. There are no words to accurately convey the world of absolute knowledge. Any attempts to coin descriptive terminology are often shunned as holistic consciousness jargon.

How did the great Yogic masters, for example, communicate their absolute knowledge? Delving into any of the Eastern writings gives us a partial explanation. Metaphors, riddles, koans, and haikus were used to translate mystical experience into rational linguistics. This poetic language, which is sometimes infuriatingly illogical, is an attempt to describe a world of opposites, incongruencies, and inconsistencies. The realm of inner space doesn't follow the same laws as left-hemisphere-dominated reality. A few examples follow:

> There the eye goes not,
> Speech goes not, nor the mind.
> We know not, we understand not
> How one would teach it. [9, Kena Upanishad, as quoted therein, p. 29]

> You can make the sound of two hands clapping.
> Now what is the sound of one hand? [9, Mu-Koan, as quoted therein, p. 49]

> The contradiction so puzzling to the ordinary way of thinking comes from the fact that we have to use language to communicate our inner experience, which in its very nature transcends linguistics. [9, D. T. Suzuki, as quoted therein, p. 45]

Many self-assessment tools are suggested throughout this book. All of them are intended to add to nurse's and client's knowledge of themselves and others. Self-awareness suggests more than a thinking approach to new experience and information. It implies sensing, feeling, valuing, and judging an experience. Since holistic practitioners do not accept the split of the body, mind, and spirit, all awareness exercises are expected to stimulate integration of sensations and feelings in all aspects of the person's life.

Awareness of sensations, attitudes, and postures in the self leads to awareness of them in others. A connectedness of feeling or oneness with humanity sometimes occurs during awareness exercises. Most methods for increasing self-awareness focus on sensitizing people to their senses, trusting their perceptions, getting in touch with feelings and their external expression. Changing and heightening awareness in oneself then gives people the confidence to change what happens to them. They begin to feel and express a belief and confidence in themselves and their intuitions and exercise control over their lives.

Body, Mind, and Spirit Awareness

Awareness of the body is an important aspect of self-awareness. Self-awareness and the term "body work" go hand in hand. One is prerequisite to the other. The term is really a misnomer because body therapists view the body as the mirror of the mind and spirit, and they see the mental and spiritual facets of a person as interconnected and reflected in the body. In later chapters, nurses will learn that the way the body is incorrectly taught to function—for example, walking, posture, and breathing—reflects a certain mental attitude about oneself and can cause serious damage years later. A prevalent attitude which holistic practitioners are struggling to change is the separation of persons from awareness of their bodies. One of the major thrusts of the self-help and holistic movement is re-establishing the unity of the body, mind, and spirit. Our Western culture teaches us to suppress pain, emotion, and symptoms. Illness is seen as negative, a punishment and betrayal by the body. Techniques for changing this attitude will be suggested later in this chapter.

A return to awareness and enjoyment of the body requires an active conscious attempt to experience taken-for-granted acts, such as looking at the body and touching it, eating thoughtfully, and enjoying sexual activity. Self-awareness and self-responsibility may have to begin with an active assuming of it through language. Some examples are: "I have overworked myself and lost track of the warning signals." "I have let my nutrition and relaxation slide for other priorities." "I have sickened myself and need to look at what my goals really are."

Nurses and clients ask amazing miracles of medical science. They attribute powers to healers that may go beyond their capabilities. A healer cannot replace the healer within the client.

Awareness should be distinguished from knowledge in that it occurs in the present, whereas knowledge is the storehouse of information packed into our memory banks. Awareness involves standing outside ourselves and noting our own behavior. When we can view our actions somewhat objectively, we can choose to act or change consciously or continue in the same habit pattern.

Meditating or doing a progressive relaxation exercise such as the one mentioned in Figure 6–19, can help a person become more aware of each part of the body and how it feels. Sometimes an uncomfortable feeling will be observed in a place where it has never been noticed before. This does not mean that the tension or sensation never existed; it merely means that attention wasn't directed to it. Almost any part of the body can be isolated, observed, studied, tensed, and relaxed. Some people have become very adept at isolating very specialized muscle groups for particular problems, such as the frontalis muscle for migraine headaches.

Journals

One method frequently being used in holistic health and illness care is journal writing. Keeping a journal is one of the best tools for developing self-awareness and responsibility for health and any other aspect of life the person may choose. Jungian psychologists (see Chapter 4) have always made extensive use of dream journals and logs as a device for encouraging introspection, recollection, analysis, and commitment to a thought, feeling, or opinion in writing.

Many journal formats exist and can be chosen based on the client's intent and goals. Two types will be described in this text. Nurses should attempt keeping a journal or log to determine the effectiveness of the technique for themselves. As with other self-assessment techniques suggested in this text, it is recommended that the nurse self-experience a method, then try it on a friend or colleague before attempting it in his or her own nursing practice.

Ira Progoff suggests the Intensive Journal as a technique for focusing inwards, relaxing the left hemisphere, and allowing phrases, images, and memories to arise on their own. [42] This method is described in Chapter 6.

A journal format is suggested in this section. Try it. How would you use this exercise with clients? Did the exercise allow you to reorder your priorities? spend more quiet time with yourself? stimulate you to be nicer to yourself?

The feeling of displacement which is commonly expressed by nurses and clients alike may stem from not taking the time to reflect on life's events which often bombard them at a furious rate. Journal writing provides the experience of tasting life twice. Often the second time around, an insight or "shiver of catharsis" one hundred times stronger may occur. [15]

Layers of experience may need to be compared, combined, and contrasted in order for cyclic patterns to emerge. A journal can cause the writer to find some meaning and significance to behavior. New meanings, values, and interrelationships arise when thoughts and feelings are recorded. A journal forces the writer to discriminate from the wealth of random thoughts, and to organize, edit, and choose the most important of them. Through this process, defining and resolving of issues and problems can occur.

An advantage of keeping a journal is that a new level of creativity is often discovered. Once loosely hanging thoughts have been committed to writing, other possibilities for the mind to explore may arise.

A journal is somewhat like a diary except that it focuses not so much on the vivid account of external events, but on the internal thoughts, feelings, and motives behind them. The actual writing and organization will be simplified if a specific book is set aside for the purpose of journal writing. Ideally, entries should be made after a thought or event occurs, but often several entries per week are a good beginning.

The commitment of keeping a journal is a big one. If it is being used as a tool for changing some lifestyle elements, it may be an indicator of the level of motivation of the person. Taking time to write may in itself be the only time some clients allow themselves to self-evaluate and self-nurture. Journal keeping is a step on the path to self-awareness, self-responsibility, and self-care.

Some themes which may stimulate introspection and the search for meaning underlying behavior that have worked for some people are described in the table on pages 39–40.

Freedom and Responsibility

It is not uncommon in obtaining a health history for a holistic nursing practitioner to hear comments such as "That flu bug just got me," or "I got hit by a car." By the same passive stance a client will attribute wellness or regaining health to a doctor or a pill. In this respect the self-responsibility movement is not well served by the English language. Even the word "patient" embodies this passive, helpless attitude.

Rollo May described the daily struggle to be free as requiring responsibility

SUGGESTED JOURNAL TOPICS

1. *Time Perspectives.* This section can be used to help make contact with life processes through time—from the past into the present and toward the future. Stepping stones (bridges from where we were to where we are or hope to be), intersections (roads taken and not taken), and memories may be noted.

2. *Techniques for Growth.* Experiences and techniques that nurse and client deliberately decide to use. Also, other unplanned experiences or situations that are helpful in the ongoing growth process, that can be repeated intentionally, as techniques.

3. *Hangups.* Personal weaknesses or limitations of which nurse and client are aware and on which to work. Particular emphasis can be placed on the methods which can be used to overcome them. Recorded also may be any strong negative reactions to other people as they may clarify unrecognized and projected problems.

4. *Peak Experiences.* Any "high" or "deep" experiences of peace, joy, love, expansion, awakening, etc., and their circumstances and effects.

5. *Emotional Awareness and Catharsis.* This section can contain the reflections on, and expression of, feeling in all aspects. This can also be a place to "let off steam," to express on paper feelings that might otherwise be bottled up or expressed in a harmful way to another person.

6. *Subpersonalities and Identification.* Reflections on various subpersonalities and their interactions, and following the development and harmonization of the major ones the nurse and client may presently be working with. What personality elements are the nurse or the client working to *dis*identify from their experience or sense of personal identity?

7. *Dreams.* Description of night dreams, which are most easily recorded immediately upon awakening. Description of daydreams. Also, the content of dreams and any associations, feelings, and interpretations which might occur.

8. *Imagery.* This may include images which come spontaneously, or those that occur during the purposeful use of guided imagery techniques. They may be recorded in writing and/or through drawings. It is important to record the *feelings and associations* felt in response to the images (or to specific aspects of an image, such as its form, color, etc.), that have meaning and a tentative interpretation, if possible. Particular attention should be given plans to "ground"—to express in everyday life—whatever insights may have been gained from them. Also recorded here are fantasies, stories, situations, and quotations which have special meaning and which may serve as seeds for further imaginative work.

(continued)

9. *Meditation.* Noted here are deeper thoughts, thinking about specific ideas, issues, or questions as well as any "formal" meditation along the lines of some specific approach. Included, perhaps, are the central "see" ideas of reflections, the direction of thinking, any insights and intuitions, and other related results of effects obtained.

10. *Bright Ideas.* The heading speaks for itself. Many have found that simply having a section called "Bright Ideas" seems to make the ideas come.

11. *Dialogue with the Body.* Engaging in dialogue with the body, or with a part of it that has special relevance for the nurse or client at a particular time. It is especially helpful to use this technique with a part of the body that has been causing difficulty or of which the person is ashamed. Carry on a conversation with the body part—talk to it and let it talk to you—and write down the conversation. Allow the conversation to emerge, don't force it. This technique of inner dialogue can begin with the person speaking directly to the particular area to apologize, resent, or appreciate. In time, the person begins to speak from the body part, to express its needs and wants. Sometimes a body part experiencing "disease" or pain can be seen in a creative way as a chance to change, to appreciate, or to put less stress on itself.

for one's self and one's existence. Self-responsibility involves more than the instinct of self-preservation on a biological level. It requires that an individual actively go about fulfilling one's destiny. This involves informed choice. [30, p. 171]

When persons choose to take responsibility for every aspect of their lives, they cannot blame anyone else for imposing control on them. On the other hand, they do not indulge in guilt or self-pity. When persons choose self-responsibility, they choose a certain self-discipline which reinforces a particular value system. If a person takes responsibility for creating a healthy lifestyle, everything that person does is directed toward or away from that goal. [30, p. 173]

The person who is in the process of integration takes responsibility for everything he feels, thinks, and believes. He has developed an ethical system for his life. He develops social graciousness and experiences passion, tenderness, and suffering, not because he feels he should or needs to, but because he wants and chooses to. [22, p. 270]

Abraham Maslow has described the self-responsible person as self-actualized in his theory of personality. Self-actualized people take responsibility for others as well as for themselves and have a finely developed sense of awareness and a capacity for pleasure.

Exercises in Taking Responsibility

Gestalt therapy helps people discover how to integrate the fragmented parts of their personality within a sound framework of self-awareness and self-responsibility:

Give away your personal faculties of discernment, of evaluation, of self-reference, and you lose your integrity (your wholeness). Take responsibility for your every thought, your every feeling, your every action. [14]

When adversities occur, self-blame, helplessness, or inadequacy are not acceptable excuses to someone who is self-responsible. Nurses and clients can change an unfortunate situation and/or an attitude about a particular incident. A popular Gestalt exercise in verbally taking beginning responsibility for actions is called "I can't, I won't, and I try":

Everytime you hear an "I can't" coming into your thoughts or conversation, substitute "I won't." If that's too difficult try, "I can't right now." Instead of "I'm not able to," say "I'm not willing to." Instead of "I'm unable to," "I'm unwilling to." As you practice this exercise you will become more sensitive to others using "I can't" to cover up what's really happening with them or to disown responsibility.

"I try" or "I tried" is another phrase that says someone else didn't want me to make it or I should be pitied. Substituting "I did it" or "I didn't do it" is at least a verbal way of taking charge of your life. [10, p. 31]

Examples of nurses or clients not taking responsibility for their actions follow:

"I've been on diets most of my life, but I just can't lose weight."

"I know I need to cut down my smoking, but I can't right now until exams are over."

"I tried to research this idea in the library, but all the books were checked out."

Another exercise to help clients and professionals get in touch with their responsibility is called "Owning your I."

How often do you use the pronoun "I" in conversation? Do you often substitute the pronouns such as "you," "we," "it," when you really mean "I"?

Comments like, "She is really a hostile client," or "It appears that the whole group turns off whenever she enters it," may really be a cover-up for "I really feel she doesn't like me," or "I feel uncomfortable in the group when she's in it."

What about our interactions with clients? How often have we heard comments from practitioners like "*It's* time for your routine Pap Smear," instead of what we really mean: "*I think you* . . ." or "*Most people* feel this is a worthwhile prenatal group," as a substitute for "*I think*."

Recall or make up some typical "I" statements of your own. Do you take responsibility for your actions and opinions? In the following nurse-client interaction, the nurse does not take responsibility for her true feelings:

Nurse: (*Verbal*)	We've really got to get working on that, Joan. Haven't you read the studies on the relationship between weight and coronory artery disease?
Meaning/Interpretation: (*Unspoken*)	I have difficulty with fat people and I think you'd look a lot more attractive thin.

Problem: The nurse is superimposing her goal on Joan. She is covering her real meaning with a paternalistic, intellectualized statement. The nurse needs to "own up" to her own feelings on obesity. If she can't get by them honestly, maybe she shouldn't be counseling overweight clients.

ROLES

We are beginning to describe a certain kind of holistic nurse—one who is self-aware, self-acceptant, and self-responsible. We are defining the holistic nurse's role as conscious and caring as she engages in deliberate preventive and generative interactions with a client, family, or community aimed at high-level wellness within the context of that client's individual life situation.

What other qualities of the holistic nurse's role can be deduced? The nurse as teacher, counselor, listener, friend, observer-participant, and facilitator of the client's own self-healing abilities are a few. (The role of nurse as healer is described in Chapter 3.)

Roles stereotypically attributed to nursing—such as the mother-surrogate or handmaiden role—will not be discussed in detail. The mother-surrogate role is often brought into play in pathological situations in which clients are involved in an immobilizing health event which renders them dependent and causes them to regress for a period of time. In such situations, it is often therapeutic for a nurse to temporarily take the role of mother-surrogate.

The handmaiden role is of historical significance in nursing and is still operant in some nursing settings. Traditionally, the handmaiden is identified as a person/nurse who satisfies any need without complaint or question. Clear definition of the expanding role of nursing in relation to other health professions has changed this once prevalent image of nursing.

A brief discussion of the structure of roles will assist the nurse in working with clients and coworkers. A *position,* or status, is a place in a system of social classification recognized by a community. Each person occupies multiple positions:

Adult—Male—Father—Teacher
Adult—Female—Mother—Nurse
Adult—Female—Voter—Student

Position or status is acquired in different ways. It can be *ascribed,* that is, related to factors in which there is little leeway for change, as in sex or age.

Position or status can also be *achieved* dependent on prerequisites or on a contract—such as in marriage or employment. Examples of achieved status include those of nurse, wife, teacher, voter, or member of an organization. Status can also be *adopted,* as in the role of the moralist, the judge, etc. Finally, status can be *assumed,* as in those statuses taken on in games or the psychotherapeutic and teaching/learning techniques of role play.

Each position has a role and, in fact, the two terms are often used interchangeably. *Role* is defined as a pattern of wants and goals, beliefs, feelings, attitudes, values, and actions which members of a community expect should be characteristic of the typical occupant of a position. The behaviors of a role are learned intentionally, by instruction, and incidentally, by observation. The nurse role is learned by both methods. [44]

Society specifies the behaviors of each role. Each participant knows what behavior to expect of other persons in the role. Roles specify what the individual must do, to whom he has obligations, upon whom he has rightful claim, and the duties and obligations, as well.as the rights, of the position. [44]

Complementary and Symmetrical Role Relationships

Role relationships may be considered complementary or symmetrical. No value is attached to either type. In a symmetrical relationship both people express the same types of behavior. Information, gifts, and sentiments are traded equally. Symmetrical behaviors appear to be brief, unstable, and always changing with one party winning or losing—or getting the last word. An example is when two nurses compare their day's experiences with clients. [5, p. 6]

In complementary relationships (for example, nurse-"patient," parent-child) the relationship is not equal, and both participants recognize one person as the dominant figure who directs and gives, while the other submits, receives, and takes. This is not a good or bad condition and it is constantly changing within the relationship. A balance in which neither a complementary nor a symmetrical type of relationship takes precedence is considered optimal.

The classic example of an all-complementary relationship is seen in the sexism present in health-care roles of women clients and nurses that often result in inequality, feelings of incompetence, powerlessness, and hopelessness. The result has frequently been inadequate health-care services, incompetence, and malpractice in women's health care. [5] Problems occur when both parties do not consent to their assigned roles, resent them, and begin an increasingly negative downward spiral in the relationship. This is termed *discrepancy*. [5, p. 8]

Sometimes the receptive role is one that allows the client a form of dignity and control. Again, the nurse has no idea of the meaning of illness for that person. Although the focus of this text is wellness health behavior, it is helpful to observe the role of the sick person since it is from this behavior that the word patient derives its meaning, and clients do cycle in and out of illness situations.

The Sick Role

The sick role was theoretically explained in 1958 by sociologist Talcott Parsons. The sick role had some universal qualities:

1. Sick persons were not responsible for their illnesses. They were not their fault.
2. Sick persons were not expected to heal themselves without professional assistance.
3. Sick persons were temporarily relieved of their normal family, occupational obligations. [27]

In return for these exemptions, sick persons were expected to:

1. declare illness as undesirable;
2. do everything to recover from illness;
3. undergo diagnosis and treatment by cooperating and collaborating with medical professionals to cure or effectively manage the disease. [27]

The Good Patient

The role of the "good patient" is outlined as:

> totally cooperative;
>
> trusting the doctor implicitly and not questioning the reason or purpose of testing or therapy;
>
> not being curious;
>
> not having emotional relations who demand explanations;
>
> controlling tensions—being stoical about pain;
>
> being a thorough and accurate observer of symptoms and an accurate historian of the past;
>
> having a bodily disease which can be diagnosed and cured. [7, p. 42]

With these models as guides, it is no wonder that the role of the medical professional has acquired the social-control function that it has in our society. That health, illness, and medical activities now comprise 20 percent of the Gross National Product of the U.S. and that clients are reimbursed for getting sick—*not* for staying well—is not surprising.

Changing The Sick Role To A Well Role

In these roles, how can "patients" become clients? With roles that are defined thus, patients obediently present themselves, offer their symptoms, passively undergo the treatment regimen, and suffer any untoward effects silently. In a predictable fashion, the doctor, nurse, and health professional see themselves as having the power and sole responsibility for making the "patient" well. It is a difficult role for both parties to play. Patients claim the doctor didn't make them well as the incidence of malpractice suits goes ever higher, and the doctors complain that patients don't comply to the therapeutic regimens prescribed. It has been estimated that the compliance rate for clients who take long-term medications for chronic diseases averages 50 percent. [27] Once out of the institutionalized "control" of the physician, perhaps clients find a way to act out their defiance and anger by manipulating and/or eliminating their medications.

The role of the health professional is one of specialization, which creates its own bureaucracy, language, and self-interest. The state of the medical world is not necessarily the state of the rest of the world. It is very difficult for professionals to look at their world dispassionately. On the other hand, professionals feel lay people are inadequately prepared to deal with some of the complexities of health-care issues.

The role of the professional is characterized by autonomy, protection from encroachment, control of production, application of knowledge, and a code of ethics. The complementary role of the client, according to Reeders, is—not surprisingly—characterized by receptivity, limited information, and a large potential for error in communication due in part to language barriers. [43]

Realistically, a health professional is trained to look at conditions, groups of symptoms, and recommended protocols for situations fitting certain criteria. This simplifies a very complex task. Unfortunately, the uniqueness of individuals and recognition of their own effect on their health is often lost. Professionals have answers and diagnoses for problems which represent an *average* picture of a certain condition. It is the client's responsibility to share their unique perspectives with a professional who is receptive to that information and who uses it in an individualized plan of care.

The word *consumer* is often used instead of the word *client* because it was felt this might make the health-care establishment more sensitive to the person who pays the bills, that is, the client—who pays directly or through his insurance premiums. It has been hoped by some that consumerism would attack health-care issues with the same militance that it did the environmental and business sectors. This would require more than courage, for, in fact, the real consumer who dictates the fees and payments of the health-care system is not the client, but rather, the physician. Approximately 75 to 80 percent of health-care expenditures are determined by physicians, not by clients. [27] The physician is responsible for generating the hospital's revenues. An insurance company will reimburse almost all costs legitimized by a physician. Preventive measures, health promotion and education, and most holistic approaches are not covered by third-party payment. Test cases contesting these practices are attempting to set precedents for holistic and preventive health measures reimbursement.

With the push of consumerism and with the focus on preventive health and competition in the late sixties and seventies, clients have begun to find themselves in a buyer's market for some services that are not emergency or crisis medical-care-oriented. In wellness care, the motivation and follow-up is controlled by customers who can afford to shop around to get the best health promotion programs they can. The power for following a prescribed program rests squarely with the consumer. This is a radical role shift for health practitioner and client alike. Once the consumer moves out of the institutional setting, those roles that have been determined by the institution—doctor, nurse, patient—are no longer useful.

In the primary-care setting, for example, the nurse's role no more resembles that of a handmaiden than does the consumer's role resemble that of a supplicant. The health-care hierarchy and power structure is not only changing from the grass roots up but from the upper level decision makers downward. The nature of power and change and the participation of the lay person in decision making will be discussed in more depth in Chapter 10.

One way of changing the all-complementary role pattern between health care giver and taker has been the institution of the client/advocate role. This is often played by a nonhealth person who is employed by a health-care agency to perform certain functions which facilitate understanding of the communication between health professional and client. Nurses have often served as client advocates and will probably continue to do so. There is some question about the nurse-advocate role regarding whether the client is really building *his own* advocacy and assertiveness skills or merely allowing the nurse to practice hers.

Health practitioners who are self-aware regarding their own roles can teach clients to assume more self-responsibility in their own health care. This process begins with the first contact with the client. The health assessment should incorporate and attach value to the clients' sharing of information and self-knowledge.

Clinical Examples and Research

A striking clinical example of using the self-responsibility process to self-heal is the work reported by Stephanie and Dr. Carl Simonton of Forth Worth, Texas. The Simontons' special area of interest is oncology—the study of tumors. They, like the "Type-A" researchers described in Chapter 5, draw a personality type that they think predisposes a person to cancer.

The Simontons support the "surveillance theory" of cancer which proposes that cancerous cells are always present in the human body but are controlled by the immune system. An unusually stressful event coupled with the cancer personality triggers a failure in the immune system and the subsequent spread of cancer cells.

The Simontons believe that an exploration of the question, "Why did I need my cancer in the first place?," and an honest recognition of the "secondary gains" of the disease is the first step towards taking responsibility for one's cancer. This is *not* equivalent to blaming oneself for "getting" cancer. [25] The Simontons assist their clients to move from the role of helpless victim to active participant. Even the location and type of cancer can have a particular meaning for the client.

The rest of the Simontons' approach involves meditating and visualizing the tumor in a way the client can understand. The client may see the cancer as a snake, for example, and healthy cells as a dragon doing battle, as illustrated in Figure 2–1.

Criticisms of the Simontons' work are aimed at the validity of their studies and at the selectiveness of their screening procedures. Concern has also been expressed that clients who might be helped by other methods of treatment (for example, chemotherapy, radiation therapy, etc.) will see the Simonton method as their sole hope and ignore other possibilities. In fact, the Simontons work with clients who have been referred from other oncologists who use standard treatments as well as newer approaches.

The Simontons operate the Cancer Counseling and Research Center and have published a self-help guide to overcoming cancer called, *Getting Well Again,* in which positive expectancies and psychological self-awareness and self-care are advocated for health maintenance in well persons, but especially for the cancer client.

Some of the subject areas covered in their book are the link between stress, illness, personality, and cancer; a whole person model of cancer recovery; par-

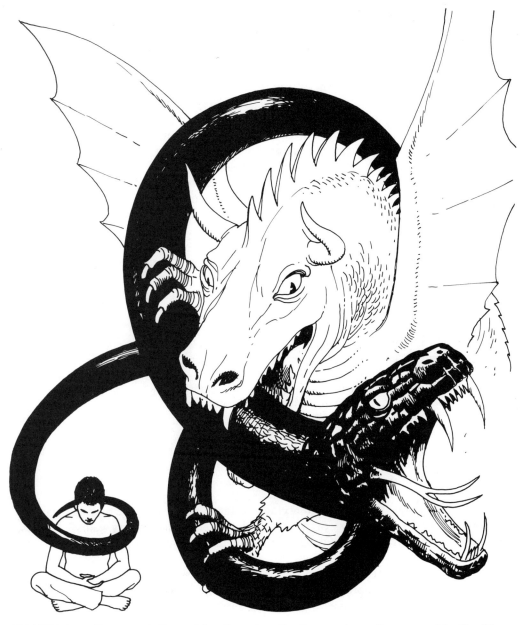

FIGURE 2-1 Representation of healing visualization such as those used in the Simontons' Technique

ticipating in one's own health; the benefits of illness; learning to relax; the value of positive mental images; and visualizing recovery. [52] The area of cancer appears to be illness-oriented when in fact so much of cancer screening and detection embody preventive health practices. The actual diagnosis, treatment, and rehabilitation of cancer is fast becoming infrequent, episodic, acute care with nonhospitalized follow-up. The client is often in need of generative nursing care that utilizes innovative techniques which require reprogramming not only the client, but also the family's and community's negative images surrounding cancer.

Susan Sontag does a beautifully sensitive job of describing cancer as it is viewed in American society today—that is, as a mark of doom, a punishment, or a symbol of someone "not sufficiently sensual or in touch with their anger." [55] Chapter 3 will touch upon the example of cancer as an expanding area for holistic nurses who utilize caring, touching, and healing processes with clients.

When strong external forces such as weather, other people, and uncontrollable events prevail, the individual can choose or not choose to participate. Not choosing to take responsibility can take the form of a verbal excuse, blaming someone else, or avoiding a decision through illness or accident.

Mechanic cites some studies which link discomforting life events and subsequent viral respiratory complaints of a minor nature. The effect of the respiratory complaint is not sufficient to warrant absenteeism from work or social obligations, but it achieves that end regardless. Suggestions regarding causality included the following:

1. The stressful life event contributed in some form to the incidence of infection.
2. The viral respiratory condition itself caused a significant source of stress and weakened the person's incentive to go to work.
3. The condition served as an excuse to relieve distressful obligations and helped avoid social sanctions for nonperformance of responsibilities.
4. The condition allowed the person to justify to himself his failure to adequately meet social responsibilities.
5. The client couldn't differentiate clearly the source of his distress and attributed it to the viral respiratory condition.
6. Or, all of the above reasons. [31]

The phrase "there are no accidents" takes on a whole set of new meanings when seen in the context of what psychiatry terms "secondary gains," that is, psychological reasons why people develop illnesses other than the primary reason given.

In a fascinating study on the treatment of acne vulgaris, a psycholinguistic self-responsibility approach was utilized, that is, changing the words, statements, behaviors, and mental images clients had surrounding acne:

1. Clients were asked to consider acne merely as another common human behavior rather than as a disease.
2. Clients were shown that when irrational (negative) statements were made to them by themselves or by others, their response was to feel "picked on," which was accompanied by itching and picking on acne lesions.

3. The clients were shown that the operant hypothesis guiding their "psycholinguistic therapy" would be that any thought pattern or contributory behavior of the "picked on" variety, if it could be eliminated, would improve the acne. [12]

Other than the usual health history and physical examination, extensive attention was paid to clients' postures and facial expressions. Experiments were performed to convince the client that body language effected mood and vice versa. Ending sentences with an upbeat tone was given value, for example.

Clients were given a crash course in self-responsibility for health. They were told that they were in charge of their lives and that nothing they did in their lives was done without their consent. Words such as "should," "must," "have to," "ought to," and "got to," were words that implied their motivation and destiny was in someone else's hands.

Clients were taught to see events merely as "happening," not as directed to them. If something unwanted or untoward occurred, they were helped to alter their perception or personalizing of the experience.

At the conclusion of the therapy, the clients were told that the brain is patterned by everything that happens to it, and that introducing a new way of naming and looking at things is not a small task. It takes up to two years of practice to really change habitual behavior patterns. It requires constant vigilance to triumph over a lifetime of "picked on" thoughts and behaviors. The author's conclusion is that if disease is in fact a modifiable behavior, as his acne study proved, then there is no such thing as an untreatable disease. [12]

The approach to taking responsibility for health is understandably controversial. The author states in a 1978 introduction to a reprint of his original article that he really wanted to substitute cancer for acne as the case study in question, but that would have been tantamount to professional suicide at the time. [11] Today, many holistic practitioners are utilizing this self-responsibility precept in their everyday work with both terminally ill and healthy individuals.

SELF-CONTROL AND SELF-HEALING

One of the most influential concepts of self-control has centered around internal versus external control of reinforcement, called locus of control. Locus of control is a measurable concept in psychology, as well as a timely idea to help explain current social concerns and problems.

Locus of Control

The concept of external or internal locus of control was formulated in 1966 by Rotter, although the initial research was conducted in 1955. Locus of control is one major concept within a conceptual framework of Social Learning Theory. The major question behind Social Learning Theory is how choices are made by individuals from the variety of potential behaviors available to them. How can people be expected to act given certain kinds of situations and reinforcement? One thesis is that learning and performance in specific situations are different when subjects perceive that they control the contingency between behavior and reinforcement and when they perceive that they lack such control. [41]

In 1966, Livran, Rotter, and Crowne refined a scale which measures the relative degree of internal versus external control in certain situations. The scale has a certain degree of reliability and validity in predicting how a person will react when faced with certain sets of choices. (The Rotter Internal-External Control Scale (I-E Scale) is found in the appendices.) Mean scores in 1966 ranged from 5.48 to 10.00 out of twenty-five possible items. The higher the score, the more external the belief. A high-scoring individual whose belief is largely in an external control would perceive the result of an action to be contingent upon luck, chance, fate, under the powerful control of others, or as totally unpredictable.

A person who believes that an event is based on their own personality characteristics and behavior is evidencing internal control. [46] They would probably have a low I-E score.

The applications of internal versus external control are not difficult to imagine. The degree of internal control, for example, would certainly help an holistic practitioner to formulate a learning program based on self-responsibility for health. It is possible to have a large degree of internal control in regard to a job situation but not in regard to health, for example. The I-E Scale attempts to weigh different life areas so that the person can evaluate areas that need work. Internal control appears to be consistent with greater attempts at coping or gaining mastery over environment. This mastery appears to be attained through more efforts at acquiring information, retaining it, ferreting out gaps in information, and using the information to reinforce a belief.

"Internals," as they are sometimes called, seem to be more effective at controlling their destiny and at self-control and self-discipline. It is possible that internals are more likely to be cautious and engage in less risky behaviors than externals because they believe that they do indeed control the outcome.

There is evidence that internally controlled people not only attribute self-control over events to themselves but also to the behavior of others. An internally controlled nurse might see smoking or overeating as more of a conscious attempt at self-destruction in a client than would an externally controlled colleague. This would have important implications for a caring therapeutic relationship. The nurse needs to evaluate herself for strong values about events such as this one. How will these values effect her relationship with a client?

Response to stress is a pivotal concept to be explored in Chapters 5 and 6. External control individuals see forces outside themselves as responsible for their fate. Their response is likely to be one of resignation to the inevitable—for example, accidents, sickness, life-threatening events. Internally controlled subjects not only suffer high negative arousal—anxiety symptoms, increased heart rate, etc.—but they are also less likely to report anxiety and are more defensive about admitting it. As we shall see in Chapter 5, this type of individual would be at risk for disorders stemming from chronic stress.

Physicians and nurses in a Tubercular Rehabilitation Hospital were asked questions similar to the following:

1. How good is the patient's understanding of the details of his own illness? (diagnosis, prognosis, and progress)
2. How good is the patient's understanding of the nature of TB in general? (its causes, cure, and prevention)

Clients were asked:

1. When you receive a new treatment, medication, or test, does someone explain it to you in advance?
2. Do you think you are informed enough about your illness and how you are getting along?

Forty-three pairs of internal-external white male clients were matched for occupational status, education, and ward placement. The internals were found to know more about their condition, to be more inquisitive with doctors and nurses about their diagnosis and situations, and indicated less satisfaction with the amount of information they were getting from hospital personnel. [51]

Can locus of control help predict which type of therapy or growth experience will best suit clients? Smith showed that clients who sought psychotherapy to resolve an immediate acute life crisis showed a significant decrease in externality as they learned more effective coping techniques in therapy. [53]

It has also been demonstrated by Foulds (1971) that experiences in an atmosphere of acceptance and unstructured group exploration and expression facilitate a sense of internal control. Internally controlled clients are more likely to choose an analytic or nondirective Rogerian therapist (see Chapter 3), whereas externals prefer a behavioristically oriented one (see Chapter 9). [17]

In summary, externals are characterized as powerless, fatalistic, alienated, normless, as experiencing anomie and loss of personal control, and as professing a belief in luck and chance occurrences. Externals must live in a world beset upon by overcrowding, pollution, unresponsive governments, authoritarianism fear of control by government, specialists, or technocrats. [41, p. 171] They would need help accepting the self-responsibility ethic and might benefit from assertiveness training.

Lefcourt has indicated that development of methods which foster internal control will be in demand as individualism and privacy become more of an apprized value in our culture. Along with these values are generated more loneliness, discontent, and personal misery among those less advantaged and less equipped to cope with life and societal stress. [28] Development of internal control becomes a matter of survival.

People who have no sense of internal control think of themselves as pawns of fate or as unlucky. They make mental self-statements such as:

"It's meant to be and can't be changed."
"It's meant to be and shouldn't be changed."
"It's meant to be and only . . . can change it." [22, p. 267]

Self-responsible persons are concerned with "being" now. They allow themselves and others to grow. They set realistic goals and have a purpose in life.

The Placebo Effect

The placebo effect mentioned in Chapter 1 merits a closer look. Jerome Frank, a researcher, sees it as a tangible symbol of the physician's power. "The physician validates his power by prescribing medication, just as a shaman in a primitive tribe may validate his by spitting out a bit of blood-stained down at the proper moment." [18]

The psychophysiological mechanism involved in the placebo effect is still a mystery. The most important factor is the belief of the healer and healee in each other and in the placebo. It would seem that an externally controlled client would respond more favorably in these cases, but this is not necessarily true if the healer and the healee are the same person. This has not been borne out by research studies, but anecdotal accounts and testimonies would lead us to believe that self-healing can involve the placebo effect.

Dr. Carl Jung, the psychiatrist, has theorized that disease is a creation of the unconscious mind. In order to achieve healing it is necessary to establish a connection between the client's conscious and unconscious minds. Jung feels the two can be linked through the image-making power of the mind. These images are messages as well as symptoms that can be called up and understood through the technique of "active imagination." The goal of the following exercise is self-healing or wholeness:

> Take the unconscious in one of its handiest forms, say a spontaneous fantasy, concentrate on it, and observe its alterations. This fantasy is a real psychic process which is happening to you personally. If you recognize your own involvement you enter into the process with your own personal reactions, just as if you were one of the fantasy figures, or rather, as if the drama being enacted before your eyes were real. [33]

Not only is the placebo documented as effective in the treatment of angina pectoris, rheumatoid arthritis, pain, hay fever, headache, cough, peptic ulcer, and essential hypertension, but it also enhances an overall feeling of wellness in clients. [4]

Symptoms can be looked at as an individual's attempt at a profound self-healing process. [35] This is termed a "healing crisis" by some holistic practitioners. It is seen as a positive opportunity for individuals to develop themselves, to modify their lives, and to change and grow.

How many nurses have experienced in their own lives or in the lives of their clients a complete reversal in attitude following an illness or symptom? Even terminal illness can be viewed as a chance to grow.

When people feel that they are active participants in their own health, they no longer see themselves as "victims" or as receivers of care. Based on what we have read about the power of belief systems, placebo effects, and so on, the unconscious creates what is expected or believed. This is not unlike a self-fulfilling prophecy. [39]

Self-Hypnosis and Autosuggestion

Another aspect of programming the unconscious mind which may be responsible for many healings is autosuggestion and self-hypnosis. As with any of the self-healing techniques, self-awareness and reflection are prerequisites. If there is a particular problem—for example, self-confidence—then it must be defined. The suggestion to the unconscious mind is in the form of an affirmation or positive statement. A way to speed up the process is to picture it as already completed, for example, "I am secure and self-confident."

T. X. Barber submits that a "hypnotic trance" is not necessary to control pain, to experience amnesia and age regression, to experience the content of nocturnal dreams, to control skin temperature, increase visual acuity, or to control allergic responses. [2]

Barber's *Training in Human Potentialities* involves the use of experimenter/model demonstrations, and in a typically cognitive behaviorist manner, it requires a return demonstration for evaluation. A typical session is presented in Figure 2-2.

FIGURE 2-2 Modeling a relaxation experience

Reprinted with permission from T. X. Barber, N. P. Spanos and J. F. Chaves, *Hypnosis, Imagination, and Human Potentialities* (New York: Pergamon Press, 1974).

> I introduce the training in relaxation by speaking to the subject along the following lines:
>
> Most individuals are so busy living their daily lives that they rarely, if ever, allow themselves to experience total relaxation. In fact, it is questionable whether most individuals know how to relax. This is unfortunate because the ability to relax completely is very useful in our daily lives. Once we have learned to relax, we are able to remain calm and at ease in many situations that normally produce anxiety or tension. For instance, many individuals become tense or anxious when they meet new people, when they are in a strange or new situation, and when they feel that they are being judged by others. Also, individuals who are alcoholics or who are obese or who cannot quit smoking become tense and anxious when they have not had alcohol or food or a cigarette for a period of time. Some individuals also have specific kinds of fears; for instance, fear of riding in an airplane, fear of heights, or fear of narrow spaces. If these individuals could learn how to relax, they could control their anxiety, tension, or fear. An important fact that has been emphasized by behavior therapists is that anxiety and tension are incompatible with physical and mental relaxation. If a person lets himself relax, he can control or block the anxiety, tension, or fear. In fact, many of the useful effects that are attributed to yoga, hypnosis, Zen, and transcendental meditation appear to be due to the relaxation that is produced by each of these techniques.

(continued)

I next state that I will now model for the subject, showing him how to relax. I introduce the modeling demonstration as follows:

I will now show you how to relax. To get rid of distractions, I will first close my eyes. Then I will think to myself that I am becoming very relaxed. I will tell myself that my arms are relaxing, my legs are relaxing, my eyes are relaxing, all parts of my body are relaxing. I will then imagine that I am floating on a soft cloud and that my body feels very, very relaxed. I will continue telling myself that I am completely relaxed and I will imagine scenes, such as floating softly on smooth water, which will make me feel more and more relaxed.

I then model for the subject, demonstrating how to relax. After a few minutes, I open my eyes, report what I was thinking and imaging during the period of relaxation, and then ask the subject to try relaxing in the same way. I may give the subject several practice trials during the session, asking him to relax for longer and longer periods of time. Before the subject leaves, I usually ask him to continue practicing the relaxation technique at home and try to use what he has learned about relaxation in his daily life whenever he begins to feel anxious or tense. [2]

FIGURE 2-2 (continued)

Basically, curing or healing means self-curing or self-healing in the sense that the organism itself becomes active. External interference or other measures can only provide conditions for a cure, not the cure itself. Healing processes can take place only in integrated overall systems that are able to regulate themselves; here we may note that there is more than an etymological relation between the words ''heal'' and ''whole.'' [49]

Psychic self-healing often conjures up occult images, when in fact it encompasses many different ways of triggering a universal ''relaxation response'' that promotes health and healing. (The physiology of this response, which has been well researched and documented, will be elaborated on in Chapters 5 and 6.)

Any type of visualization can effect a person's health for better or worse. A healing visualization can be as simple as seeing a symptom or ailing body part as grey and then breathing into that body part or symptom.

Some people enjoy mentally visiting a favorite place, real or imagined, such as a beach, the mountains, or any place connected with good feelings of happiness and warmth. By placing themselves in that healing place and by sensing all the feelings, sights, sounds, and smells about it, they can create an internal environment conducive to health and healing. Visualization has been successfully used to relieve intractable pain, to improve vision, and to restructure negative images surrounding childbirth. [48] Visualizing a blue-white light or aura around the body has been used as a protection against physical, mental, and bacteriological harm, although these claims have not been substantiated by research. A simple method of psychic healing follows:

PSYCHIC HEALING MADE SIMPLE

1. Relax the body completely—in bed just before falling asleep is best.
2. Count backwards from five to zero, visualizing each number three times.
3. At the count of 0, you will see within the 0 a picture of the cause of the difficulty—you will know it when you see it.
4. Erase the picture and substitute an image of yourself or your client in perfect health. This can be found on the reverse side of the 0. It is not unusual for this to take place while dreaming. [33]

A mental self-care responsibility technique, called Rational Self-Counseling, takes a neobehaviorist approach to maintaining emotional health. The therapy was formulated by Albert Ellis based on the learning theories of Skinner, Mowrer, Rotter and others. Rational Self-Counseling sees negative emotions as irrational thinking which can be logically discussed and resolved. Dependence on alcohol and drugs is seen as a waste of time and as an inefficient way of dealing with stress. [26]

The technique is highly directive and involves some assumptions:

Emotional disorders result from and are not the cause of irrational thinking. Distorted thinking creates havoc with the mind, the nervous system, the entire body. Someone or something doesn't upset us; our own perceptions, evaluations and emotional responses upset us.

The individual is solely responsible for his behavior because only he can produce thought, perceptions, and evaluations.

Our value systems can be changed to limit our energies to the kind of thought that is useful and functional rather than self-defeating.

People can do various things with their thoughts. They can discontinue thoughts that are leading nowhere, they can change thought patterns that have gone on for years, they can change a thought whose only reason for existence is that it has never been questioned and has become a habit. Destructive cues can be extinguished such as:

"It's 6:30 and time for a drink;
I must have a cigarette with my drink."

"Should" and "ought" are not sufficient reasons for doing something. Dwelling on "If only I" or "It should have been" this or that is not a meaningful statement because if the correct conditions had existed for something to happen, it would have happened. When correct conditions exist, then an event will occur; therefore, everything is always as it should be.

Statements to and about yourself by you are very important in shaping your attitude about yourself. If you make a mistake, that does not make you an idiot. [26, p. 15]

Five rules for rational self-analysis have been formulated:

1. Is thinking based on objective reality or on subjective opinion, that is, facts or feelings?
2. Is what is contemplated life-preserving?

3. Is what is contemplated goal-producing?
4. Will this action make the person feel better; will it help them avoid significant personal conflict?
5. Will this action make the persons in authority (parents, teachers, police, employer, wife, etc.) feel better about them?

If three of the five rules can be answered positively, chances are the contemplated action is rational. [26, p. 15]

The following formula is used to analyze interactions and to employ rational self-counseling to everyday situations:

Section A: This is where the objective facts are presented. This should not contain opinions.

Section B: This consists of thoughts, attitudes, and beliefs relating to Section A. These are usually irrational emotional statements which people tell themselves to maintain a negative upset state.

Section C: In a few words, feelings are described, usually in terms of an emotion (for example, fear, pity, anger, etc.).

Section D: This contains a rational response to each statement in Section B, following the terms stated in the five rules for rational self-counseling. [26, p. 16]

An example of a nurse using Rational Self-Counseling following an unsuccessful interaction with a client follows:

Section A: In discussing a vegetarian client's nutritional practices, I forgot to ask for a five-day-diet diary to analyze what they know and are already doing for themselves.

Section B: 1. How dumb I am!
2. Why didn't they give me a piece of paper with it all written out?
3. Doesn't that client know he should come with that information?

Section C: Anger, Depression, Decreased Self-Esteem.

Section D: 1. "I'm dumb" is: not true and based on insufficient data. This was an oversight that won't happen again. Thinking about it only makes me feel bad about myself.
2. If a diet formula were all written out, they wouldn't need me to provide the interaction and interviewing skills.
3. Blaming the client is irrational and based on insufficient data and on a subjective impression.

Rational self-counseling has been used to help people clarify their values, improve interpersonal interactions, cope with stress, and to make and adhere to rational lifestyle choices. It represents effective use of a yang, left-hemisphere-dominated rational approach which works for some people.

INTERPERSONAL SELF-RESPONSIBILITY

The whole world of self-awareness, consciousness, and self-responsibility is filled with spiritual-phenomenological (the study of external and internal phenomena) language which often distorts rather than clarifies. As nurses, we are called upon to describe phenomena and data gained in a transactional relationship in which the information is perceived, sensed, collated, and suddenly "known" or "put together" in a way that makes sense to ourselves and to the rest of the health-care team.

Nurses have been encouraged in the past to refrain from subjective opinions and judgments about clients in their recording and reporting. Subjective reporting is often accepted only in such areas as journal keeping or in a verbal report.

Awareness and participation in a nurse-client interaction is what Paterson terms the intersubjective realm. [36] It often defies description. A client tells the nurse he is experiencing a variety of stressful life events and is responding with insomnia. A clinical definition of insomnia does not touch the fear, aloneness, and desperation that the client is experiencing in the early morning hours. A metaphoric, literary portrayal of his experience may be one way of communicating his feeling about his health problem. It should be added to the report and care plan.

What is the importance of becoming self-aware of another person's problem or life situation? It helps keep the nurse attuned to each client as a unique feeling individual with problems that are often a first-time frighteningly challenging experience for him. Instead of responding to the "exam-time jitters" diagnosis superimposed on a stressed student-client, the self-aware nurse perceives this as a highly singular important event for this client. If it is important enough to require her presence at the clinic, it is of value to the nurse. A stereotypical response such as "She just needs reassurance and/or a tranquilizer," is highly inadequate when seen in the context of self-awareness. Only through our own becoming self-aware and getting in touch with our bodies, our feelings, and ourselves can we effectively share with our clients in a collegial relationship.

The nurse must try to view the world through the clients' eyes, imagine the kinds of alternatives the clients might choose from in coping with that world, support their decision-making process, and accept the client regardless of the objective outcome of a situation.

Contracts

The kinds of contractual agreements and relationships that stem from a therapeutic relationship based on self-responsibility are well characterized in Figure 2-3, which describes a sample consumer/therapist contract. Various self-care-oriented community groups have used this contract as a model for their own health-care arrangements.

A contract is defined as "an agreement between two parties for the doing or not doing of some definite thing." [19] The types of contracts commonly used between health professionals and clients are outlined by Blake and Morton:

> *Acceptant Contract:* In an atmosphere free of judgments, the patient is helped to sort out problems in a self-reliant manner. The intention of the acceptant contract is to establish a helping relationship. [*The author has found techniques of active and passive listening and supportive counseling effective in this mode.*]
>
> *Catalytic Contract:* The patient is assisted in collecting further data with which to test and reinterpret his perceptions. The patient is not told what to do, but may

FIGURE 2-3 A sample consumer-therapist contract

Reprinted with permission from Sally Adams and Michael Orgel, "Through the Mental Health Maze," (Washington, D.C.: Health Research Group, 1975). (Available from Health Research Group, 2000 P St. N.W., Washington, D.C. 20036; $3.25)

(1)
(2)
(3, 4)

(5)

(6)
(7)

(8)

(9)

(10)

(11)

(12)

I, *Mr. Client,* agree to join with *Ms. Therapist* each Thursday afternoon from May 1, 1975, until June 5, 1975, at 3 P.M. until 3:50 P.M. During these six 50-minute sessions we will direct our mutual efforts towards three goals:

1. enabling me to fly in airplanes without fear
2. explaining to my satisfaction why I always lose my temper when I visit my parents
3. discussing whether it would be better for me to give up my full-time job and start working part-time

I agree to pay $30 per session for the use of her resources, training and experience as a psychotherapist. This amount is payable within 30 days of the session.

If I am not satisfied with the progress made on the goals here set forth, I may cancel any and all subsequent appointments for these sessions, provided that I give Ms. Therapist 3 days warning of my intention to cancel. In that event I am not required to pay for sessions not met. However, in the event that I miss a session without forewarning, I am financially responsible for that missed session. The one exception to this arrangement being unforeseen and unavoidable accident or illness.

At the end of the six sessions, Ms. Therapist and I agree to renegotiate this contract. We include the possibility that the stated goals will have changed during the six-week period. I understand that this agreement does not guarantee that I will have attained those goals; however, it does constitute an offer on my part to pay Ms. Therapist for access to her resources as a psychotherapist and her acceptance to apply all those resources as a psychotherapist in good faith.

I further stipulate that this agreement become a part of the medical record which is accessible to both parties at will, but to no other person without my written consent. The therapist will respect my right to maintain the confidentiality of any information communicated by me to the therapist during the course of therapy. In particular, the therapist will not publish, communicate, or otherwise disclose, without my written consent, any such information which, if disclosed, would injure me in any way.

| _____ | _____ | _____ |
| Date | Name | Name of Professional |

arrive at a better awareness of the problem and how to handle it through exposure to new information or new techniques of problem solving.

> . . .the nurse can fulfil her responsibility to the patient by providing him with the necessary information which will enable him to make a sound decision on his own. He should be informed of the consequences of each alternative open to him. [19]

Confrontation Contract: The patient is challenged to reexamine his thinking and assumptions and to select new, more effective actions. This contract may lead to threatened reactions.

Prescriptive Contract: The prescriptive contract is frequently seen in medical practice and may occasionally be used by nurses in crisis or emergency situations. In this mode the patient is told what to do to rectify the situation. The prescriptive contract involves issuing prescriptions and recommendations.

Contracts will vary according to the nature of the problem and the terms acceptable to both nurse and patient. The type of contract and the mode of intervention may change as circumstances change. [19]

Evidence exists that the client who is involved in planning, goal setting, and decision making is more likely to internalize the new health behavior, and that this internalization is more conducive to *permanent* behavior change than is mere compliance. [19; Kalisch, 1975, Dyer, 1973, and Green, 1976, as quoted in Harris, p. 56]

Share Care

The concept of ''share care'' is well demonstrated in a Women's Healthing Model developed by Bermosk and Porter of the University of Hawaii in which clients and ''facilitators'' (clinical nurse specialists) mutually negotiate and sign a share-care agreement (see Figure 2–4). If the agreement is not serving either party, it can be renegotiated, changed, and/or terminated. Clients find themselves practicing, not merely listening to, the philosophy of self-responsibility.

Contracting for grades has long been used in education and is finally making its way into health care. Contracting for wellness goals spelled out clearly and in behaviors that tell client and practitioner that progress is occurring is an important part of the self-responsibility process.

Groups Encouraging Self-Responsibility

Groups which allegedly foster self-responsibility have multiplied by the hundreds in the last decade. They carry names such as human potential, personal growth, and encounter groups. Attempts to evaluate their effectiveness have thus far been inconclusive, with some yielding little or no positive effects. Many ''therapies'' are protective of their methods and clients, which makes controlled research even more difficult.

Some popular self-improvement organizations have been defined in Chapter 1. Three prototypical groups that are supported by a body of literature and that have stood the test of time are described in Figure 2–5. Any group which en-

FIGURE 2-4 Statement of agreement form

Reprinted with permission from Loretta S. Bermosk and Sarah E. Porter, *Women's Health and Human Wholeness* (New York: Appleton-Century-Crofts, 1979), p. 138.

STATEMENT OF AGREEMENT
REGARDING SHARING OF HEALTH CARE

We, _____*Jane D.*_____ (client)
and _____*Doris S.*_____ (facilitator)
agree on the following health care goals for_____*Jane D.*_____

    1. Have vaginal infection clear up
    2. Learn more about my body and how it works
    3. Learn what to do to stop having so many sore throats
    4. Go to the "Stress Management" class

I, _____*Jane D.*_____ (client) understand my part in achieving the goals of health care and agree to participate in the following ways:

    1. Follow the medication instructions for 3 weeks
    2. Don't wear tight jeans
    3. Stop scratching
    4. Refrain from intercourse until the pain and itching stop
    5. Attend the "Stress Management" class
    6. Check **Our Bodies, Ourselves** out of the Center Library
    7. Return to Center if problem is not clearing in one week, or if unable to keep agreement

I,_____*Doris S.*_____(facilitator) agree to participate in achieving the goals of health care in the following ways:

    1. Initiate the mutual record of health care today and encourage Jane D. to write her comments
    2. Be available for questions and discussion by phone. Give Jane D. the specific hours that I'm at WHM.
    3. Give Jane D. enrollment card for class on "Stress Management"
    4. Inform Jane D. about new class being formed on "Women's Health and Human Wholeness."

I understand that this health care agreement is not legally binding and that my keeping this agreement is my own responsibility, and that if this agreement is not kept, the goals as stated above may not be achieved. If the health care plan is not satisfactory, it is my responsibility to return to the WHM and work out another plan.

_____ (client)
_____ (facilitator)

1 copy to client
1 copy to client's record

FIGURE 2-5 Three self-improvement groups

Reprinted with permission from the Esalen Catalogue, Fall 1978, p. 33.

Encounter

The ground rules of encounter are that participants be open and honest in a group setting, and that they avoid mere theorizing and talk instead about their feelings and perceptions. There is often an emphasis on eliciting emotions which lead to positive or negative confrontations rather than away from them. The focus of encounter is to explore interpersonal relations. Over the past years, encounter has evolved into a direct approach incorporating several related disciplines to achieve its aims. Techniques and insights gained from gestalt, sensory awareness, bioenergetics, massage, movement, and structural integration are all part of Esalen's encounter groups today.

Gestalt

Gestalt Awareness Training is a theory and approach to personality integration first developed by Fritz and Laura Perls, though new styles and methods are being developed by other leaders. The goal of the training is to assist the participants to utilize excitement and awareness and to develop responsibility. Excitement—to have life energy freely available and flowing, not blocked. Awareness—to be conscious of energy and where it flows; to have action accessible to consciousness, not happening mechanically. At times, everyone in the workshop may work simultaneously with some awareness exercise, or in interaction with each other. More traditionally, a fair amount of time will be spent with participants working individually with the leader. The starting point for such individual work is whatever is here and now of most involving concern for the organism; a fantasy or dream, an interaction with another person, a memory, or a physical posture. "Problems" are welcome as starting points, if they are truly present and not merely verbally presented. In keeping with Gestalt emphasis on personal responsibility, the leader usually leaves the initiative for such work with the participants. The assumption is made that participants are not "patients" but are persons responsible for their own life decisions.

Psychosynthesis

Psychosynthesis is a psychological and educational approach for recognizing and harmonizing the many, often conflicting, elements of our inner lives. It is a developmental process based on a positive conception of man/woman within an evolving universe. Starting with each person's existential situation as he or she perceives it, personal growth is organized into a process aiming at the integration of personality and the emergence of an effective unifying center of being and awareness, the Self. The practical work of psychosynthesis

(continued)

> chooses in each situation the appropriate progressive activities among many techniques and methods available. Some of these are: guided imagery, movement, self-identification, creativity, gestalt, meditation, training of the will, symbolic art work, journal keeping, ideal models, and development of intuition. The emphasis is on fostering an ongoing process of growth that can gain momentum and bring about a more joyful, balanced actualization of one's life. [13]

FIGURE 2-5 (continued)

courages continuing dependence on a demigod or prophetical leader will not be discussed, since self-reliance and responsibility are the ultimate goals of the holistic health movement and holistic nursing.

Specific groups that assist their followers in achieving high levels of spiritual wellness through religious means cannot be covered in this chapter, but are discussed in some depth in Murray and Zentner's *Nursing Concepts for Health Promotion.* [32] It is recognized that any cultural or religious belief system can dramatically alter or potentiate the use of placebos, hypnosis, and psychic healing methods. The belief system and religious persuasion of the client should always be assessed and understood before the nurse attempts to use any of the techniques mentioned in this text. Philosophical and spiritual perspectives on life and health can be found in such classics as Martin Buber's *I and Thou,* Teillard de Chardin's *The Phenomenon of Man,* Paul Tillich's *The Courage To Be,* and in countless others. Paterson and Zderad, in *Humanistic Nursing,* have listed many more resources for further study. [36]

Assertiveness Training

The role of patient advocate is one which nurses have always played, but it is appropriate only when the clients are unable to articulate their own needs. In a situation in which a client is powerless, this advocacy may be necessary. As soon as the responsibility for asking informed questions, expressing wants, needs, complaints, and dislikes can be assumed by the client, it should be shifted. The nurse then becomes a support person and colleague to an educated and assertive client.

Both nurses and clients are becoming more assertive through assertiveness training workshops. Assertiveness involves changing habitual roles and ways of acting and reacting. One of the major tasks in any assertiveness training group is to identify a list of rights such as the ones listed in the appendices at the end of this book. An assertive client or nurse respects his or her own rights and the rights of others.

Once students, nurses, and clients know their rights they can recognize when they are being ignored or negated. With the proper support—a group, organization, or union—they can begin to state their feelings when a right is abrogated. Anger, negative assertion, and aggressive behavior are discussed and role played in a group. Practicing support and giving and receiving positive comments is considered important.

Increasing awareness of self and others includes identifying areas in which behavior is habitually compliant and passive as well as situations in which unnecessary aggression is a pattern. It is important for nurses and clients to examine these aspects of self-responsibility which will influence the effectiveness of their communications and interpersonal relationships. Specific assertiveness exercises are included in Chapter 6.

Self-Care in the Nurse-Client Relationship

What about the impact of self-care on the role of the nurse and client? Is there a role for the nurse? What role function does it entail? In Chapter 6, the self-care movement is discussed as one method advocated for individual and community coping with the stress associated with life in a highly complex technological environment. Here, self-care will be approached from the point of view of self-responsibility, with the emphasis on the role of the nurse and client.

Self-care is described by Lucille Kinlein, an independent nurse practitioner, as a concept which recognizes and emphasizes the inherent human attribute of individual domain over one's actions. [23] Nursing, then, is assisting persons in their self-care practices in regard to their status of *health,* which incorporates body, mind, and spirit—not *illness*—which is the focus of medicine. A nursing approach based on self-responsibility begins with the self-care practices that clients articulate, not the ones the nurse thinks they should be practicing.

Kinlein views the nurse as an extension of the client and his needs, not as a physician extender involved in carrying out orders which facilitate the diagnosing and treating of disease. The nurse-client relationship is formed around the goal of self-care in improving states of health. The client is the primary decision maker seeking out the unique expertise of the nurse and other resources. [24]

COMMUNITY SELF-DETERMINISM

The "Medicalization" of Life

Ivan Illich, in his scathing attack on modern medicine, accuses the American health care system of "medicalizing" every aspect of life, thus depriving individuals, families, and communities of their own ways and cultural methods of handling crises, life events, and even death.

One striking example by Illich of the medicalization of life is the medicalization of old age. [21] With 28 percent of the American medical budget expended on the 10 percent of the population who are over 65 and the projected increase in that population of 3 percent a year, one has only to calculate the costs in the years to come. The "solution" to caring for the aged with multiple degenerative disorders appears to be taking them from their communities, cultures, and support networks and placing them in institutions to await their fate alone.

Institutionalization of the aged deprives them of their dignity and self-control, and deprives society of their valid contributions. The kibbutz system in Israel has demonstrated that a valid social role is as important to good health as is an easy access to medical care. The plight of the aging is an example of the outcome of negating a whole group's sense of self-responsibility and independence. An innovative self-help group called SAGE (Senior Actualization and Growth Exploration) is attempting to meet this need. (It is described further in Chapter 6.)

One heartening study based on encouraging patient responsibility in a nursing home was conducted by Judith Rodin and Ellen J. Langer of Harvard. [45] Ninety-one elderly patients were randomly selected and divided into an experimental responsibility-induced group and a control group. The responsibility group was given a plant and told they were responsible for its care. The control group was told that the staff would care for their plants.

Nurses and physicians were asked to rate the responses of each group for eighteen months. The experimental responsibility group was found to have a significant increase in alertness, behavioral involvement in activities, improvement in health status by 25 percent, and a decreased mortality rate—half of the control group's—over an eighteen-month period. It was felt by the researchers that assuming responsibility for a single plant caused generalized feelings of increased competence in day-to-day decision making where it was potentially available. [37, as cited in Pelletier, p. 210]

Other studies support the process of individual and group responsibility to a job, task, person, or group, etc., as a determinant in health status and longevity. The implications for holistic nurses are clear in both illness or wellness situations, institutional or community settings: *A feeling of responsibility for self is a basic life process and must be protected and nurtured.*

Summarizing the self-responsibility ethic, Illich has said that success in health is "in large part the result of self-awareness, self-disciplined inner resources by which each person regulates his own daily rhythm and actions, his diet, and his sexual activity." [21]

Community and Government Policies
Encouraging Self-Responsibility

Surprisingly enough, the American medical establishment is not as opposed to self-responsibility as one would be led to believe:

> Many people mistakenly believe that health care is synonymous with medical care. Health is, to a large degree, a matter of personal responsibility that must be exercised within the limits of genetic endowment. As a general rule medical care has relatively little impact on health measurements that supposedly reflect health, such as morbidity, longevity, growth and development are not measures of the quality of medical care being received. [54, Journal of the American Medical Association, May 24, 1976, p. 2327, as quoted in Somers]

In Public Law 94–317, The National Consumer Health Information and Health Promotion Act of 1976, the Federal Government went on record as recognizing:

1. the crucial roles of individual information, responsibility and behavior in determining personal and national health status;
2. the responsibility of government to provide the necessary information and assistance to enable the individual to protect his health. [54]

Any new health policies and programs must be based on two premises, according to Public Law 94–317:

1. Responsibility for health rests primarily with the individual, not with government, not with physicians or hospitals, or any third-party financing program. Meaningful national health policies must be directed to increasing rather than eroding the individual's sense of responsibility for his own health and his ability to understand and cope with health problems.
2. If the individual's responsibility is to be effectively discharged, it must be supported by social policies designed to provide them with essential environmental protection, health information, and access to health care when needed. [54]

The 1970s have been acknowledged as the "me" decade, focusing on self-awareness and development. Some have carried the self-responsibility ethic to extremes, as in the case cited by Leon Kass:

All the proposals for National Health embrace, without qualification, the no-fault principle. They, therefore, choose to ignore or to treat as irrelevant the importance of personal responsibility for the state of one's own health. As a result, they pass up an opportunity to build both positive and negative inducements into the insurance payment plan, by measures such as refusing or reducing benefits for chronic respiratory disease care to persons who continue to smoke. [Leon Kass, as quoted in *Health Pac Bulletins* (January/February 1978), 11.]

Obviously, placing blame for all illnesses and accidents on a person's lack of self-responsibility is as useless an exercise as claiming that all illness is caused by microbes. Penalizing undesirable health behavior is an ineffective teaching/learning strategy at best, as Chapter 9 demonstrates. One alarming point of statements like the one mentioned above is that a whole group of self-responsibility advocates appear to be ignoring the social and cultural determinants of individual behavior as significantly influencing lifestyles. It is very convenient (and cheaper) for insurance companies, industry, and government to support this interpretation of the self-responsibility ethic. It can also serve as a rationale for reducing expenditures in the areas of human services (for example, health, education, welfare). The 1980s should include some community, occupational, and governmental accountability and accessibility, as well as individual responsibility.

Self-responsibility can be supported by a public policy which creates and maintains the conditions under which Americans are most likely to optimize their health potential. Self-responsibility extends to the planning of an environment in which people and things live harmoniously, not in competition. This means more stringent environmental legislation and enforcement. It means a continued emphasis on zero population growth and improvement of the quality of life for the disenfranchised. Nurses have a personal and professional role in all these areas.

From a national community standpoint, what can be done to motivate individuals to optimize their health and to want to create a sense of purpose in their lives? National leaders should help provide people—especially youth—with opportunities for individual and group challenge and goal achievement which stimulate a sense of self-responsibility.

It is no secret that individuals have lost faith in big government and big business. The political climate is ripe for programs offering a return to self-reliance. Self-responsibility cannot be legislated, but it can be stimulated by an environment which gives value to self-reliant individuals. Holistic nursing is part of that environment.

REFERENCES FOR CHAPTER 2

[1] Sally Adams and Michael Orgel, "Through the Mental Health Maze," (Washington, D.C.: Health Research Group, 1975).

[2] T. X. Barber, N. P. Spanos and J. F. Chaves, *Hypnosis, Imagination, and Human Potentialities* (New York: Pergamon Press, 1974), pp. 109–26.

[3] Mary Morgan Belknap and others, *Case Studies and Methods in Humanistic Medical Care* (San Francisco: Institute for the Study of Humanistic Medicine, 1975).

[4] Herbert Benson and H. O. Epstein, "The Placebo Effect, A Neglected Asset in the Care of Patients," *JAMA*, 232, no. 12 (June 23, 1975), 1225–27.

[5] Loretta S. Bermosk and Sarah E. Porter, *Women's Health and Human Wholeness* (New York: Appleton-Century-Crofts, 1979).

[6] Eric Berne, *Games People Play* (New York: Grove Press, 1964), p. 178.

[7] Anita Blau, Laura Hively, and Naomi Remen, *The Masculine Principle, The Feminine Principle, and Humanistic Medicine* (San Francisco: The Institute for the Study of Humanistic Medicine, 1975).

[8] Harold H. Bloomfield, "Holistic: The New Reality in Health," *New Realities,* II, no. 1 (Fall 1978), p. 15.

[9] Fritjof Capra, *The Tao of Physics* (Boulder, Colo.: Shambhala Publications, 1975).

[10] Victor Daniels and Laurence Horowitz, *Being and Caring* (Palo Alto, Ca.: Mayfield Publishing, 1976).

[11] Wallace C. Ellerbroek, "Language, Thought, and Disease," *The CoEvolution Quarterly* (Spring 1978), 30–38.

[12] Wallace C. Ellerbroek, "Hypotheses Toward a Unified Field Theory of Human Behavior with Clinical Application to Acne Vulgaris," *Perspectives in Biology and Medicine* (Winter 1973), 240–62.

[13] Esalen Catalog, Fall 1978, p. 33.

[14] Esalen Catalog, April-July 1979, p. 3

[15] Nancy Evans, "The Journal as a Self-Recording Device," *Quest* (November-December 1977).

[16] Tom Ferguson, "Working in the Period Log," *Medical Self-Care,* no. 4 (1979), 13–14.

[17] M. L. Foulds, "Changes in Locus of Internal-External Control: A Growth Experience," *Comparative Group Studies,* no. 2 (1971), 293–300.

[18] Jerome Frank, *Persuasion and Healing* (New York: Schocken Books, 1961), p. 66.

[19] Janet Harris, "Advantages of the Nurse-Patient Contract," *Nursing Papers,* 10 (Summer/Fall 1978), 56–59.

[20] Holly Hutchings and Louise Colburn, "An Assertiveness Training Program for Nurses," *Nursing Outlook* (June 1979), 394–97.

[21] Ivan Illich, *Medical Nemesis* (New York: Bantam Books, 1976).

[22] Muriel James and Dorothy Jongeward, *Born to Win* (Reading, Mass.: Addison-Wesley Publishing, 1971).

[23] M. Lucille Kinlein, "The Self-Care Concept," *AJN*, 77, no. 4 (April 1977), 598–601.

[24] M. Lucille Kinlein, *Independent Nursing Practice with Clients* (Philadelphia: J. B. Lippincott, 1977).

[25] Jonathan Kirsch, "Can Your Mind Cure Cancer?" *New West*, 2, no. 1 (January 3, 1977), 40–45.

[26] Paul Knipping and others, "Rational Self-Counseling in a Variety of Applications," *Health Values: Achieving High-Level Wellness*, 1, no. 3 (January/February 1979), 11–16.

[27] John Knowles, *Doing Better, Feeling Worse* (New York: W. W. Norton & Co., 1976), p. 15.

[28] Herbert Lefcourt, *Locus of Control* (Hillsdale, N.Y.: Lawrence Erlbaum Assoc., 1976), p. 3.

[29] George Leonard, "The Search for Health: From the Fountain of Youth to Today's Holistic Frontier," *New West*, 2, no. 1 (January 3, 1977), 14–15.

[30] Rollo May, *Man's Search for Himself* (New York: W. W. Norton & Co., 1953).

[31] David Mechanic, "Stress, Illness, and Illness Behavior," *Journal of Human Stress*, 2, no. 2 (June 1976), 4.

[32] Ruth B. Murray and Judith P. Zentner, *Nursing Concepts for Health Promotion*, 2nd ed. (Englewood Cliffs, N.J.: Prentice-Hall, Inc., 1979).

[33] Irving Oyle, *The Healing Mind* (Millbrae, Ca.: Celestial Arts, 1975), pp. 62–63.

[34] Michael Parenti, *Power and the Powerless* (New York: St. Martin's Press, 1978), pp. 114–17.

[35] Talcott Parsons, "The Sick Role and the Role of the Physician Reconsidered," *Millbank Memorial Foundation Quarterly*, 53, no. 3 (Summer 1975), 257–78.

[36] Josephine G. Paterson and Loretta I. Zderad, *Humanistic Nursing* (New York: John Wiley & Sons, 1976).

[37] Kenneth Pelletier, *Holistic Medicine* (New York: Delacorte Press, 1979), pp. 209–10.

[38] Kenneth Pelletier, *Toward a Science of Consciousness* (New York: Dell Publishing Co., 1978).

[39] Kenneth Pelletier, *Mind as Healer, Mind as Slayer* (New York: Dell Publishing Co., 1978), p. 33.

[40] Fritz Perls, *Gestalt Therapy Verbatim* (Lafayette, Ind.: Real People Press, 1969), p. 100.

[41] E. J. Phares, *Locus of Control in Personality* (Morristown, N.J.: General Learning Press, 1976), p. 25.

[42] Ira Progov, *At a Journal Workshop* (New York: Dialogue House Library, 1975).

[43] L. G. Reeder, "The Patient-Client as a Consumer: Some Observations on the Changing Professional-Client Relationship," *Journal of Health and Social Behavior*, 13, no. 4 (December 1972), 406–12.

[44] Paulette Robischon and Diane Scott, "Role Theory and Its Application in Family Nursing," *Nursing Outlook*, 17 (July 1969), 52–57.

[45] J. Rodin and E. J. Langer, "Long Term Effects of a Control-Relevant Intervention with the Institutionalized Aged," *Journal of Personality and Social Psychology*, 35, no. 12 (1977), 897–902.

[46] J. B. Rotter, "Generalized Expectancies for Internal versus External Control of Reinforcement," *Psychological Monographs*, 80, no. 1; whole no. 609 (1966), 1.

[47] Anne Kent Rush, *Getting Clear* (New York: Random House, 1973).

[48] Mike Samuels, *Seeing With the Mind's Eye* (New York: Random House, 1975).

[49] R. E. Schaefer and others, *Toward a Man-Centered Medical Science*, vol. 1 (New York: Future Publishing Co., 1977), p. 73.

[50] Gary Schwartz and D. Shapiro, *Consciousness and Self-Regulation*, vol. 1 (New York: Plenum Press, 1976).

[51] M. Seeman and J. W. Evans, "Alienation and Learning in a Hospital Setting," *American Sociological Review*, 27, no. 6 (December 1962), 772–83.

[52] O. Carl Simonton and Stephanie Matthews-Simonton, *Getting Well Again* (Los Angeles: J. P. Tarcher, Inc., 1978).

[53] R. E. Smith, "Changes in Locus of Control as a Function of Life Crisis Resolution,"

Journal of Abnormal Psychology, 75, no. 3 (June 1970), 329–32.

[54] Anne R. Somers and Herman R. Somers, "A New Framework for Health and Health Care Policies," papers on the National Health Guidelines: Conditions for Change in the Health Care System (Washington, D.C.: U.S. Government Printing Office, 1977).

[55] Susan Sontag, *Illness as Metaphor* (New York: Random House, 1977), p. 24.

Chapter 3
caring

CHAPTER OUTLINE

A. Caring
   1. Defining the Process and Ingredients of Caring
   2. Humanistic Caring in the Helping Relationship
   3. Encouraging the Feminine Principle in Health Care
   4. The Caring Relationship in Nursing
B. Intrapersonal Caring
   1. Caring for Self
   2. Centering
C. Interpersonal Caring
   1. Communicating Caring Through Touch
      a. Eastern touch therapies
      b. Laying-on-of-hands healing
         (1) Sensing and photographing energy fields
         (2) Therapeutic Touch—a healing meditation
   2. Self-Transcendence Through the Transpersonal Relationship
D. Community Caring
   1. The Need for Caring in an Uncaring System
   2. Hospice Movement
   3. Alternative Birthing
   4. Nurses in Transition

CHAPTER OBJECTIVES

1. Define caring and its eight ingredients as they relate to the helping relationship.
2. Compare Milton Mayeroff's caring with Carl Rogers's humanistic idea of a therapeutic relationship.
3. Describe the feminine principle in health care and receptive caring.
4. List three methods of caring for self.

5. Explain the importance of touch in human development and interaction.

6. Discuss Therapeutic Touch in relation to laying-on-of-hands healing and energy fields.

7. Review the necessary conditions, the five phases, and the five observable short-term effects of Therapeutic Touch.

8. Describe transpersonal psychology as a development and application of humanistic thought.

9. Cite two examples of caring movements in the community.

CARING

Caring is the interactive process by which the nurse and client help each other grow, actualize, and transform towards higher levels of well-being. Caring is achieved by a conscious and intuitive opening of self to another, by purposefully trusting and sharing energy, experiences, ideas, techniques, and knowledge. Caring incorporates several major approaches and theories—the feminine principle in health and illness, humanistic philosophy and psychology, and the holistic helping and healing relationship.

Caring is a difficult process to research and even more challenging to teach. Some nurse educators feel that caring is an inborn ability which can be developed by the individual but which cannot be taught. The same has been said of healing. It is our goal here to contest those beliefs by exploring the ingredients and components of the ethereal caring and healing processes and by then demonstrating ways in which nurses can apply caring healing principles to themselves and others. In the words of Sally Hammond, "We are all healers." [14]

Caring, taken in the sense of satisfying the basic physical needs of clients, has been an inherent part of nursing since the Crimean War. It is this aspect of caring which is still addressed by the all too familiar statement, "Nursing has *always* cared for the whole person." We will assume that professional nursing care is meeting the basic physical needs of clients. Achieving proficiency in specific bedside nursing skills is not the concern of this book. Traditional bedside nursing is one small nurturative portion of the larger process called caring.

The caring process is one which all health professionals share and is the focus of all efforts aimed at high-level wellness. The caring—often termed therapeutic— relationship is the *medium* through which all wellness goals are achieved. It is to obtain whatever special qualities or outcomes of the caring relationship that the client comes to the nurse or "professional." If the client were continually functioning at the highest level of self-care, consulting the health professional would not be necessary. Something about the caring process between the client and the nurse makes it different and desirable at this moment on the health-illness continuum.

What is this "something" that makes up the caring process in nursing? How can it be differentiated from the caring of a lover, a friend, a relative, or another professional? A description of the caring process and caring in nursing follows.

Defining the Process and Ingredients of Caring

Milton Mayeroff, a philosopher, first attempted writing his thoughts on caring in the *International Philosophical Quarterly* in September 1965. His refined dissection and examination of the caring process was published in 1971 and is deceptively simple in length and organization. [23] Many of Mayeroff's thoughts strongly parallel work by the humanistic psychologists Carl Rogers, Erich Fromm, and Rollo May. One major difference in Mayeroff's exposition is the detailed description of the ingredients of caring—knowing, alternating rhythms, patience, honesty, trust, humility, hope, and courage. [23]

Knowing involves many kinds of knowledge. Mayeroff distinguishes direct experimental knowing—actually applying or doing something—from secondhand, indirect "book knowledge." Explicit knowing is being able to articulate the knowledge about someone or something, for example, "I hear you saying you're angry." Implicit knowing is sensing information but being unable to express it. An example could be as simple as the "uh-hmm," the "I understand," or the nonverbal nod which can signify countless words.

Intuitive knowing can be considered direct knowing in that suddenly knowledge or feeling is "sensed" in a manner not obtainable by normal means. This kind of knowledge has been downplayed in an era of discrete scientific determinations. Intuitive methods of gaining information—for example, "psychic" assessment data gathering—are being given more credence and are being utilized by many holistic practitioners.

Knowing a person in a caring relationship means acknowledging his or her strengths and weaknesses and recognizing his or her needs, goals, and wishes. If the nurse admits the different ways of knowing another human being, and becomes sensitive both to rational and intuitive knowledge about a client, she will have the first requisite of a caring relationship. *Professional* knowing requires the nurse to have additional knowledge about health and illness, human behavior and development, communication, and problem solving.

Alternating rhythms is a phrase which Mayeroff uses to describe the capability for taking different perspectives or points of view on a problem. Being able to see clients and their problems from varying positions is a difficult skill to master. Seeing the self or other as he sees himself or a problem takes more than understanding. Alternating rhythms means the ability to look at a situation from a broader point of view, to see a critical incident in its proper historical perspective, and to look at the long-term ramifications of a decision. Nursing experience does not negate the importance a health incident may have for an individual. On the other hand, living firsthand and vicariously through certain health situations and crises gives the nurse the advantage of seeing a health problem as a client sees it, and yet of being able to step back and look at it from an overall nursing point of view.

Patience enables nurses to allow themselves and clients the space to grow in their own time and in their own way. [23, p. 12] One of the most difficult tasks for nurses is to allow clients to make their own decisions and to set their own goals. Lip service has been paid to *mutual* goal setting. If nursing involves teaching wellness health behaviors, it needs to incorporate Carl Rogers's philosophy of learning:

I have come to feel that the only learning which significantly influences behavior is self-discovered, self-appropriated learning. [31, p. 276]

Patience "is not waiting passively for something to happen but a kind of participation with the other in which we give fully of ourselves." [23, p. 12]

Patience in caring requires allowing an elderly client ten minutes to walk to an exercise class instead of passively riding for two minutes in a wheel chair. Letting a child learn through structured trial and error may be part of a nurse's advice to an apprehensive mother. Patience may mean accepting total rejection by a client who is suffering from grief or loss. The nurse's professional interaction is characterized by conscious patience as clients struggle on their own—not the nurse's—path to wholeness.

Honesty is a positive quality that encompasses more than simply not lying. It begins with being honest about one's *own* thoughts, weaknesses, and motivations before those of the client are approached. A student nurse honestly examines the reasons for choosing nursing and for wanting to help a client. The nurse is also honest about differentiating her goals from those of the client.

Both Mayeroff and Rogers see honesty as a genuineness or realness in regard to the nurse's own feelings about clients and what they are saying or doing. If the nurse is able to identify and accept feelings—even negative ones—about the client and still express them in a caring manner, then she has reached another level of honesty, one that is viewed as an essential part of a therapeutic relationship.

Honesty has a real sense of the present associated with it. It involves feeling and understanding an experience with the client, stepping inside the client's shoes, and seeing the world through his eyes. This "empathic understanding," as Rogers terms it, is differentiated from sympathy, in which the client's entire identity and problems are taken on as one's own.

Distinguishing empathy and sympathy invariably leads to the caring ingredient, humility, which is more than not being arrogant or pretentious. *Humility* prevents the enthusiastic "helper" from overwhelming clients with sympathy and understanding—in a sense, smothering them with concern. When this kind of paternalism occurs, it may mean that the nurse has identified so strongly with the client or a client problem that she intends to solve it her way, because it has become her cause and the nurse's ego is now invested in the outcome.

Humility, according to Mayeroff, prevents an overreaction of sympathy by helping the nurse to realize that her "particular caring is not in any way privileged." [23] Thus, clients are not "mine" or "yours," but rather, individuals from whom we always have something to learn and whom the nurse cannot control.

David Brandon captures the essence of humility in caring in this verse:

If only
I could throw away
The urge
to trace my patterns
in your heart
I could really see you
        [4, p. 47]

Trust is probably the most fundamental ingredient in any relationship. It is related to honesty and patience in that it allows the nurse to experience a client as a distinct self-determining person, not as an extension of the nurse's will, and also as one who needs a safe, supportive environment in which to grow.

Trust is the ability to take a risk and to make that "leap into the unknown" with a client. [23] Recalling an early injection or a first gynecological exam can help the nurse reexperience that frightening element of uncertainty and distrust with which a client comes to a health care situation. Add to that basic fear of opening oneself to another, a negative health care experience, and establishing trust may be one of the biggest goals to achieve in the nurse-client relationship.

Trust can be established in the most minute ways, such as by fulfilling a simple commitment to send a client some additional information in which they have indicated interest. Reliability and honesty help establish trust in the beginning phases of the nurse-client relationship. Without a basic foundation of mutual trust, the caring relationship is destined for failure.

Hope is an ingredient of caring which maintains the desire to continue caring. Hope is not constantly thinking of the future; it sees the present moment as "alive with possibilities." [23, p. 19] Nurses are constantly dealing with chronicity and recurrent health problems. For example, despite all efforts, a three-year-old returns two weeks after initial treatment with another sore throat or ear infection. Hope helps the nurse help herself—and the exasperated mother—to see other alternatives and opportunities to try new approaches, to learn from the illness experience, and to strengthen mother-child bonds.

Caring takes *courage*. It's difficult to care for angry, hostile, unattractive, or abusive clients. It takes courage to disagree with a client or a colleague. Encouraging a person to do something that is uncomfortable or inconvenient, adhering to professional ethics and values, defending a person's rights, offering alternatives to orthodox methods of treatment, expressing what one is feeling, or restating to a client what he is saying or doing—all these things demand courage from the nurse.

As with self-responsibility, caring begins with self-caring. Mayeroff states, "Only the man who understands and appreciates what it is to grow, who understands and tries to satisfy his own needs for growth, can properly understand and appreciate growth in another." [23] One of the major theses of this book is that holistic nursing needs to be self-experienced and to be self-applied in order to use it with others. Most of the humanists cited later in this chapter will support this view.

Studies on child abusers have indicated that they were rarely nurtured in their family relationships. Therapy often focuses on allowing the parents to experience, sometimes for the first time, being loved, held, and cared for. The premise of psychoanalyst Willard Gaylin's treatise on caring states:

> In order for each successive generation to fulfill its potential for becoming caring individuals, they must be treated in a caring way. We must be made to feel lovable in order to be loving. The degree to which we are nurtured and cared for will inevitably determine the degree to which we will be capable of nurturing and caring. [13, p. 51]

It is especially important that nurses feel safe and secure both in themselves and their nursing roles in order to create that same supportive environment with clients. It is for this reason that self-responsibility is a prerequisite to the caring/healing process. Just as a nurse-healer in poor health should not be healing another, a nurse who is suffering from a lack of self-confidence, adequacy, power, and independence will experience difficulty encouraging these qualities in the caring relationship.

In caring for a client the nurse provides the genuine excitement, delight, and admiration that comes from knowing the personal struggle a client has endured in order to achieve a goal. This "positive regard" helps the client to have more trust in his ability to set and achieve other possible aims. A true and expressed appreciation of what the client has done for himself encourages him to try again.

A delicate balance should be struck between the nurse who sets herself up as the agent of approval and the one who leaves the client totally to his own devices. Until total self-responsibility has been achieved, the nurse helps the client make his or her own decision by providing information, offering alternatives, and pointing out potential consequences.

Humanistic Caring in the Helping Relationship

What Mayeroff has stated in philosophical but simple terms is echoed by the Humanistic Movement in psychology, education, medicine, and nursing. A review of the development of American psychology may help us understand the two major schools of thought on the study of human behavior.

Behaviorism began in the 1920s with Thorndike's animal conditioning experiments and has been identified ever since with the physical sciences and the rational analytical approach which studies behavior largely in an objective reductionistic fashion. Data and conclusions are stated largely in quantitative terms—a good example of left-hemisphere-dominated yang masculine principle thinking.

At about the same time, another group of behaviorists, led by Erich Fromm, viewed human behavior from a holistic perspective and attributed value to subjective experience and feelings. This camp called themselves the phenomenologists, and they believed in the unknowable spiritual aspects of human beings.

The phenomenological approach gave rise to the Humanists, who were led by William James and Abraham Maslow, the father of humanistic psychology. Maslow's major contribution to humanistic theory development was his theory of human motivation, which has served as the basis for a theoretical framework in the helping professions—especially nursing—for the past fifteen years. Maslow proposed the hierarchy of human needs pictured in Figure 3-1, which will be reviewed in Chapter 9.

Humanistic psychology has been called "The Third Force" because it has been established as a viable alternative to orthodox Freudianism (see Chapter 4) and objective behaviorism. Maslow himself was initially a behaviorist, but he found the available theories of human behavior lacking in regard to mental health and

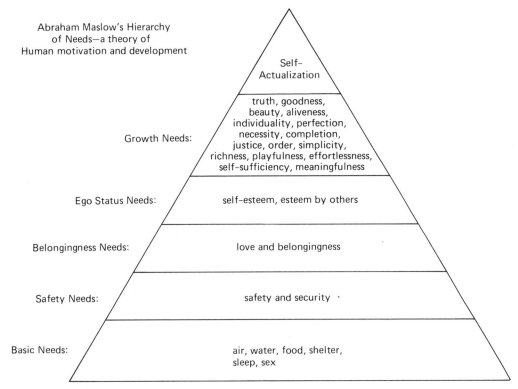

Abraham Maslow's Hierarchy
of Needs—a theory of
Human motivation and development

Self-Actualization

Growth Needs: truth, goodness, beauty, aliveness, individuality, perfection, necessity, completion, justice, order, simplicity, richness, playfulness, effortlessness, self-sufficiency, meaningfulness

Ego Status Needs: self-esteem, esteem by others

Belongingness Needs: love and belongingness

Safety Needs: safety and security

Basic Needs: air, water, food, shelter, sleep, sex

FIGURE 3-1   Abraham Maslow's hierarchy of needs
Adapted from Abraham Maslow, *Motivation and Personality* (New York: Harper & Row, 1954).

wholeness. Great attention had been paid to neuroses and psychoses in psychology, but very little had been focused on what constituted the "farther reaches of human nature." [21] Since Freudians were fixated with the unconscious and behaviorists with objective observations of animal experiments, Maslow felt the subjective experience of humanity was being ignored and invalidated. Studying the "average" individual was not a true indicator of what levels of development were possible for individuals. Maslow was to propose his theory which incorporated high-level wellness as a goal of psychological health.

Finally, Maslow was a critic of the mechanistic atomistic approach of breaking human nature into pieces for study. Maslow felt that human beings were systems in which each part related to another, and that the interrelationships and the whole were essential to any analysis of human behavior. Maslow supported the holistic or Gestalt approach that the whole is more than the sum of its parts and that human nature is made up of wholes or patterns. His theory of motivation is explained in more detail in Chapter 9. What is important to our present purposes is that Maslow felt that the highest level of need gratification to be achieved was self-actualization. This term has been adopted by most followers of the humanistic, human potential movement. The self-actualized person has gone beyond basic physical, safety, security, belongingness, and ego needs. Maslow describes self-actualization as "the desire to become more and more what one is, to become everything that one is capable of becoming." [20, p. 92] Some characteristics of persons who are moving toward or achieving self-actualization are subjective "feelings of zest in living, of happiness or euphoria, of serenity, of joy, of calmness, of responsibility, of confidence in one's ability to handle stresses, anxieties and problems." [22, p. 157]

In summary, humanistic psychology sees human beings as integrated, with the capacity to think, feel, evaluate, solve problems, and assume responsibility for self and others. It supports efforts to cope, self-explore, and to discover unknown potentials. [7, p. 13]

Behaviorists and humanists should not be placed in total opposition to each other. As with yin and yang and the masculine and feminine principles, they are different facets of a unifying whole. Brewster Smith points out that many applied behaviorists and behavior modification proponents employ humanistic strategies and reality-based philosophies and techniques with their clients. [34, pp. 27–36] Humanists, on the other hand, have been known to use behavioral and instrumental gimmicks to achieve therapeutic goals. The lines between the two sides are blurring considerably.

Encouraging the Feminine Principle in Health Care

In the autumn of 1972, the program in humanistic medicine was begun by the Institute for the Study of Humanistic Medicine at Mt. Zion Hospital and Medical Center, San Francisco, to deal with practitioner-client problems relating to the specialization of medical care, in which increasing focus was placed on technology in health care and authoritarianism in the health care establishment. The program still attempts to prove that contemporary scientific medicine can be integrated with human caring, full respect for the responsibility of the patient, and with concerns such as the meaning of illness and how the patient's values affect his or her health. The program has tried to address problems of more effective communication, mobilization of untapped resources within clients for health behavior, and the definition of alternative and more sensitive treatment methods for health situations, especially those with psychosomatic components. [1, p. 10]

One of the major philosophical constructs held by the Institute for the Study of Humanistic Medicine is the feminine principle in health care. (Recall Figure 1–3 in Chapter 1.) The masculine and feminine principles of Oriental medicine are represented as two opposing tendencies, but they should be viewed as different facets of the whole person. We all have masculine and feminine characteristics. Medicine has long been dominated by the masculine mode in which the health practitioners define and formulate the problem and the plan of therapy. Curing or healing is attributed to the health practitioner or to a specific therapeutic regimen. In reality, clients only use these things or people to heal themselves.

Curing is a major focus of health care, but Madeline Leininger, a nurse researcher/educator, points out that "caring acts and decisions make the crucial difference in effective curing consequences. Therefore, it is caring that is the most essential and critical ingredient to any curative process." [6, Leininger as quoted therein, p. 14]

In the feminine mode, a client's illness is not "managed" or "controlled" as it is in the active masculine principle. [30] Feminine principle caring is receptive, not passive—that is, "to take in, meet with, experience." [30, p. 54] The feminine principle guides the nurse in recognizing and respecting the special meaning of the disease in the focus of the life situation and goals of the client. The nurse and client discover and enrich each other's experiences through shared experience. [30, p. 54]

An exercise that can help the nurse take note of masculine and feminine principle qualities in a routine health examination is demonstrated in Figure 3–2. Obviously, certain aspects of the masculine principle are desirable in health care, however, the goal is to incorporate more of the feminine characteristics.

Active caring is associated with curing; receptive caring with "healing." In curing, the health practitioner bears the heavy burden, but in healing, the responsibility is shared as clients restore themselves to health and wholeness with support and guidance.

The Caring Relationship in Nursing

From our discussion thus far, it becomes obvious that caring—with its major ingredients—and humanism—with its supporting theories—supposes a dynamic conscious interactive process. *Health* caring incorporates some additional background and experiences which shape caring for a client. The depth and quality of caring is defined by a set of values or guideposts which set standards of behavior or certain expectations for clients to have of nurses and for nurses to have of themselves.

A *value* is a special form of belief within one's own total belief system about how one ought to behave and the end state of existence which is or is not worth attaining. [7, Rokeach as cited therein, p. 179] Examples of value statements are: Health is better than illness; Pain is bad, its relief is good; Death should be prevented at all cost, and life should be sustained at any price.

Values cannot be seen, but rather, they are inferred from people's behavior—what they attach value to, what they say they believe in, and the choices they make under varying conditions. [7] Values may be consciously felt, articulated, or unconsciously held. They serve to clarify the purpose and meaning of life, and they set standards of culturally acceptable behavior. [7] Given a variety of opportunities on which to act, values can be viewed as standards against which one evaluates directionality and risk taking. [7] Recognizing and clarifying one's own values is an essential obligation of any professional helper. Failure to do so can cause one to embrace prevailing systematized beliefs that perpetuate dehumanizing practices. [7]

There is considerable disagreement about how to go about teaching and learning caring humanistic values in nursing. Some educators feel that to incorporate humanities in nursing education will ensure a caring nurse. Others feel caring can be added into the job setting through continuing education with an emphasis on humanistic values. This author advocates values clarification and education as soon

	MASCULINE PRINCIPLE	**FEMININE PRINCIPLE**
Client History	Verbal/articulate	Nonverbal communication
	Rational thought	Feelings
	Content of words	Ways things are said, tone of voice, body language
	Parent/child interaction	Adult/Adult interaction
Health Exam	Technological and laboratory assessment	Intuitive assessment methods
	Detached, decisive, efficient	Empathic touch
Problem Statement	Intellectual/analytic	Intuitive
	Isolation of an illness diagnosis	Gestalt (the whole picture of client's life situation)
	Discounting of symptoms and complaints not verifiable by clinical assessment	
Plan	Knowledge	Wisdom
	Decisive power	Compassion
	Will/strength	Concern with lifestyle and meaning of illness for the individual client
	Suppress symptoms Eradicate disease	Illness viewed as an opportunity for creative change.

FIGURE 3-2 Masculine and feminine qualities in a routine health examination

Adapted from Anita Blau, Laura Hively, and Naomi Remen, *The Masculine Principle, the Feminine Principle and Humanistic Medicine* (San Francisco: Institute for the Study of Humanistic Medicine, 1975), p. 99.

as possible, with humanistic nursing values education and ethics integrated throughout the nursing curriculum. (Methods for encouraging humanistic values are discussed in Chapter 9.)

Nurses need immediately to begin clarifying, expressing, and comparing their values in relation to health situations. In Chapter 4, a scheme for analyzing nursing moral dilemmas will be described. Nurses need to be clear about their own value system in order to respect the value systems of their clients. The ingredients of patience, trust, and courage in caring, if truly practiced, will help nurses to accept belief systems different than their own.

How do nurses operationalize humanistic caring with clients who indicate a desire to modify certain lifestyle elements? New values need to be articulated, discussed, and proved more contributory to healthy living—as the client perceives it—than old ones. If the client incorporates a new and different value it will often be some time before the corresponding health behaviors may change. (Chapter 9 explores a Health Belief Model which is being used to predict changes in values and behaviors based on teaching/learning experiences.)

The caring relationship as described by Rogers has been alluded to. It also has ingredients that strongly resemble those of Mayeroff's caring ingredients and some of the characteristics of Gibbs' Trust Model [29] (compared in Figure 3-3):

1. Helpers are genuine or real in their relationships with clients. They do not suddenly don another role with clients or say something "appropriate" even if they do not feel it. Rogers calls it "congruence" when helpers describe experiences as they see and feel them.
2. Helpers feel and express "unconditional positive regard" for the client. This attitude is characterized by warmth and acceptance. Positive regard requires helpers to do something that a concerned friend would not do—reflect without judgment, any feeling, attitude, or value the client throws out. If a client expresses anger, hate, love, fear, etc., the helper accepts it openly without making a judgment about the behavior and without trying to change it. This is true patience and trust in the basic tendency of the client to move toward wellness and self-actualization. Rogers states that research verifies the effectiveness of this technique.
3. Helpers are characterized by empathic understanding or by being able to see the world as the client sees it as well as from the outside nursing perspective. If helpers can grasp the client's experience without losing their own identity, then change is likely to occur. [31, pp. 61–63]

The changes one nurse experienced as she evolved toward a humanistic nursing approach have been described by Paulen, a clinical nurse specialist working with oncology patients, and included the following:

1. She changed her approach from patient-client centered to person centered.
2. She changed her concept of self from nurse-professional to person-nurse-professional.
3. She became open, honest, and caring, and shared how she felt in the here and now of the interaction, that is, sad, helpless, hopeful.
4. She gave up control over the other's situation (the professional attitude of knowing what is best for the person) and accepted the patient's decisions about alternatives in the patient's health care and lifestyle.
5. She validated what the other person might be feeling, and checked out her observations and impressions with the other, making a statement that the other could confirm or deny, talk about now or later, but which let the other know of her interest, concern, and caring. [2, p. 104]

ROGERS'S THERAPEUTIC RELATIONSHIP	MAYEROFF'S INGREDIENTS OF CARING	GIBBS' TRUST MODEL INTERDEPENDENCY-BUILDING STRATEGY
Genuine, real, congruent	Honesty	Open, two-way communications, with wide sharing of important, sensitive information (*Step 2*)
Unconditional positive regard	Humility Trust Courage Honesty Hope	Person sets own goals, participates in making decisions (*Step 3*) Self-control, interdependence (*Step 4*)
Empathic understanding	Alternating rhythms Patience Courage Trust	Acceptance and trust of others, understanding, empathy (*Step 1*)

FIGURE 3-3 A comparison of three approaches to the caring relationship

The caring relationship in nursing is unique in comparison to other helping professions. Holistic nurses work with clients in their totality—body, mind, and spirit. Nurses, along with physicians, physical therapists, and a very few others, are licensed to touch. Beyond medicine, nurses live health as well as illness experiences with clients. Nurses maintain an intensity and duration of contact rarely experienced by anyone other than a family member. The intimacy, or the potential for it, in the caring nurse-client relationship is truly privileged as is much of the confidential information the nurse becomes privy to.

The possibilities for knowing, being with, caring, and sharing are limitless in the nurse-client relationship. The dangers of betraying trust or of not fulfilling a commitment are equally possible. The caring nurse is experiencing, valuing, reflecting, and conceptualizing the theory of nursing in every interaction—a heavy responsibility. The nurse is then sharing this with a client who needs that knowledge and synthesis.

Paterson and Zderad have listed twelve nursing behaviors that reflect one nurse's attempt to apply caring in nursing:

1. I focused on recognizing patients by name, being certain I was correct about their names, and using their names often and appropriately. I also introduced myself. Names were viewed as supportive to the internalization of personal identification, dignity, and worth.

2. I interpreted, taught, and gave as much honest information as I could about patients' situations when it was sought or when puzzlement was apparent. This was based in the belief that it was their life, and choice was their prerogative as they were their own projects.

3. I verbalized my acceptance of patients' expressions of feeling with explanations of why I experienced these feelings of acceptance when I could do this authentically and appropriately.

4. When verbalizations of acceptance were not appropriate, I acted out this acceptance by staying with or doing for when appropriate.

5. I expressed purposely, to burst asunder negative self-concepts, my authentic human tender feelings for patients when appropriate and acceptable.

6. I supported patients' rights to agape-type love relationships with others: families, other staff, and other patients.

7. I showed respect for patients as persons with the right to make as many choices for themselves as their current capabilities allowed.

8. I attempted to help patients consider their currently expressed feelings and behaviors in light of past life experiences and patterns, like and unlike their current ones.

9. I encouraged patients' expression to better understand their behavioral messages and to enable me to respond overtly as therapeutically as possible.

10. I verified my intuitive grasp of how patients were experiencing events by questions and comments and being alert to their responses.

11. I attempted to encourage hope realistically through discussing individual therapeutic gains that could be derived from patients' investment in therapeutic opportunities available to them.

12. I supported appropriate patient self-images with as many concrete "hard to denies" as possible.*

* Reprinted with permission from Josephine G. Paterson and Loretta T. Zderad, *Humanistic Nursing* (New York: John Wiley & Sons, Inc., 1976), pp. 107-08.

INTRAPERSONAL CARING

Caring For Self

Caring for self involves attending to the body, mind, and spirit aspects of health. As many as 70 percent of doctor visits have been termed "unnecessary," and the average family of four now sees a doctor more than twelve times a year. [37, p. 1] The competent physician, in response to these visits, reassures the client or advises measures that are basically over-the-counter or home remedies. [37, p. 1] Such statistics support the trend toward self-care, which is one emerging aspect of caring for self. The self-care movement supports a belief in one's own or the client's ability to assume control over normal function and minor deviations from wellness, rather than habitually consulting the professional before looking at self.

Self-care has also been described by psychologist Yetta Bernhard as the process by and through which self-respect, self-worth, and self-liking are developed. Self-care is realized intrapersonally and then through relationships with significant others, family, and community. Self-care does not exploit another and maintains the right of independence and interdependence in a significant relationship.

Self-care asks:

What can I do for myself?
What can I do for you?
To what purpose?
At what cost? [3]

Creating a belief in one's own self-care, self-healing ability takes trust, courage, and patience. Self-care involves the ability to calm and center oneself, listen to body-mind-spirit messages, and counsel self. Distinguishing and describing symptoms and comparing them with healthy norms takes practice. Gathering mind-spirit information involves the intuitive realm. Messages from the unconscious right-dominated hemisphere require guiding the body and the mind through some meditative technique that works for the individual.

Centering

Centering usually means finding a place to be alone to listen to oneself for ten to thirty minutes. Creating a comfortable time and place to center is half the task. Once the nurses or clients have performed a centering exercise, and have seen the beneficial effects, they will be more willing to make—not give up—time for this form of self-caring. Centering is also the preliminary step to any form of healing of others. (Centering is merely another form of relaxation or meditation, as described in Chapters 2 and 6.)

Daniels and Horowitz suggest an exercise called "Following your breath," described on p. 83.

No matter what form of centering is used, it might be helpful to record in a journal or notebook the feelings and sensations experienced while meditating. Any changes in perception or behavior patterns, not necessarily occurring during the

FOLLOWING YOUR BREATH

Continue to breathe normally just as you have been. Center your awareness in your chest and feel your breathing and the movement of your body from the inside as you breathe. Let your breathing be your consciousness.

Notice how shallow or deep your breathing is, how tense or relaxed your chest, and whether you are breathing with your stomach, your chest, or both.

When your breath is halting and irregular, and when you momentarily stop breathing entirely, just notice that. When you remember to, check to see what you were thinking of a moment before that might have provoked the tinge of anxiety that caused you to stop breathing regularly.

If you don't try to control or direct your breath, but stay aware of it, eventually it will slow down and become more regular and rhythmic by itself.

As you pay attention to your breathing, various ideas will come into your mind. Each time you notice an idea beginning to form, you have the choice of thinking about it or of keeping your attention on your breathing.

Often you'll find that your attention has drifted away from your breathing. When this happens, take note of where it has drifted to and ask yourself whether that's an important matter for you to think about. If so, you can jot down a word or two in the pocket notebook you keep beside you when you meditate (if that's not distracting for you), and then return your attention to your breathing. If not, pick up your attention from wherever it's drifted to and bring it back to your breathing. Or if you want to think about an important matter right then, instead of saving it until later, you can go ahead and do that. With time and practice, you can develop the ability to pick up your attention and bring it back to your breathing or other object of concentration each time it drifts away. [12, p. 286]

meditation, should be noted. Differences in muscular tension, sleeping, eating, and playing habits should be documented. Insights or new ways of looking at problems may occur. Keeping a record of alterations in lifestyle can help nurse and client to develop their own beliefs in meditation or centering.

INTERPERSONAL CARING

Some of the intrapersonal aspects of the caring relationship have been examined. These can all be applied to the nurse-client relationship. Caring for self has been emphasized as a prerequisite to humanistic caring for others.

The humanistic nurse might be well described by the Personal Orientation Inventory (POI) devised by Shostrum in 1966. [17, Shostrum as cited therein] The inventory measures self-actualization as described by Maslow. A caring nurse scoring high on the inventory would be inner-directed, independent, self-supportive, freely expressive of feelings, possessing a high sense of self-worth, self-acceptant in spite of weaknesses, and having a positive capacity for intimate contact with others. (The predictable phases of the therapeutic relationship with clients and groups will be described in Chapter 10.)

Communicating Caring Through Touch

How is caring communicated in the nurse-client relationship? Obviously, verbal communication is of some import and will be discussed in Chapter 7, but one of the most basic and universal practice components of nursing is the use of touch. Touch is used in nursing to perform fundamental skills as well as to establish a therapeutic relationship with clients, although not usually purposefully. As with the other life processes in holistic nursing, touching in caring is a conscious deliberate act directed toward a goal.

Research shows that touch is the first and most fundamental means of communication. [39, Barnett as quoted therein, p. 72] Touch influences perceptual and cognitive functions in human development, and represents an all-pervasive, positive attribute of interaction. [39, p. 76] Frequency of touch affects metabolism, intestinal motility, endocrine and muscular systems. It has been viewed as a stabilizer and facilitator of interactions between individuals and is correlated with self-actualization. It enhances liking of self, an awareness of one's body, a sense of closeness with others, and healthy biologic development of one's sexual identity. [39; Boderman '72, Burnside '73, Casper '65, Frank, 1957 as quoted therein, p. 78]

Eastern Touch Therapies

The therapeutic use of touch in caring as a powerful healing tool has fallen into disuse in the twentieth century with the advent of technology, scientific research, and modern medicine. Anything as personal, subjective, and unscientific as touching is difficult to examine rationally in a controlled experiment.

Acupuncture, acupressure, Jinshin Jyutsu, Reiki, and shiatsu make use of touch and massage in healing, and certain Eastern cultures use healing massages to effect cures and health. Polarity balancing is a touch technique that assesses the life force currents that flow through a trained helper's hands to release blocked energy that is often reflected in the body as illness or pain. [28] Figure 3–4 demonstrates a polarity therapist's suggestion for relief of tension headache. (Some specific touch therapies are described in Chapter 6. See the appendices for a moving description of one person's use of touch and massage to communicate caring. [32])

Laying-on-of-Hands Healing

The laying-on-of-hands is considered a form of psychic healing. Psychic healing has been defined as conducting and channeling the superconscious energy which

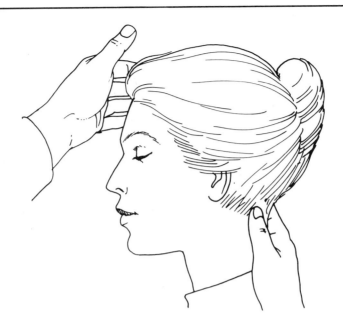

First, rub your hands briskly together and "feel your own energy."
Next, gently touch the palm of your right hand to the back of the person's neck.

Hold your left hand one half inch away from your subject's forehead.
Ask the subject to take ten deep breaths and let each one out with a
sigh. The subject's breathing will "increase the feeling of life-force
that you will feel in your hands." If that doesn't happen, have the subject repeat the breathing again.

Your hands should be left in place as long as you can feel a strong
energy transference. Within three to five minutes, claims Gordon,
most headaches will be gone or greatly relieved. When finished, he
reminds, shake your hands forcefully, and wash them in cold water to
remove static energy.

FIGURE 3-4 Gordon's treatment for tension headaches

Adapted from Bea Pixa, "Laying on of Holistic Hands," *San Francisco Sunday Examiner and Chronicle,* March 4, 1979, p. 4.

is the source and intelligent center of all life. [15] Some people can heal through
meditation or prayer; for others, it is an act of imagining or visualizing a person as
well and whole. Psychic healing is characterized by a spirit of humility and by a
feeling of unity with all other beings. It is a sense of being free of personal pride,
desire, or ambition.

Anne Kent Rush demonstrates an extremely simple healing exercise that can be performed with a friend or client:

> You can channel healing energy through your body. It seems to be particularly strong through your arms and hands. To experiment, simply place your right hand (palms down) on any spot on a friend's body which is tense or sore. Place your left palm on any other part of their body. (One especially good position is to have your hands opposite each other—that is, your right hand, say for stomach pain, on the stomach and your left hand opposite it on the back.) Close your eyes and relax your body. Center yourself and begin "exhaling" out your palms. You can also try imagining that the tension is moving from your right hand toward your left and dissipating. After five minutes or so, slowly take your hands away and ask your friend if any of the soreness or tension has gone. [33, p. 279]

Laying-on-of-hands healing has become identified more closely with nursing since the doctoral research of Dolores Krieger, a nurse-educator-healer at New York University. Her book, *The Therapeutic Touch,* summarizes her findings and experiences with the technique and describes a step-by-step centering, sensitizing, assessment and healing process which she has been practicing for over nine years. [19]

Krieger's position is that therapeutic touch healing is a natural human potential and can be performed by anyone in good health who has the intention of healing. The human body is seen as an "open" system always engaged in energy exchange. Therapeutic Touch is a specific transfer of energy directed and modulated in a therapeutic manner. [19] A subsequent section in this chapter will explore Krieger's work in more depth.

Sensing and photographing energy fields

Thelma Moss and Kendall Johnson of the UCLA Neuropsychiatric Institute, have used radiation photography to examine the "energy field" around the body. [25] The Russian technique of Kirlian photography has captured healers and meditators in the process of centering and focusing. Kirlian photography is a method of high-voltage photography which produces an image of energy fields or auras that surround the bodies of all living things and change with a person's emotional, mental, or physical state. The process was discovered by a Russian, Kirlian, and has been refined by scientists in the United States and Russia. [25] It is speculated by some that this technique may contribute to understanding the basis for how acupuncture, psychic phenomena, and "laying-on-of-hands" healing work. [25] Figure 3–5 demonstrates a Kirlian photograph. Kirlian photography demonstrates that centering and healing are real events that can be documented through objective technological means.

Another electroluminescent method similar to Kirlian photography has been developed by Rumanian scientists, and is produced on radiological films. Electronography quantifies electron emission, electromagnetic field effect around the biological organism, and ionization in the proximal electrical area which shows the adherent gas ion layer plus free gasions. [36]

William Tiller, a Stanford University Ph.D., attempts to explain the scientific rationale behind healing. He describes three major structural levels present in the

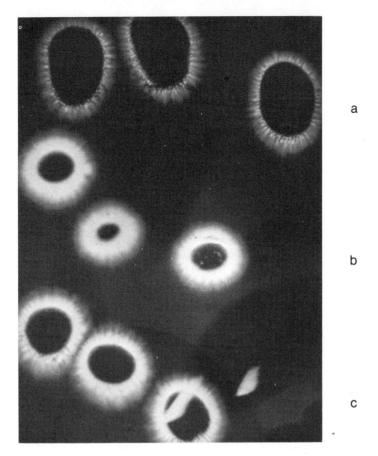

a

b

c

FIGURE 3-5 A Kirlian photograph of a healer's fingertips (a) before, (b) during, and (c) after a healing episode

From Dolores Krieger, *The Therapeutic Touch* (Englewood Cliffs, N.J.: Prentice-Hall, Inc., 1979), p. 11.

human being—the chemical level, the conventional energy field level (for example, electromagnetic), and the nonconventional energy field level embedded in a frame of mind which is embedded in a frame of spirit which is part of a larger "divine." [36, p. 46] Tiller theorizes that homeostasis at the biochemical level requires homeostasis at all levels, whereas disruptions in one level flow through to the others. [36]

According to Dr. Tiller, what we can expect from science is a set of logical, consistent, step-by-step assumptions and relationships. Einstein's theory of relativity questioned this lineal type of thinking and changed our definitions of time and space. We are on the brink of looking at reality and energy in a new way. Some new sets of conclusions can be drawn:

1. There are new energies which have never been dealt with before in physics.
2. Human beings have within their organisms sensory (or extrasensory) capacity for cognitions of these energies.

3. Time, space, and matter are all mutable. Certain people are able to transcend their fixed location in time (precognition). Some people can alter their location in space (remote viewing). Some people can dematerialize and materialize objects. If a few people can do these things, others can do them.

4. Whatever appears to be reality as perceived through the five physical senses, is not the only reality.

5. Techniques of sensing this other reality are being developed yearly as the photographic methods mentioned above indicate. [36, p. 46]

When practitioners use touch, acupressure, reflexology, or massage, they are working at the electromagnetic field level. All healing takes place in the untended energy fields as well as at the rudimentary chemical level. [36, p. 49] Dolores Krieger, also a neurophysiologist, cites the electrical conductance of the neuromuscular system which follows the biophysical principle that there must always be a field to carry the charge in electrical conductance. She describes the work of Harrold Saxon Burr at Yale University which measures L-fields or "fields of life" which change and cause concomitant changes in physical and mental states of clients. [19, p. 44]

Therapeutic Touch—a healing meditation

Therapeutic Touch as described by Dolores Krieger is basically a healing meditation in that the process involves centering and maintaining that center throughout the healing process. Some basic assumptions described in Eastern literature must be made before performing Therapeutic Touch:

1. Human beings are open systems in constant flux, and they experience input, throughput, and output of energy.

2. The healthy person has an excess of *prana* (Sanskrit for "vigor") and the ill person has a deficit.

3. A transfer of energy can occur from a healthy person who intends to help or heal to a healee. [17, p. 786]

The actual Therapeutic Touch takes only fifteen to twenty minutes and varies according to the sensations the healer picks up which tell her to terminate.

Three conditions exist in order for the nurse to become a helpful healer: (1) intentionality, (2) motivation in the interest of the healee not to heed the ego of the healer, and (3) the ability to confront oneself and the willingness to do so. [18]

Krieger has outlined five phases of Therapeutic Touch. They are:

1. Centering oneself.

2. Making an assessment of the healee. (See Figure 3-6.)

3. "Unruffling" the field.

4. Directing and modulating the energy.

5. Recognizing when it is time to stop. One stops when there are no longer any cues; that is, relative to the body's symmetry there are now no perceivable differences bilaterally—between one side of the field and the other—as one scans the healee's field. [19, p. 69]

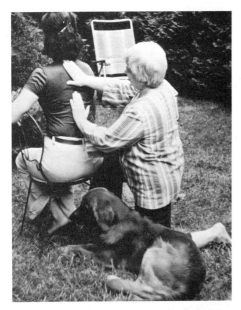

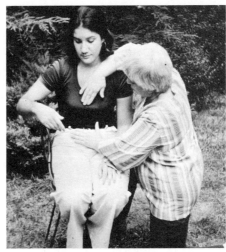

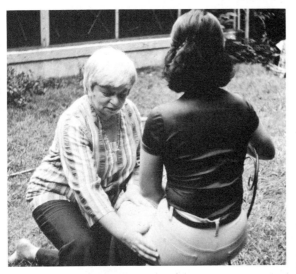

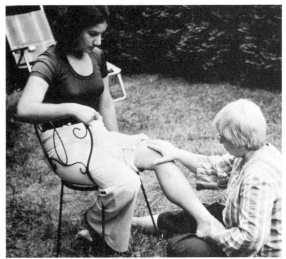

Energy is what fills the universe
Energy is what comes and goes
Consciousness is what defines the energy
Under that consciousness we're each
in touch with all of it.

Open yourself to absolutely anything that
gets thrown at you
Including death and life—
Open all the way
Don't worry about picking out the important stuff
Just let it all get thrown at you
and the important stuff
will be what hits you
All you have to do is not shut anything out.

FIGURE 3-6 Assessing the healee in Therapeutic Touch

Poems reprinted from Paul Williams, *Das Energi* (New York: Electra Books, 1975). Reprinted with permission from Dolores Krieger, *The Therapeutic Touch* (Englewood Cliffs, N.J.: Prentice-Hall, Inc., 1979), pp. 62–63.

As with most interactive caring techniques, Therapeutic Touch is a skill and requires a sensitivity which needs to be practiced initially with supervision and feedback. There are many exercises and awareness games designed to help the nurse-healer discover healing potential and create a belief system. It is *not* a prerequisite that the healee have a belief in this form of touching. The healer can practice healing self as well as others.

Therapeutic Touch is only one example of the healing use of touch being researched and used by holistic nurses. Many other methods exist and can yield the same observable effects. Some other cultural healing methods will be mentioned in Chapter 8.

Holistic nurses can evaluate the effects of Therapeutic Touch by observing any or all of the following:

Objective Observations:
1. Lowering of the healee's voice;
2. Slowing and deepening of the healee's respirations;
3. Peripheral flush of the skin, especially in areas specifically treated.

Subjective Observations:
4. Generalized feeling of warmth expressed;
5. Spontaneous verbal response—a sigh or comment, "I feel relaxed." [18]

What scientific data has been gathered on healing through laying-on-of-hands? The literature cites research with a well-known healer by Sister Justa Smith who demonstrated changes in enzymatic levels in test tubes subjected to laying-on-of-hands healing. [17, p. 787] Krieger's research demonstrated changes in mean hemoglobin values of patients subjected to Therapeutic Touch. Many more valid studies will need to be conducted, however, before laying on of hands becomes an accepted adjunct to orthodox healing methods.

The implications of laying-on-of-hands for current nursing practice are exciting. Many nurses and other professionals are seeking out these techniques, learning them, and practicing them on clients in acute care, long-term, and outpatient settings. Some methods can be incorporated as part of a routine massage or daily nursing care, for example, while others require a more specific position, place, and method. It is important that both nurse and client feel comfortable with the technique and, as in meditation, do not actively force healing to occur. Although untoward effects are almost negligible, the nurse needs to be familiar with the particular procedure and its guidelines. We are not unlike our ancestral healers experimenting with a force that is not fully understood. What *is* understandable after experiencing a healing with a client is the warmth, closeness, and mutual trust that is established. The accompanying physiological signs are often dramatic, but are not a necessary component of a healing episode. The advice in Figure 3–6 is well-taken by beginning holistic nurses.

Self-Transcendence Through the Transpersonal Relationship

Closely tied to the healing experience is that self-transcendence often described as being an outside-of-body phenomenon and at the same time as a feeling of oneness with the client, healee, and/or the universe.

The transpersonal world is filled with religious healers and psychics who attribute their powers to something beyond themselves—to a divine power or spirit. Whether it be from a philosophical or religious position, nurses are encouraged to recognize that all human beings possess the ability to project themselves beyond their current existence or predicaments. Some people choose to spend a significant percentage of their time in the transpersonal world—for example, as do some groups of Zen monks. Others have tried to induce transpersonal experiences artificially, through drugs. Singular transcendent experiences have been described by meditators, athletes, and dying clients.

A branch of humanistic psychology which devotes itself to the perceptions, experiences, and behaviors associated with the spiritual unconscious realm is termed transpersonal psychology. A group of psychologists organized and began publishing their own research and observations on transpersonal topics in the *Journal of Transpersonal Psychology* in 1968.

Anthony Sutich, founder of the journal, describes Transpersonal Psychology as a recognition, acceptance, and realization of such states as illumination, mystical union, transcendence, and cosmic unity. [9] Transpersonal psychotherapy is not directed toward pathology, but rather toward the expanding of consciousness in which the client is encouraged to discover and integrate transpersonal experiences.

Transpersonal therapists believe that each human being has impulses toward spiritual growth, a lifelong process that goes beyond self-actualization. Transpersonal therapy defines three stages on the path to transcendence: identification, disidentification, and self-transcendence. Commonalities exist between these stages, the nurse-client relationship, and the path to mutual growth.

1. *Identification*. In this first stage of awakening, the client gets in touch with the body, with feelings, with *deep* feelings, and with deep intuitions which influence his or her choices. This first step could be compared to taking responsibility for self. Involved in self-responsibility is the expression of negative feelings and antisocial impulses. This process of self-discovery goes on within the structure of the safe, supportive caring relationship. Through the helper's listening, clients begin to listen to themselves. Internal awareness is stimulated through meditative practices which encourage a receptive rather than an active manipulative mode of consciousness. One of the major learnings is that the client is the subject rather than object, the center of consciousness, who is capable of choice and free will and who is able to transcend past conditioning, no matter how negative. [9]

2. *Disidentification*. Paradoxically, disidentification involves divesting oneself of traditional roles, activities, and possessions. Ego gratification becomes less important; being has more value than doing or achieving. The Eastern attitude (mentioned in Chapter 1) of human suffering which stems from clinging to persons and things is solved by an increased detachment and a decreased need for possessions.

3. *Self-transcendence.* This is characterized by the qualities of acceptance, wisdom, tolerance for ambiguity, and the ability to play with opposing ideas. Self-transcendence in the nurse would not mean losing the ability to care and be involved; rather, it would mean being able to be truly present with clients in *their* situations without imposing the nurse's desire for a specific outcome on the client. [9]

An important idea, reinforced by Carl Jung, Ram Dass, and others, is that a helper cannot take someone beyond where he or she has been. The client initially responds as the helper responds, and learns to listen as the therapist listens. [9] Thus, the more spiritual growth the nurse has gained, the better able he or she is to help clients on their paths to self-transcendence.

COMMUNITY CARING

Community caring should center around the community's own helping process rather than imposing an outside helping system on a community. How can professional and voluntary helping be used to expand the community's own caring capabilities?

One federally-funded example—the neighborhood health center movement of the late sixties—attempted to act on the community self-control concept, but it experienced problems when very few skilled health professionals could be found within the community. Importing health practitioners and administrators seemed contrary to the idea of community control. Some neighborhood health projects succeeded even with professional helpers from the "outside," and eventually community control was assumed.

The secret to community control and outside helpers may lie once again in Rogerian-type nondirective leaders who do not set themselves up as experts, but who place value on the indigenous skills and resources of the community. Help focuses on community development—that is, on developing ways for community members to express and articulate needs, goals, and methods. The function of the helper is to listen, to provide guidance when requested, and to summarize and express general wishes indicated by the group. [4]

The Need for Caring in an Uncaring System

Some suggestions for bringing the caring back into health care have been proposed. One of the biggest criticisms that health professionals face is that clients often become depersonalized and dehumanized as soon as they enter the health care system. One major problem nurses face is the technical bureaucracy of medicine which robs both nurse and client of a satisfying and effective caring/healing relationship. The nurse becomes a time manager and efficiency expert who executes orders and directs paraprofessionals. The desire for interpersonal contact which initially motivated students to choose nursing has been lost in a move towards specialization and technology.

Nursing care is suffering the symptoms of fragmentation, lack of continuity, and the subjective feeling by clients that competent caring is being placed at the bottom of the priority list. Touch and caring humanistic values need to be reincorporated into standardized nursing care plans. The caring process in nursing attempts to encourage a philosophy in which the dignity and the growth potential of the client are respected and nurtured.

Hospice Movement

Two examples of caring in action in the community will be mentioned here. When humanistic values cannot be incorporated into the current health care system, alternatives such as hospice and alternative birthing are being offered outside that system.

The hospice movement began in 1967 when Cecily Saunders, a British physician, opened the doors of the St. Christopher's Hospice to the terminally ill. Hospice is a concept that has grown into a movement synonymous with humanistic caring for the dying and their families.

Hospice began as a place, but now the focus of the idea is on home care if that is at all possible. Rather than to remove the dying person from living and his loved ones, a program is developed for each client that incorporates tender, loving care and visits by a home care team trained in comfort, care, and pain management techniques. Extensive counseling is available to the family, and the role of the helper is seen as facilitator for the person's own support systems.

The hospice movement is an excellent example of a creative alternative to institutionalized care for the dying. How does this apply to the wellness end of the spectrum? The answer is because hospice deals with the entire well family from the first contact on. After the client dies, the family in crisis becomes the focal point for follow-up counseling, listening, nurturing, and referral.

Families experiencing real or potential loss describe the hospice worker in terms such as: "It was like a guardian angel coming in to support me just when I thought I couldn't stand it anymore," and "They helped me realize the last lesson my mother taught me—how to die," and "It was really an incredible experience—I'm not afraid anymore."

The hospice movement is often voluntary and self-supporting. Health professionals usually donate their time because they believe in hospice and want families to have some choice about where and how they die. Today there are over 350 home care teams throughout the world.

Hospice volunteers find that self-control over their environment is a very important need of clients in health care and dying care. For the client to have his personal possessions, loved ones, pets, plants, etc., is often more important than around the clock medical supervision.

Just as with alternative birth centers and home deliveries, the thrust in hospice is self-determinism with support from and participation of family and friends. Life events traditionally handled within the community—before they became "medicalized"—are being brought back under the auspices of the intrapersonal, interpersonal, and community systems.

Alternative Birthing

Another concept based on individualized humanistic health care is the alternative birth center which combines the warmth and caring of home delivery with the safety of modern medical backup. Although still within the confines of the hospital environment, labor, delivery and recovery take place in one room—a contemporary bedroom, often with double bed, couch, carpeting, stereo, and whatever personal items the expectant mother cares to include. Family and friends may attend the birth and mothers may choose to keep their babies with them rather than to have them in a nursery.

A group of San Francisco Bay Area nurses with maternity training and experience have banded together to encourage parent-infant bonding. Bonding is a process which begins at birth in which close physical contact between mother and child promotes health through a variety of psychobiological mechanisms and provides the basis for optimum development of the child (see Chapter 4). The nurses are on call to stay with the mother, father, and baby for several hours following birth. The service has become overwhelmingly popular as parents respond to genuine competent caring and education. [35]

Some hospitals feature not only natural childbirth but also the Leboyer method, often called "birth without violence." Birthing is seen through the baby's eyes as dimmed lights, soothing music, a warm bath, and a massage greet the infant.

Home births with midwives in attendance are on the upsurge, and it is predicted that one in twenty births in California will be home deliveries in the near future. [35] California state law recognizes only a registered nurse (RN), certified by the American College of Nurse Midwives and working under the supervision of a medical doctor (MD), as a nurse-midwife. Only 66 percent of midwives meet this criteria, and most of those work with clinics and hospitals. [33] Despite the illegality of home births, some parents are willing to risk a potential problem rather than to give up their right to a warm and joyous family experience. Alternative health care examples abound as consumers struggle from the grass roots up to gain more control over their health and the care they receive.

Nurses in Transition

How are nurses handling the frustration and confusion that inevitably accompanies the shift in roles brought about by such holistic humanistic innovations in health caring as described in this chapter? A San Francisco Bay Area group called "Nurses in Transition" is one attempt to deal with these personal and professional changes. The group hopes to "collectively learn new ways to channel our healing energy, starting with healing ourselves. The support network we have formed meets regularly and publishes a newsletter. The group is giving us the strength to speak out about health issues." [24] Groups such as these are helping nurses and clients to articulate their needs and rights to humanistic professional caring and to self and community determinism.

REFERENCES FOR CHAPTER 3

[1] Mary M. Belknap and others, *Case Studies and Methods in Humanistic Medical Care* (San Francisco, Ca.: Institute for the Study of Humanistic Medicine, 1975), pp. 27–29.

[2] Loretta S. Bermosk and Sarah E. Porter, *Women's Health and Human Wholeness* (New York: Appleton-Century-Crofts, 1979).

[3] Yetta Bernhard, *Self-Care* (Millbrae, Ca.: Celestial Arts, 1975), pp. 26–29.

[4] David Brandon, *Zen in the Art of Helping* (New York: Dell Publishing Co., 1976).

[5] Rick Carlsen, *The End of Medicine* (New York: John Wiley & Sons, 1975), pp. 63–64.

[6] Barbara A. Carper, "The Ethics of Caring," *Advances in Nursing Science,* 1, no. 3 (1979), 11–29.

[7] Jane E. Chapman and Harry H. Chapman, *Behavior and Health Care* (St. Louis: C. V. Mosby Company, 1975).

[8] Neil Chesanow, "Is It Time To Take Psychic Healing Seriously?" *Family Health* (August 1979), 22–28.

[9] Frances V. Clark, "Transpersonal Perspectives in Psychotherapy," *Journal of Humanistic Psychology,* 17, no. 2 (Spring 1977), 69–81.

[10] Arthur W. Combs and others, *Helping Relationships* (Boston: Allyn and Bacon, Inc., 1973).

[11] L. L. Curtin, "The Nurse as Advocate," *Advances in Nursing Science,* 1 (April 1979), 1–10.

[12] Victor Daniels and Lawrence Horowitz, *Being and Caring* (Palo Alto, Ca.: Mayfield Publishing Co., 1976).

[13] Willard Gaylin, *Caring* (New York: Avon Books, 1976).

[14] Sally Hammond, *We Are All Healers* (New York: Ballantine Books, 1973).

[15] Christina Ismael, *The Healing Environment* (Millbrae, Ca.: Celestial Arts, 1976), pp. 116–17.

[16] Jean Jenny, "A Humanistic Strategy for Patient Teaching," *Health Values: Achieving High-Level Wellness,* 3, no. 3 (May/June 1979), 175–80.

[17] Dolores Krieger, "Therapeutic Touch: The Imprimatur of Nursing," *AJN,* 75, no. 5 (May 1975), 784–87.

[18] Dolores Krieger, Therapeutic Touch Workshop, conducted at San Francisco State University Department of Nursing, March 17–18, 1978.

[19] Dolores Krieger, *The Therapeutic Touch* (Englewood Cliffs, N.J.: Prentice-Hall, Inc., 1979).

[20] Abraham Maslow, *Motivation and Personality* (New York: Harper & Row, 1954).

[21] Abraham Maslow, *The Farther Reaches of Human Nature* (New York: Penguin Books, 1973).

[22] Abraham Maslow, *Toward a Psychology of Being,* 2nd ed. (Princeton, N.J.: D. Van Nostrand Company, 1968), pp. iii–v.

[23] Milton Mayeroff, *On Caring* (New York: Barnes & Noble Books, 1971).

[24] *New Dimensions/Common Ground* (San Francisco: Baha-uddin Alpine & Sherman Chickering, Copublishers), no. 20 (Summer 1979).

[25] Irving Oyle, *The Healing Mind* (Millbrae, Ca.: Celestial Arts, 1975), pp. 86–91.

[26] Josephine C. Paterson and Loretta T. Zderad, *Humanistic Nursing* (New York: John Wiley & Sons, 1976).

[27] E. Mansell Pattison, *The Experience of Dying* (Englewood Cliffs, N.J.: Prentice-Hall, Inc., 1977).

[28] Bea Pixa, "Laying on Holistic Hands," *San Francisco Sunday Examiner and Chronicle,* March 4, 1979, p. 4.

[29] Adina M. Reinhardt and Mildred Quinn, eds., *Family-Centered Community Nursing* (St. Louis: C. V. Mosby Company, 1973), pp. 139–44.

[30] Anita Blau, Laura Hively, and Naomi Remen, *The Masculine Principle, The Feminine Principle, and Humanistic Medicine* (San Francisco: Institute for the Study of Humanistic Medicine, 1975).

[31] Carl Rogers, *On Becoming a Person* (Boston: Houghton Mifflin Co., 1961).

[32] Enid Rubin, "Touching and Saying Goodbye," California Living Magazine, *San Francisco Sunday Examiner and Chronicle,* May 8, 1977.

[33] Anne Kent Rush, *Getting Clear* (New York: Random House, 1975), p. 279.

[34] Brewster Smith, "Humanism and Behaviorism in Psychology: Theory and Practice," *Journal of Humanistic Psychology,* 18, no. 1 (Winter 1978), 27–36.

[35] Mary Spletter and Ellen Sherberg, "If You're Having a Baby," California Living Magazine, *San Francisco Sunday Examiner and Chronicle,* February 5, 1978.

[36] William Tiller, "Creating a New Functional Model of Body Healing Energies," *Journal of Holistic Health,* III (1978), 43–50.

[37] Donald M. Vickery and James F. Fries, *Take Care of Yourself* (Reading, Mass.: Addison-Wesley Publishing Co., 1977), pp. 1–10.

[38] Jean Watson, *Nursing: The Philosophy and Science of Caring* (Boston: Little Brown, 1979).

[39] Sandra J. Weiss, "The Language of Touch," *Nursing Research,* 28, no. 2 (March-April 1979), 76–80.

Chapter 4
human development

CHAPTER OUTLINE

CHAPTER OBJECTIVES

1. Define terminology related to the human development process.
2. List the universal underlying principles of human growth and development and be able to apply these to developmental tasks across the lifespan.
3. Identify the theories which have contributed to the body of knowledge surrounding growth and development and name those that are particularly significant to the holistic health movement.
4. Differentiate self-image, self-esteem, self-ideal, and body image.
5. Describe two human potential growth movement philosophies which support development of self.
6. Describe three examples in which an understanding of human development is essential information for nurses.
7. Assess one's own level of psychosocial development using two of the methods mentioned in the chapter.
8. Discuss the role of the nurse in intrapersonal, interpersonal, and family developmental critical periods.
9. Illustrate some applications of human development theories in the community as demonstrated in specific programs.

One of the most fundamental processes for nurses to understand and use in health and illness caring is human development. A sound knowledge and application of human development theory enables nurses to predict age-specific areas of expected growth in a client as well as to prevent potential stage-related hazards to wellness. Knowing normal developmental tasks and bench marks, the nurse can quickly help clients and families to detect deviations from normal and can pinpoint groups particularly at risk for certain problems.

Chapter 4 will define basic human development terminology and will scan a few prominent theorists and recent research, particularly in the heretofore uncharted area of middle and late adulthood. Some principles of human development that relate to philosophical holism and current ideas about human potential and self-actualization will be articulated. Intrapersonal, interpersonal, and community applications of holistic approaches based on the human development process will be reviewed.

The human development process incorporates preventive, nurturative, and generative nursing activities. Each developmental stage brings with it potential hazards and periods of stress. The nurse is keenly aware of age and stage-related lags and crises and helps clients and families prepare for and prevent those occurrences. Human development requires nurturing and caring behaviors of the holistic nurse. Creative and generative strategies are devised to help clients meet stage-related transitions openly and to view them as opportunities for continuing growth and change. The holistic philosophy and human potential movement espouse and encourage the belief in ongoing movement toward perfection, wholeness, and self-actualization.

Infant and early childhood development have been examined thoroughly for over fifty years, and clear ideas of minute developmental tasks and activities have been formulated and validated by countless experiments. Early, middle, and late adulthood had been neglected until the last decade, at which time psychologists decided to study their own developmental stage from a developmental perspective. The results of these adult growth studies are just beginning to reach professionals and lay people alike. Some of the ideas are controversial but exciting and open up an entirely new area of application for nurses, psychologists, and other helping professionals. Even more encouraging is the discovery that the stereotype of aging as a depressing journey towards death in which human beings are gradually divested of their dignity, self-esteem, and intellectual processes, is shown to be patently untrue.

TERMINOLOGY AND BACKGROUND

Life Span, Life Course, Life Cycle, and Life Structure

Those who study human development have created their own terminology to describe their observations and have constructed certain universal principles to explain the process of growth in humans. The terms life span, life course, and life cycle have been defined by researcher Daniel Levinson as follows:

1. *Life span* is a category that indicates the interval from birth to death. [34, p. 6]
2. *Life course* refers to the flow of the individual life over time—the patterning of specific events, relationships, achievements, failures, and aspirations. [34, p. 6]
3. *Life cycle* incorporates the ideas of a process as well as the notion of seasons. The process is a journey from birth to death but includes all the influences which shape the nature of the journey. Seasons are the series of periods or stages within the life cycle. [34, p. 42]

The *life structure* is the basic pattern or design of a person's life at a given moment, and it includes the person's sociocultural world (that is, class, religion, ethnicity, family, political system, and occupational structure, all of which modify a person's life).

The self is a complex patterning of wishes, conflicts, anxieties, and ways of resolving or controlling them. It includes fantasies, moral values, and ideals, talents and skills, character traits, modes of feeling, and both conscious and unconscious thought and action. A person's participation in the world is another part of the life structure, as well as how people interact in the world, through relationships and through their roles as citizens, workers, lovers, parents, friends, group members, or leaders.

Human Development, Growth, Maturation, Learning, and Holistic Philosophy

Perhaps the most overly used term is that of *development* itself. It has often been used to describe growth changes that are normally predictable increases in size or complexity, as well as those changes that occur as a result of maturation and learning. In this text, development incorporates both definitions. *Maturation* does *not* mean maturity, but rather, it refers to physiological, genetically programmed growth, which unfolds at a fixed rate regardless of environmental influences. An example of maturation is the readiness of the musculoskeletal system and motor coordination in a child about to begin walking.

Inherent in the concept of maturation is genetic endowment. For example, it is still impossible to alter the genetic make-up of individuals once they have been conceived. It will soon be technologically possible to engineer the genetic make-up of a person prior to fertilization; but the bioethical ramifications of such manipulations are tremendous and will be debated for years to come. In the meantime, great strides have been made in determining some chromosomal abnormalities in the amniotic fluid—the fluid in which the fetus floats. This poses a moral dilemma for parents who can opt to abort an abnormal child or who can use the remaining months of pregnancy to prepare for the lifelong changes a special child will cause in the family situation.

Motivation and *learning*—the processes by which behavior is initiated in response to a need—are two determinants of human development that can certainly outweigh the effects of heredity—sometimes to a great degree. Excellent examples of individuals who are triumphing over genetic endowment are seen in cases of physical impairments, brain dysfunctions, or chronic diseases in which persons learn to manage their disabilities and maximize their own levels of wellness. (Chapter 9 will address the learning process in more detail.)

The holistic health movement has been very active in the area of maximizing human potential. Some methods, such as Gestalt, have been described in Chapter 2. The underlying belief in the tendency of human beings to grow toward wholeness and perfection is held by almost all holistic practitioners. In 1926, Jan Christian Smuts, the father of holism, described his philosophy of human development in *Holism and Evolution:*

> The holistic nisus [striving] . . .is the guarantee that failure does not await us,
> that the ideals of well-being, truth, beauty and goodness are firmly grounded in

the nature of things . . . .Wholeness, healing, holiness—all expressions and ideas springing from the same root in language as in experience—lie on the rugged upward path of the universe, and are secure of attainment—in part here and now, and eventually more fully and truly. The rise and self-perfection of wholes in the whole is the slow but unerring process and goal of this holistic universe. [1, Smuts as quoted therein, p. 89]

In 1933, Smuts was joined by Alfred Adler, who developed a concept of personality that involved a basic striving toward completion, superiority, or evolution. Carl Rogers restated Adler's idea in what he called the "formative tendency."

Smuts, Adler, and Rogers's progressive ideas were in opposition to the popular systems theory idea of entropy or deterioration espoused by Bertalanffy. The humanists were grounded in the biological and behavioral sciences, whereas the closed systems approach is rooted in physics. This author supports an optimistic perspective on the development of humankind that echoes Adler's sentiments:

The development of man . . .is subject to the redeeming influence of social interest, so that all his drives can be guided in the direction of the generally useful. The indestructible destiny of the human species is social interest . . .Man is inclined toward social interest, toward the good." [1, Adler as quoted therein, p. 92]

Body Image, Self-Concept, Self-Esteem, and Self-Ideal

A major developmental concept which incorporates the three categories of body, mind, and spirit is *body image,* which is part of the overall *body concept* that includes a person's perceptions and knowledge about his body's appearance, boundaries, limits, and inner structures. Body image has been defined as a Gestalt or unified pattern for organizing sensory input. It has a physiological basis and is composed of physical, psychologic, and social experiences. The body image not only includes an individual's personal and psychologic investment in the body and its parts, but it also has a meaning for the individual in society.

Bioenergetics therapist Alexander Lowen goes even further in defining the relationship of people to their bodies, stating that each person is his body. No person exists apart from that body in which he has his existence and through which he expresses himself and relates to the world around him. The body expresses who one is and how he is in the world. The more alive the body is the more the person is present in the world, while the exhausted, drained body affects the people around it. [35] Nurses need to recognize this fact when caring for ill clients. As Chapter 7 demonstrates, the image the body conveys is often a far more accurate indicator of what is really going on with a client than is anything that he may verbalize.

Fisher and Cleveland demonstrated as early as 1956 that a client's body image is related to the site of cancer. [33] One type of body image visualizes the skin as a strong and protective barrier; an opposing view sees it as permeable and easily penetrated. The researchers concluded with valid and reliable test results that an individual's unconscious image of his body is an index to aspects of his personality which can influence the site at which he develops physical symptoms. [33]

The body image begins to develop at birth from the moment tactile and other perceptual stimuli are received and registered from the environment. Figure 4–1 sketches the development of the body image through childhood. One of the major developmental stages in which body image changes are experienced is adolescence. Teenagers not living up to their self-ideal often spend months or years discrediting their bodies and attempting to alter themselves beyond recognition. If the conflict is not resolved, the adolescent may suffer from a distorted body image and lose touch with reality.

Adulthood usually sees individuals' body images falling into line with socially acceptable stereotypes. A positive self-image is advised and sought after—thus leaving a market open for miraculous self-improvement schemes. Middle and later adulthood often presents a midlife crisis in terms of body image for men and women, as overweight and gradual decline creep into the picture people have of themselves. In aging, body image is often presented in a very unfavorable light. All physical signs of aging are considered by society to be negative, so that even an older person with a healthy body image faces problems.

Nurses need to remember that any alteration in body image, no matter how slight—for example, acne, pregnancy, eye glasses—can be devastating to a person's image of himself or herself. If the normal tactile and kinesthetic feedback a person is accustomed to is removed because of accident, illness, or other losses that person can truly lose an essential sense of himself in the world.

Let's draw our attention now to other common terms often confused with body image—self-image or concept, self or ego, self-esteem, and self-ideal.

Self-image or concept includes a person's perceptions of his ego, his nonbody images—such as spiritual, emotional, and intellectual make-up—as well as the body image itself, a major component of this self-image. *Self-esteem* is the individual's judgment of how he measures up to his self-ideal and to the standards of others. *Self-ideal* is Freud's equivalent of the "superego," that is, the individual's vision of how he should be and behave. If a person's self and self-ideal are drastically different, the person will have low self-esteem. *Self* or *ego* will be expanded later in the chapter; for now, simply know that it refers to everything that makes up the person—body, mind, and spirit, as the person sees them. For example, an infant sees only part of the body and none of the mind or spirit aspects of self.

Levinson sees the structure of society as reflected in the self. Each person's life gives evidence of society's wisdom and integration as well as its conflicts, oppression, and destructiveness. The self is a critical factor that forms and transforms each individual's world. [34]

The first psychologist to view the life cycle in stages was Else Frankel-Brunswick in the 1940s. [45] She was also the first to devote more attention to adult development rather than to that during the first decade of life. Part of the fixation on early childhood development stemmed from the principle that basic traits, attitudes, and behaviors are formed during infancy and early childhood. This doctrine arose from the Freudian belief that adult development was merely a continuing replay of all the conflicts of early childhood and infancy and that behavior change was virtually impossible.

Some attention will be paid to certain random ages and stages; however, this

Infant	Toddler (1-3 years)	Preschool (3-6 years)	School Age (6-12 years)
Unable to differentiate body from other objects in the environment (e.g., hand vs. rattle).	Able to differentiate between self and the environment.	Interested in one's own identity, "I."	Sense of industry vs. inferiority period.
Attitude toward own body: bites fingers, hands, or toes.	Due to increase in physical growth, toddler experiences modification in body image.	Identifies with parental model.	Learns how to interact socially with peers.
Develops trust relationships which contribute to further development of positive self-concept.	More aware of significant others.	Increased growth of language, intellectual, and motor skills.	Increased development of sex role identification.
	Developing a sense of autonomy.		Further development of intellectual skills by testing them against peers.
	Learning mastery over environment through development of: basic motor skills language skills bladder-bowel mastery.		Increasing concern with how others see one's body.
			Growing knowledge about the body and how it works.

FIGURE 4-1 Stages of body image development during childhood

Adapted with permission from Sharon L. Roberts, *Behavioral Concepts and Nursing Throughout the Life Span* (Englewood Cliffs, N.J.: Prentice-Hall, Inc., 1978), p. 271.

chapter is primarily a review of selected developmental theories. Applications to holistic nursing and presentation of material relevant to holistic practitioners will be emphasized here.

PRINCIPLES OF HUMAN GROWTH AND DEVELOPMENT

The holistic view of development and aging, then, is as a progressive, positive growth process that is moving in the direction of wholeness. Since the psychological and spiritual aspects of human development are valued, the gradual decrease in physiological function attributed to aging is seen as less important than the overall growth of the person. Decline can be minimized through lifestyle modification and a positive mental set. Certain principles of human growth and development have been hypothesized, observed in operation, and tested (Figure 4–2). Periodically reviewing these principles as you read this chapter will help one to focus on the universality and individuality of human development.

Developmental Tasks

The last principle in Figure 4–2 involves two important concepts—developmental tasks and ages and stages. The term "developmental task" was first used by Havighurst to describe a task that takes place at or about a certain period in the life of the individual. Successful achievement of this task leads to happiness and success in later tasks, whereas failure leads to unhappiness in the individual, disapproval by the society, and difficulty with later tasks. [28, Havighurst as quoted therein, p. 5]

Stages

Dr. Lawrence Kohlberg has validated this notion of stages through longitudinal studies and he recognizes stages by the following characteristics:

1. Stages are "structured wholes" or organized systems of thought. Individuals are consistent in levels of moral judgment.
2. Stages form invariable sequences. Movement from stage to stage or within a stage is always forward. Individuals don't skip stages.
3. Stages are considered hierarchical—that is, reasoning at a higher stage presumes lower stage thinking. The tendency is to function at the highest stage available. [30]

MAJOR THEORIES AND NEW RESEARCH

Since the field of developmental psychology includes many theories based on intuition, observation, and valid research, it will be necessary to isolate only a few major ones that have embodied a holistic perspective or that were historically necessary to the growth of an important idea.

1. The direction of growth occurs from the head end to the foot. (*cepalocaudal sequence*)

2. Growth progresses from the central parts of the body that mature earlier and function before those located nearer the periphery. (*proximodistal sequence*)

3. The trend of the direction of growth proceeds from mass to specific activities. (*differentiation*)

4. Development follows a definite, orderly, sequential, and predictable pattern. (*maturation*)

5. Development comes from both maturation and learning.

6. Every individual follows a definite pattern of growth and development; each individual does so in his own style.

7. During infancy and early childhood basic attitudes, traits, lifestyles, behaviors, and patterns of growth are formed; these can be modified in later life.

8. Each phase or stage of life has characteristic traits that are typical of that phase and must be completed for further development to occur.

FIGURE 4-2 Principles of human growth and development

Adapted from Doris C. Sutterly and Gloria F. Donnelly, *Perspectives in Human Development* (Philadelphia: J. B. Lippincott, 1973), p. 226; and from George Kaluger and Meriem F. Kaluger, *Human Development, the Span of Life* (St. Louis: C. V. Mosby Co., 1974), pp. 1-10.

Four terms recur throughout this section. They are *philosophy, concept, principle,* and *theory.* Brief definitions follow:

A *philosophy* is a set of values and beliefs about how one ought to live one's life.

A *concept* is a symbol that represents a set or series of common attributes.

A *principle* is a fundamental or predictive statement derived through reason or experiment about why something exists or occurs.

A *theory* is a broad comprehensive set of statements that attempt to predict experiments in science. A theory may or may not be verified.

Infant and Early Childhood Development

Sigmund Freud

Historically speaking, Sigmund Freud merits attention as the founder of psychoanalysis—the process of investigating the conscious and unconscious determinants of behavior. Knowledge of Freudian concepts is essential to the study of human development because of its emphasis on the stages of psychosexual development (see Figure 4-3). Freud dealt largely with neurotic clients, therefore his view

Freud's Stages of Psychosexual Development	Erikson's Eight Stages (Crises) of Human Development
Oral	Infancy: Trust vs. Mistrust
Anal	
	Toddlerhood: Autonomy vs. Shame
Phallic	
	Early Childhood: Initiative vs. Guilt
Latent	
	Middle Childhood: Industry vs. Inferiority
Genital	
	Adolescence: Identity vs. Identity diffusion
Young Adulthood	
	Adulthood: Intimacy vs. Isolation
Adulthood	
	Middle Age: Generativity vs. Self-Absorption
Maturity	
	Old Age: Integrity vs. Despair

FIGURE 4-3   Freud's and Erikson's stages of human development

of psychological well-being was slightly biased. Freud proposed a useful structure for analyzing behavior, however; he saw it as a dynamic relationship between the id, the ego, and the superego. Freud's model and ideas are useful because they laid the foundation for other theorists, such as Jung, Rank, and Adler, and the neo-Freudians Sullivan, Horney, and Fromm. Not all developmental psychologists were as absorbed with personality development as the Freudians. Others, such as Piaget and Gesell, were assessing childhood behavior, particularly cognitive and language development.

Arnold Gesell

Gesell looked at early, middle, and late childhood and youth according to maturity traits and gradients of growth. Both Gesell and Piaget respected the universal quality of growth and development, but they placed high value on the development of the individual self. Gesell, in particular, made it clear that the ages and stages were only approximate "zones" in which certain traits or behaviors would occur rather than exact moments in time. Nurses need to discern the *range* of normal for a developmental task as well as to assess individual variations within that range. For example, conscientious first-time parents may need reassurance if their child has not achieved a specific task by a specific time.

Erik Erikson

Perhaps the most quoted, imitated, and modeled developmental psychologist is Erik Erikson, a graduate of the Freudian Vienna Psychoanalytic School in the 1920s. In 1950 he proposed his eight stages of man (Figure 4-3).

Erikson's stages are based on the development of the self or ego. Each stage presents a problem composed of two opposites or polarities. The task is to balance the two—a notion reminiscent of the Chinese idea of balance between yin and yang, or masculine and feminine in the personality. Even though Erikson is concerned with developing certain attributes within the person—the capacity for commitment, the virtue of caring, the sense of trust—he also stresses the effect that society and culture have on that person and the response of that person to others and to society.

Erikson's stages are characterized by "crises" or critical periods in which the person is particularly susceptible to stress, but capable of greater potential and achievement. The critical periods are wrought with decisions, anxiety, times of progress and seeming failure, and backsliding. If persons finally resolve the developmental crisis, they can move on to the next stage. Erikson originally hypothesized that each stage must be completed before another can be tackled, but in reality people don't completely resolve conflicts. They recycle through old stages, especially during periods of increased stress or illness.

Trust versus mistrust is Erikson's first stage, and it lasts through the first year of development. Development of trust revolves around the quality of the maternal child relationship which provides reassurance and constancy.

Autonomy versus shame and doubt encompasses the second year of life, during which the child begins to sense his powers and the limitations society (parents) place on him. The child tests the limits and manipulates the environment within reason. It is the firm but caring attitude of the parents which helps shape his sense of individuality and independence.

Initiative versus guilt describes the toddler who explores and learns at a furious pace. It also provides an arena for guilt over "the goals contemplated and the acts initiated in one's exuberant enjoyment of new locomotor and mental power . . ." [16]

Youth and Adolescence

Erik Erikson

The next two of Erikson's psychosocial development stages place us squarely in late childhood and adolescence. Ages six through eleven mark the *industry versus inferiority* period. The child is exposed to systematic group learning; he takes responsibility for tasks and cooperates with others. Failure to achieve at this stage can affect the child's attitude toward learning and his future work ethic.

Adolescence is aptly characterized by *identity versus identity diffusion*. Identification with media-hyped models is a rampant catalyst for the rejection of more appropriate figures. "Falling in love with love" is a common attempt at an identity—even if it is projected or gained from another. The influence of cliques and peer pressure are of utmost importance. Rejection of parental concern or the acquisition of an identity through an occupation or job often occurs. Adolescence is the time to test, reject, and adapt a personal set of values, to become independent, and to move successfully into adulthood. The chances of a full-blown identity crisis are high during this developmental period.

Jean Piaget

The development of moral standards is an important task which cuts across ages and stages and has intrigued psychologists for years. Piaget made an initial study of it. Through his interviews and observation, he classified the *premoral stage* (birth to ages 4–5), a period during which no obligation to rules is sensed; the *heteronomous stage,* when literal obedience to rules, power, and punishment is considered the only moral right (ages 4–8); and the *autonomous stage,* during which the purpose and consequences of rules are considered and obligation is based on reciprocity and exchange of views (ages 8–12). [30]

Lawrence Kohlberg

Lawrence Kohlberg of Harvard's Center for Moral Education has proposed non-age-specific moral stages of development by which adolescents and adults make moral judgments. He has developed a method for assessing levels of moral development based on a moral dilemma situation that involves two conflicting values relating to one or more of the following: punishment, property, role and concerns of affection, role and concerns of authority, law, life, liberty, distributive justice, truth, and sex. Figure 4–4 defines and describes these moral stages. Can you envision yourself at different levels in certain situations?

Kohlberg's method of encouraging growth from one level to another involves

1. exposure of the adolescent to the next higher stage of reasoning;
2. exposure to situations posing problems and contradictions for the person's current moral structure, leading to dissatisfaction with the current level; and
3. an atmosphere of interchange and dialogue combining the first two conditions, in which conflicting moral views are compared in an open manner. [30]

It is Kohlberg's contention that values development can occur randomly—not on a preset timetable as in other areas of growth and development—or it can be taught and learned in social institutions, such as schools. Specific methods for teaching and learning values toward health are discussed in Chapter 9.

Adulthood and Aging

The discrete traits that characterize childhood become much more subtle in the developing adult. Physical changes suddenly level off in the twenties and thirties before aging changes become obvious in middle and late adulthood. The growth and development principles that gave us rationale for all physical and psychosocial changes in childhood no longer apply.

FIGURE 4-4 (*Opposite page*) Definition of moral stages

Reprinted with permission from Lawrence Kohlberg, "The Claim to Moral Adequacy of a Highest Stage of Moral Judgment," *Journal of Philosophy*, LXX, no. 18, (October 25, 1973), pp. 631–32.

I. Preconventional level

At this level, the child is responsive to cultural rules and labels of good and bad, right or wrong, but interprets these labels either in terms of the physical or the hedonistic consequences of action (punishment, reward, exchange of favors) or in terms of the physical power of those who enunciate the rules and labels. The level is divided into the following two stages:

Stage 1: *The punishment-and-obedience orientation.* The physical consequences of action determine its goodness or badness, regardless of the human meaning or value of these consequences. Avoidance of punishment and unquestioning deference to power are valued in their own right, not in terms of respect for an underlying moral order supported by punishment and authority (the latter being Stage 4).

Stage 2: *The instrumental-relativist orientation.* Right action consists of that which instrumentally satisfies one's own needs and occasionally the needs of others. Human relations are viewed in terms like those of the marketplace. Elements of fairness, of reciprocity, and of equal sharing are present, but they are always interpreted in a physical, pragmatic way. Reciprocity is a matter of "you scratch my back and I'll scratch yours," not of loyalty, gratitude, or justice.

II. Conventional level

At this level, maintaining the expectations of the individual's family, group, or nation is perceived as valuable in its own right, regardless of immediate and obvious consequences. The attitude is not only one of *conformity* to personal expectations and social order, but of loyalty to it, of actively *maintaining,* supporting, and justifying the order, and of identifying with the persons or group involved in it. At this level, there are the following two stages:

Stage 3: *The interpersonal concordance or "good boy—nice girl" orientation.* Good behavior is that which pleases or helps others and is approved by them. There is much conformity to stereotypical images of what is majority or "natural" behavior. Behavior is frequently judged by intention—"he means well" becomes important for the first time. One earns approval by being "nice."

Stage 4: *The "law and order" orientation.* There is orientation toward authority, fixed rules, and the maintenance of the social order. Right behavior consists of doing one's duty, showing respect for authority, and maintaining the given social order for its own sake.

III. Postconventional, autonomous, or principled level

At this level, there is a clear effort to define moral values and principles that have validity and application apart from the authority of the groups or persons holding these principles and apart from the individual's own identification with these groups. This level also has two stages:

Stage 5: *The social-contract, legalistic orientation,* generally with utilitarian overtones. Right action tends to be defined in terms of general individual rights and standards which have been critically examined and agreed upon by the whole society. There is a clear awareness of the relativism of personal values and opinions and a corresponding emphasis upon procedural rules for reaching consensus. Aside from what is constitutionally and democratically agreed upon, the right is a matter of personal "values" and "opinion." The result is an emphasis upon the "legal point of view," but with an emphasis upon the possibility of changing law in terms of rational considerations of social utility (rather than freezing it in terms of Stage 4 "law and order"). Outside the legal realm, free agreement and contract is the binding element of obligation. This is the "official" morality of the American government and constitution.

Stage 6: *The universal-ethical-principle orientation.* Right is defined by the decision of conscience in accord with self-chosen *ethical principles* appealing to logical comprehensiveness, universality, and consistency. These principles are abstract and ethical (the Golden Rule, the categorical imperative); they are not concrete moral rules like the Ten Commandments. At heart, these are universal principles of *justice,* of the *reciprocity* and *equality* of human *rights,* and of respect for the dignity of human beings as *individual persons.*

Erik Erikson

Erikson's last three developmental stages still work for adults, but as in the childhood stages, the desire for more predictable behaviors and traits persists. Briefly, early adulthood, according to Erikson, is characterized by *intimacy* and solidarity *versus isolation*. Having established an identity in late adolescence, the young adult is eager to "fuse that identity with that of others." Erikson agrees with Freud that this period focuses on love, with a valued and trusted heterosexual partner, and work—the work of supporting and raising a family. To not assume the traditional roles of provider and nurturer is to risk isolation and lack of intimacy. At this point, more recent trends part company with Erikson's Freudian-influenced ideas of adult development as newer concepts of relationships and family emerge.

Young and middle adulthood present a developmental crisis—*generativity versus stagnation*—in which the concern with establishing and guiding the next generation becomes important. This can be achieved through creative work, community participation, estate building, and so on. The alternative is to slip into a meaningless, humdrum existence or preoccupation with self, which takes the forms of early invalidism and depression.

Late adulthood brings the final crisis—*ego integrity versus despair*. Acceptance of the inevitability of death and loss and a feeling of oneness with the cyclical nature of humanity are signs of this stage. A desire to pass on a legacy or wisdom occurs. Focusing on the meaninglessness of life or remorse over all the tasks never accomplished during life can lead to despair.

Carl Jung

Erikson was not the only one to make a stab at analyzing and categorizing adult development. Carl Jung had written his "Stages of Life" essay in 1930 in which he focused on the latter half of life, captured in his term "individuation." *Individuation* begins at age 40 and is a developmental process through which a person becomes more uniquely individual. As the person acquires a clearer and fuller identity, that person becomes better able to utilize inner resources and to achieve self-determined goals. The seeds of individuation are sown in childhood, grow during adolescence, and come into fruition during middle adulthood.

Jung believed that every personality contained four vital parts—thought, feeling, intuition, and sensation. Parts of these have been developed to varying degrees during adolescence and early adulthood, but it is not until middle age that the person begins to balance and develop these aspects of personality. Another aspect of the self, the unconscious, contains four "archetypes" or polarities which the person in the process of individuation seeks to balance.

The four tasks of individuation are to reintegrate the following polarities: Young/Old, Destruction/Creation, Masculine/Feminine, and Attachment/Separateness.

"Young" symbolizes birth, growth, possibility, openness, energy, and potential; "old" conjures up images of termination, stability, structure, completion, and death. The developmental task is to confront these aspects of self, to give up some while retaining others, and transforming those aspects into a new life, incorporating the new meanings of youth and age into the personality at each new stage of development. Neither polarity is seen as good or bad, because aspects of both help the personality to grow and take shape, to constantly change and improve.

The second archetype is the Destruction/Creation polarity. At midlife, the realization of death is closer and this intensifies individuals' needs to do something creative with their lives before it is too late. Unachieved dreams and unrealized potentials become more apparent. The knowledge that we can and have caused pain and harm causes guilt and despair. Ambivalence in relationships is recognized by the person who realizes the capacity for both love and hate of a valued object or person. Acceptance of this two-edged sword brings greater self-knowledge and responsibility. It is the acknowledgment of the tragic flaws in our characters which partly contributes to the resolution of the destruction/creation polarity.

The third polarity—the Masculine/Feminine—was examined in Chapter 3. In reference to our present discussion, note that nurturing the neglected feminine side of our personalities is a task of middle age, at which time sex role stereotypes are questioned and sometimes altered or abandoned.

The final polarity is Attachment/Separateness—a task which the developing person has been working on since childhood. Attachment means being engaged, involved, needed, seeking, and rooted. Separateness, according to Jung, is being able to be involved with the world of the inner self, the unconscious, that part which can be reached through meditative techniques. Separateness can stimulate growth and creativity. Becoming too separate can endanger survival in society; becoming too attached to society and the world can hinder self-development. Again, a balance between the two must be struck, and this balance will vary from one stage to another. The overall goal of balancing the archetypes is to learn to care more deeply for others and for self.

Daniel Levinson

C. G. Jung was the first to describe what is popularly termed a midlife transition when he distinguished the first half of life from the latter half. This idea has been picked up and researched by many adult developmental psychologists, among them Dr. Daniel J. Levinson and associates of Yale University.

Levinson's study focused on the early and middle adult male life cycle. The sample consisted of forty men, ages 35 to 45. Levinson's rendering of the stages and transitional periods of the adult male life cycle is shown in Figure 4-5. The cross era transition points are crucial in the life cycle. The transition periods set the tone for the era to follow, and they can determine whether future eras will be renewed or stagnant.

The developmental task, according to Levinson, is to build or change the life structure (as defined on page 99). During *structure building,* which takes six to eight years, individuals create a structure, enrich life, and pursue their goals relevant to that structure. In a *transitional period,* which lasts four or five years, individuals reassess their existing structure, explore new possibilities, change friends, jobs, marriages, or social networks, and live out different facets of themselves. [34]

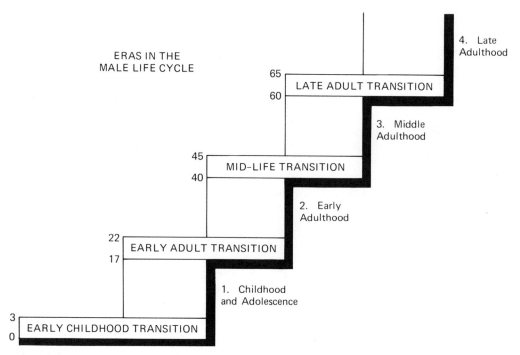

FIGURE 4-5 Eras in the male life cycle

Reprinted with permission from Daniel J. Levinson and others, *The Seasons of a Man's Life* (New York: Ballantine Books, 1978).

Other than working on building or changing their life structures, another major life task of individuals is to become more individuated, as described in Jung's theory.

Subtasks of working on the life structure involve the formation and modification of a dream, occupation, love, marriage, or family relationships; and mentoring of relationships (a *mentor* is a mixture of a good father and a friend); and the formation of mutual friendships.

Marjorie Fiske Lowenthal

Another landmark adult developmental study of 216 men and women facing transitions was conducted by a University of California San Francisco research team in 1972. The study chose certain developmental periods at four life stages—high-school seniors, young newlyweds, middle-aged parents, and preretirement people. The researchers looked at the life cycle as a series of inevitable changes which predictably occur, and they investigated whether the changes that involve role gain or role loss are potentially stressful. [36] It was shown that the anticipation of upcoming transitions serves as a stimulus to examine and even to change life goals.

An adaptation, as well as developmental, approach to life events was taken. This study was the first attempt to assess the extent to which resources or impediments fostering or hindering adaptive processes of the individual differ or resemble each other at successive stages of the adult life cycle. In other words, the study began to examine the processes of individuation and socialization at successive stages of the adult life course.

The study measured at least fifty variables related to life course transitions. The self-descriptive adjective rating list shown in Figure 4-6 suggests some life stage

FIGURE 4-6   Adjective rating list from *Four Stages of Life* developmental study

Reprinted with permission from Marjorie Fiske Lowenthal, Majda Thurnher, David Chiriboga, and associates, *Four Stages of Life* (San Francisco: Jossey-Bass, 1975).

ADJECTIVES DIFFERENTIATING EACH STAGE
FROM OTHERS OF SAME SEX * ($p < .05$)

High-School Men	Newlywed Men	Middle-Aged Men	Preretirement Men
Dissatisfied +	Cautious −	Cautious +	Ambitious −
Frank −	Cruel −	Disorderly −	Dissatisfied −
Friendly −	Dramatic +	Frank +	Hostile −
Persevering −	Hostile +	Lazy −	Reasonable +
Timid +	Impulsive +	Masculine +	Restless −
Unhappy +	Poised −	Sarcastic −	Unhappy −
	Reserved −	Self-pitying −	Uninterested −
	Restless +		
	Sarcastic +		
	Self-controlled −		
	Unconventional +		
	Versatile +		

High-School Women	Newlywed Women	Women Middle-Aged	Women Preretirement
Dependent +	Energetic −	Absentminded +	Absentminded −
Guileful +	Jealous +	Unhappy +	Assertive +
Helpless +	Warm +		Dependent −
Idealistic −			Disorderly −
Intelligent −			Dramatic −
Lazy +			Easily embarrassed −
Restless +			Guileful −
Sentimental +			Helpless −
Suspicious +			Intelligent +
Undecided +			Lazy −
			Self-indulgent −
			Stubborn −
			Suspicious −
			Undecided −

* A plus sign after an adjective indicates that this adjective is more characteristic of this stage than of others; a minus sign indicates that the adjective is less characteristic of this stage than of others.

(continued)

In the Lowenthal study, the Adjective Rating List was assembled from a seventy-item list, and adjectives were categorized as desirable or undesirable. Eighteen attributes declined systematically by stage, sixteen of which were considered undesirable. Three attributes, all desirable, increased by stage; they were: frank, reserved, self-controlled.

Lowenthal et al. state that although self-description through the stages is toward the positive and socially desirable, an increase in "rational self-limitation" occurs. A decline in the free flow and expression of physical and psychological energy is indicated. [36, pp. 63–64] Neugarten and others have connected this tendency with the psychological disengagement attributed to aging and to the realization and acceptance of death.

FIGURE 4-6 (continued)

changes in personality development. Psychological complexity was associated with a sense of well-being in the young, but at the preretirement stage, those—especially women—who had a complex view of life were the unhappiest.

Contrary to popular belief, as many young as older subjects were primarily oriented to the past. The young tended to focus on singular events, whereas the old took a broad perspective over their lives. Women reported more stressful events than men did, and that their overall stresses decreased over the life course.

A "challenged" group of men was defined as being more at risk for heart attack and stroke. These men were usually intelligent, had not developed self-protective lifestyles, and some were suffering from physical impairments. [36] These "challenged" men were more optimistic in their self-appraisals of their health than were another stressed group of men who complained about their health even though they were objectively healthier. The challenged group might be surmised to be denying both their stress and their response to it. Again, those respondents who sought and developed self-protective, stress-avoidant lifestyles seemed to age most contentedly. [36]

All middle-aged and preretirement men felt their main transition was to retirement. Two-thirds of middle-aged women felt the "empty nest" was their major transition. In discussions regarding transitions, four factors were found to influence the effect of an upcoming transition: evaluation of the transition (positive or negative), degree of planning for the transition, locus of control (mentioned in Chapter 2), and problems anticipated. [36] It could be hypothesized that preventive counseling with a client or a group would address these four areas.

Resources suggested by the study's results for stressed women included stable familial roles, emotional involvement with family, the development of a positive self-image and a feminine self-concept. All these resources helped to mediate the women's stress.

HOLISTIC APPROACHES RELATED TO DEVELOPMENTAL THEORIES AND PRINCIPLES

Although specific characteristic tasks and research regarding human growth and development have not been examined in this chapter, some holistic approaches incorporating them will be mentioned. Philosophies and methods that are particularly pertinent to nursing or that are being incorporated into nursing practice will be emphasized. Holistic attitudes are permeating all aspects of health care and human development, but especially in the areas of birthing, transitions, and aging.

Birthing and Bonding

Chapter 3 cited alternative birthing centers as an excellent example of humanistic caring in nursing. This national trend has been instituted by more than 1,000 of the nation's 6,500 hospitals. [37] The parents' own developmental needs are being supported in as natural a setting as possible, which is reshaping the entire pregnancy, labor, and delivery experience. The holistic pregnancy and childbirth process begins long before the parents make the decision about which childbirth system to use. Even if a natural childbirth method is not the one of choice, relaxation and visualization in pregnancy can change the parents' attitudes and perceptions about many of the anxiety-producing changes to come.

No matter how happy or well planned a pregnancy is, there are always negative images associated with an experience that will alter a family's life. If the parents have no past experience with caring for a totally dependent person, parenting can present a negative image. Through visualization, these images can be brought into awareness, be explored, and restructured. Meditation and relaxation techniques such as those mentioned in Chapter 6 can help parents to ready and clear their minds. Visualization makes use of this clarity so that parents can learn more about certain feelings and images and be able to create the images they want to hold. [44]

Receptive visualization can be used by parents after a relaxation exercise, during which the pleasurable and fearful aspects of pregnancy, childbirth, and caring for an infant flow through their minds. Some images will be filled with feelings of warmth and happiness, others will cause discomfort and may need to be dealt with by different methods on occasion.

Programmed visualization is a deliberate relaxation exercise. It involves picturing oneself experiencing enjoyment, health, strength, and energy in a certain situation—such as during pregnancy, during labor and delivery, or while caring for the baby.

Samuels and Samuels suggest times during the pregnancy to use relaxation for better health and well-being in both mother and baby:

1. Relax total body, especially uterine muscles and the baby throughout the day to promote circulation and well being.

2. Relax body and mind when upset, angry, or unhappy (stress hormones have an untoward effect on the baby).
3. Relax when fatigued.
4. Relax before going to sleep.
5. Relax at particular stress points during the day.
6. Relax when you feel sick or physically uncomfortable.
7. Relax a body part to anesthetize that part.
8. Relax at first sign of illness to help prevent or heal it. [44]

An example of receptive visualization in action would be to visualize oneself as happy at the thought of staying home to take care of a baby rather than to dwell on fears of being "stuck" at home; of not being able to bring in extra money by working and of having to give up things for the baby; and of being jealous of the attention the baby gets and requires.

An example of a programmed visualization would be for the mother to imagine herself and the baby as bathed in warmth and sunlight. This would channel positive energy through her and the unborn baby and keep both of them healthy and strong.

Holistic alternatives for childbirth are based on parent education, relaxation, and visualization; they include the following methods:

1. *Lamaze*—mother and father participate in labor and delivery; involves education and structured breathing exercises stimulated by a coach (sometimes the husband); drugs are not used unless necessary; baby can nurse immediately and bond with mother.
2. *Bradley*—widely taught, father is the coach; extensive parent education; relaxation and breathing; more favorable success rate than Lamaze; doctor is involved in philosophy.
3. *Other*—progressive relaxation; hypnosis; other self-systems.

In holistic childbirth the attention is focused on the baby as well as on the mother. The best known method was developed by Dr. Fredrick LeBoyer, who, as an adult, had himself participated in a human growth therapy in which he experienced the trauma of his own birth. From the pain came his pleas for making childbirth as pleasurable an experience as possible—not only for the mother, but also for the baby. The LeBoyer method uses such techniques as dimmed lighting, soothing music or hushed sounds, a warm bath and massage for the newborn infant, and placement of the newborn on the mother's stomach for immediate handling by the mother. The umbilical cord is not severed until it ceases pulsating, and suctioning is not automatically performed unless it is necessary. Neither is the baby slapped to stimulate breathing. Refraining from any active intervention is frightening at first to health professionals, but LeBoyer has both the rationale and experience to back up these changes.

The guiding principle in the LeBoyer method is to ease the transition from the uterus to the outside world so that the life of the child as it was *in utero* is maintained. This is done by maintaining a constant temperature, by not having the newborn bear weight, by maintaining the newborn in the fetal position, by fostering quiet and calm, and by embracing the infant. This philosophy, then, is translated into a deep and slow *infant massage,* which travels over the infant's back, with strokes that follow one after the other in movements that resemble waves. [32] One hand is still in contact with the infant's body as the other begins. LeBoyer describes this method as carrying the past, of the primordial slowness, the all powerful rhythm of the ocean. Although no research is available to substantiate LeBoyer's method, impressive photographs of his methods exist. Infants who are expected developmentally to smile at one-and-one-half to two months of age are smiling within twenty-four hours. As with any theory that disputes years of medical practice, LeBoyer's method still has a long way to go in the eyes of many obstetricians; but it is being increasingly pressed on them by eager prospective parents.

Another new theory that has received tremendous publicity is maternal infant "bonding," as described by Case Western Reserve Medical School pediatricians Marshall Klaus and John Kennell. Bonding is a biopsychosocial process that develops during the first hours and days of life. This period, termed the "maternal sensitive period," is characterized by the following:

Mother to Infant	Infant to Mother
Touch	Touch
Eye-to-Eye Contact	Eye-to-Eye Contact
High-Pitched Voice	Cry
Entrainment	Stimulation of oxytocin, which contracts uterus;
Time giving	stimulates prolactin (love hormone)
T & B lymphocytes	Odor
Macrophages	Entrainment (interlocking, mimicing of seeing,
Bacterial Flora	hearing, and movements in
Odor	synchrony with one
Heat	another) [29]

The initial maternal-infant bond optimizes the mother-child relationship for the years to come. Infants deprived of bonding have been shown to have less verbal interaction with their mothers in later years, and at age three-and-one-half, the "bonded" children scored fifteen points higher on an I.Q. test than did those who did not experience bonding. [44] Other facts brought to light by Klaus and Kennell are illustrated in Figure 4-7.

Fathers also experience a form of bonding called "engrossment," which involves a strong attraction to the infant, feelings of elation and increased self-esteem, and subjective statements about the "perfectness" of the infant.

The nurse's role in the bonding process is nurturative and supportive of the parents' own attempts to bond. The feeling articulated by many practitioners is that the more parents know about their baby and what to watch for, the better they will bond to that baby. [21] In some parent education groups, information is being shared about developmental tasks and assessments.

The Brazelton Behavioral Assessment Scale is a method of scoring interactive behavior in the neonate. It measures infant behaviors in sleep and wake states. The

1. There is a sensitive period in the first minutes and hours of life during which it is necessary for the mother and father to have close contact with their neonate in order for later development to be optimal.

2. There appear to be species-specific responses to the infant in the human mother and father that are exhibited when they are first given the infant.

3. The process of the attachment is structured so that the father and mother will become attached optimally to only one infant at a time. Bowlby (1958) earlier stated this principle of the attachment process in the opposite direction and called it "monotropy."

4. During the process of the mother's attachment to her infant, it is necessary that the infant respond to the mother by some signal, such as body or eye movements.

5. People who witness the birth process become strongly attached to the infant.

6. For some adults it is difficult simultaneously to go through the process of attachment and detachment, that is, to develop an attachment to one person while mourning the loss or threatened loss of the same or another person.

7. Some early events have long-lasting effects. Anxieties about the well-being of the baby who has a temporary disorder during the first day, may result in long-lasting concerns that may cast long shadows and adversely shape the development of the child.

FIGURE 4-7 Maternal-infant attachment—"bonding"

Adapted from Marshall H. Klaus and John K. Kennell, *Maternal-Infant Bonding* (St. Louis: C. V. Mosby Co., 1976), p. 14.

scale attempts to assess responses of the infant to the environment as well as his impact on it via twenty-seven scored items. The Brazelton scale also appears to be a reliable crosscultural measurement.

The Brazelton scale is just one method informed parents are using in the first few days of their newborn's life to learn more about them. Parents have the desire and ability—with some education—to assess their children, to become attuned to age- and stage-related changes and potential problems, and to use relaxation and visualization to shape their own ideas of a healthy family—thereby creating health and controlling disease through harmony of body, mind, and spirit.

In addition to giving infant massage, parents can help babies to perform yoga positions (for which their anatomy is well-suited). Some of these positions include

1. lying on the stomach, arms outstretched, head raised (*cobra*);
2. lying on the stomach, with arms, legs, and head raised (*open bow*);

3. crossing the baby's arms; and
4. very gently bringing the leg to the opposite shoulder, and shoulder to opposite leg. [44]

These positions promote flexibility, tactile discrimination, and development of balance and kinesthetic sense (the position of the body in space).

Psychosynthesis

Psychosynthesis has been discussed, and several of its techniques have been proposed, in Chapters 2 and 3. Psychosynthesis also suggests techniques for purging oneself of negative customs and critical self-analysis, and visualization techniques that evoke auditory, tactile, and other sensations, as well as visual images. All these methods are aimed at helping the individual to reach a "higher self." They can also be used for other more specific goals by nurses and other helpers.

Psychosynthesis was an attempt by Dr. Roberto Assagioli to bring together many of the theories of human development. *Psychosynthesis* is described as a method of psychological development and self-realization for those who wish to control their lives.

Assagioli's conception of the individual is divided into seven parts or levels, as shown in Figure 4–8. These parts are not hierarchical, and some levels are never reached or discovered. The goal of psychosynthesis is to unite the lower with the higher self, to achieve true self-realization and improved relationships with others. Although psychosynthesis is a developmental process, it is not connected to any particular age or stage.

The stages a person must go through to attain integration include

1. a thorough knowledge of one's personality;
2. control of its various elements through
   (a) the disintegration of useless images or complexes, and
   (b) control of the use of energies set free by ridding oneself of negative ways of thinking and reacting;
3. realization of one's true self—the discovery or creation of a unifying center; and
4. *psychosynthesis*—formation or reconstruction of the personality around the new center.

Quadrinity Process

Another holistic growth process related to psychosynthesis is the Quadrinity Process (formerly called the Fischer-Hoffman process), which is defined as a comprehensive, in-depth method of personal transformation. Individuals uncover the process of their childhood development through extensive writing and guided meditations aimed at releasing emotional trauma, anger, and fear and at promoting a discovery of one's essential identity or spiritual self. All four areas of development are explored—emotional, intellectual, spiritual, and physical.

Bioenergetics

Alexander Lowen has suggested a growth theory in his Bioenergetics energy concept. As the human organism grows, it adds layers to the personality. These layers remain alive, but ideally, they are integrated into the personality. Figure 4–9 presents these layers and the emotional task associated with each. Lowen views growth as expansion on every development level as new connections are made and experienced. As consciousness grows the person develops a widening circle of relationships (as Figure 4–9 illustrates). Eventually, as individuals develop, they become

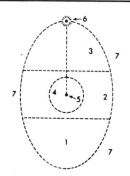

1. *The lower unconscious* (fundamental drives, dreams, and imagination of an inferior mind; uncontrolled parapsychological processes, phobias, obsessions, compulsive urges—similar to Freud's *id.*)

2. *The middle unconscious* (ordinary mental and imaginative processes. Similar to waking consciousness—not unlike Freud's *Ego* stage.)

3. *The higher unconscious or superconscious* (higher intuitions and inspirations, ethical "imperatives," source of a holistic altruistic love, genius, and states of contemplation, illumination, and ecstasy. Higher psychic functions and spiritual energies are located here.)

4. *The field of consciousness* (the part of the personality of which we are directly aware— the constant flow of sensations, images, thoughts, feelings, desires, and impulses.)

5. *The conscious self or "I"* (the center of consciousness.)

6. *The higher self* is unaffected by the mind stream or bodily conditions. It is a level of consciousness rarely reached, usually during certain transcendental experiences stimulated by yoga practices and other psychological techniques such as psychosynthesis.

7. *The collective unconscious* has to do with the individual's constant connection with humanity and the environment.

FIGURE 4-8 Assagioli's concept of the constitution of the human being

Adapted from Roberto Assagioli, *Psychosynthesis* (Baltimore, Md.: Penguin Books, 1977).

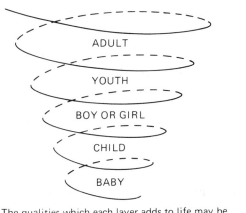

The qualities which each layer adds to life may be summarized as follows:

Baby = love and pleasure
Child = creativity and imagination
Boy or girl = playfulness and fun
Youth = romance and adventure
Adult = reality and responsibility

The layering of the personality as the human organism grows.

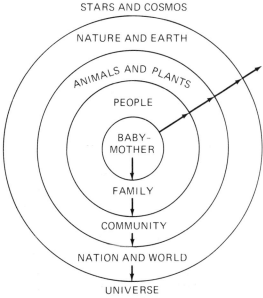

Expanding levels of development as the person interacts and incorporates more of the external world into the personality and psyche.

FIGURE 4-9 Layers of personality development: Bioenergetics

Adapted from Alexander Lowen, *Bioenergetics* (New York: Penguin Books, 1975), pp. 58 and 69.

part of the order of the earth and humanity. When they die, Lowen hypothesizes, the free energy of the organism leaves the body to merge with the universal or cosmic energy. [35]

Transactional Analysis

Transactional Analysis (TA) is a personality development theory first promulgated by Eric Berne in 1961. Its components are reminiscent of Freud's theory of id, ego, and superego and of Piaget's observations of the egocentric speech of the child and the development of socialized speech through the years. Although TA began as a psychotherapy, it has become a very popular self-help tool for solving personal and interactional problems throughout the life span, and also for educating the business and medical sectors of society.

Basically, Berne has simplified the language surrounding more complex psychological theories and has made them applicable at the intrapersonal and interpersonal levels. TA is concerned with four kinds of analysis:

1. *Structural*—the analysis of individual personality.
2. *Transactional*—the analysis of what people do and say to one another.
3. *Game*—the analysis of ulterior transactions leading to a payoff.

4. *Script*—the analysis of specific life dramas that compulsively play out. [26]

The next major section of this chapter will elaborate on structural analysis. The same section will also view transactional analysis cursorily and demonstrate its use in a nursing situation. Chapter 7 will explore transactional analysis in further detail.

The Life Review Process

Although many decremental physical changes may be seen in the aged, some positive characteristics that holistic health advocates strive for are often attained at this stage.

Butler observed not only a self-transcendent philosophy in the aged, but also concrete attempts to leave a legacy to posterity, especially to loved ones. This is often done through an oral history to a younger person, which is sometimes interpreted as repetitious reminiscing and as a sign of senility; however, nothing could be farther from the truth. The older person is attempting to confer the hard-learned lessons of life on a younger person, and although this is seemingly egocentric, it is a way of maintaining one's ego-integrity (as described by Erikson). The nurse may be the recipient of this legacy in some cases; she therefore needs to reinforce the older person's sense of self and willingness to move on to another existence or to death. The astute nurse can stimulate the life review process in a client.

The life review process as described by Butler (1963) is an active reliving of the past (in contrast to a more passive style of reminiscing). The significance to this is that it is a way of putting one's house in order, of coming to terms with past inconsistencies or "mistakes," and of preparing for the final haul. Butler has since expanded the process to include any period of crisis or transition. An active review of the past may follow from the need to resolve present life problems at any age or stage. [36]

INTRAPERSONAL APPLICATIONS

Several assessment tools are included in this section. Some of these can be applied to the young adult; others can be used on the practitioners' children and/or young siblings. Other characteristics, transitions, and tasks can be identified in parents and grandparents. Intrapersonal experience with each of the tools is recommended. Sometimes, through self- or other-guided visualization, students can imagine themselves in certain previous developmental stages, and they can watch themselves perform certain tasks and interact with significant others in those past situations. Ruth Carter Stapleton and others use the "guided meditation" technique to help clients return to early stages of development, crisis, and conflict; once there, the client relives the experience, discharges the negative emotions associated with it, and restructures the incident as he or she would like to have experienced it.

Structural Self-Analysis

Structural Analysis is a method of analyzing a person's thoughts, feelings, and behavior based on the phenomena of ego stages. [26; Eric Berne as quoted therein, p. 16] An ego state is defined as a consistent pattern of feeling experiences directly related to a corresponding consistent pattern of behavior. [26] It is the lifetime habit of reacting, replayed in situations which we interpret as requiring that mode of behavior.

Everyone has three ego states—the Parent, the Adult, and the Child. The Parent might be compared to the Superego. It consists of attitudes and behavior adopted from our own parents, such as biases and paternal, nurturing, or scolding behavior. The Adult ego state is related to the here and now; it is organized and rational—a good example of male yang-dominated thinking. The Child, on the other hand, is intuitive, impulsive, sensate, and could be compared with Freud's id or the yin hemisphere right-dominated feminine personality.

All three ego states exist in the personality and are merely different aspects of the same person. No ego state is more desirable than another. People usually flow easily and appropriately from one level to another, as demonstrated in the following example:

> *Situation*—Jim, a student nurse, has recently begun his clinical experience at the student health center. He walks into the examining room to conduct a complete health history and physical examination on a new client who seeks a pregnancy test and counseling. As he walks in, he realizes the client has been dating his best friend recently. (*Adult ego state*) He is immediately embarrassed and confused about what his role should be (*Child*); he wants to turn around and change to another client (*Child*), but he realizes that this is his assignment and that he should be adult enough to handle it. (*Parent*) However, he still has mixed feelings. (*Child*) He decides that he can be up front with his reservations and work it out with the client. (*Adult*) If they both feel comfortable with the situation, they'll continue with the exam. He can also talk it over with his instructor, if he feels the need to do so. (*Adult*)

Self-Assessment

Elder has suggested a good exercise for identifying ego states in the self:

> Think of a situation that you have been in within the last week which was enjoyable. Recall the details for half a minute.
>
> 1. How did you *feel* before, during, and after the situation you described? (*Child ego state*)
> 2. What should and might come into your mind regarding this situation? (*Parent ego state*)
> 3. What were the facts and rational thinking and behavior you engaged in? (*Adult ego state*) [15]

Figure 4–10 summarizes each of the three ego states and also details some of the attributes of each.

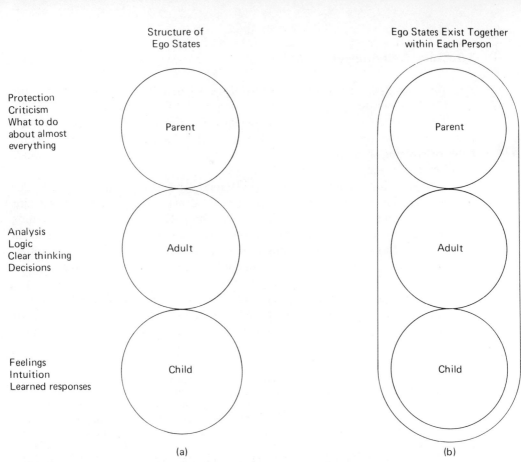

Structure of Ego States

Protection
Criticism
What to do
about almost
everything

Analysis
Logic
Clear thinking
Decisions

Feelings
Intuition
Learned responses

Parent

Adult

Child

(a)

Ego States Exist Together within Each Person

Parent

Adult

Child

(b)

FIGURE 4-10 The three-ego states: Transactional Analysis

Adapted from Eric Berne, *Transactional Analysis in Psychotherapy* (New York: Grove Press, 1961).

In addition to the many psychosynthesis tools and techniques he originated, Roberto Assagioli compiled a lengthy series of questions for each developmental level. The questions addressed to young adults, for example, are designed to help them look at the influences on their development, their families, attitudes, and values. The exercise is, in a sense, a guided autobiography. Although many people resist writing an elaborate self-history, Assagioli's questions are specific enough to encourage responses while still exploring formative relationships and experiences. A few of the questions pertaining to articulation of a philosophy follow:

1. What is your attitude toward life? What significance, value, and purpose has life for you? Are you inclined to be optimistic or pessimistic? Why?
2. What caused you to choose the subjects you are studying or the work you are doing?
3. Which aspects of the inner life are prevalent in you and which do you like most (thinking, imagination, feeling, prayer, or contemplation)?
4. What has school given or not given you? Do you think it advisable to change the methods and programs used in education? which of them? and how?

5. Are you satisfied with yourself? Do you think you can improve yourself? by what means? Would you like to receive advice in this respect?

6. What is your attitude toward the older generation, both generally and in regard to your family? Are there misunderstandings and conflicts? of what kind? How do you think they could or should be overcome? [2]

INTERPERSONAL APPLICATIONS

All intrapersonal self-assessment tools can be used in the interpersonal relationship with the client. Needless to say, the importance of the environment, family, and cultural influences that surround the developing child and adult cannot be emphasized enough. The influence of a positive bonding and parenting experience has been stressed. It has been shown that preventive, nurturing, approving, and nonrejecting parental behavior is associated with a child's belief in internal control of self and events. [42]

Nurses reinforce parental behaviors that encourage healthy development of the child, teenager, and young adult. When developmental lags or psychological problems develop, the nurse is familiar with the multitude of resources available to assist the individual and family towards wellness.

The Family

The seventh principle of human growth and development (see Figure 4–2) points out the importance of the family influence on early childhood development. Later, either a naturally occurring or chosen family continues to provide nurturance and support to the growing adolescent and young adult. Alternative family situations include communes, groups, and organizations which simulate, and in some cases, replace familial bonds that have been lost or broken. Families provide a protective cocoon around the fragile growing self, thereby creating feelings of value and self-esteem.

Some psychologists, notably Dr. Dennis Jaffe of Santa Monica, California, feel that the family is a determinant of health and illness. [25] If, for some reason, family communication is disrupted, a greater risk of illness is incurred. Dr. Jaffe specializes in family-change programs which attempt to reverse self-defeating or ineffective family interaction patterns. Even if only one family member is attempting a lifestyle change in diet or exercise, for example, the entire family is involved in the process. Family members learn to become aware of their needs, ask other members for help in meeting those needs, and feel comfortable in doing so.

One technique Dr. Jaffe uses to help families explore their backgrounds and patterns of interaction is a three generation family history which helps families to discover which family members and events have been most influential in making them who they are and in shaping their current strengths, illnesses, and difficulties. [25] Each family member writes a different history, and all the varied perceptions are then shared and discussed in a group. Sharing feelings and giving support are two goals of family-change groups.

Developmentally Related Client Services—
Women's Healthing Model

In the Women's Healthing Model developed by Bermosk and Porter, each stage of development is tied to age-linked health services which incorporate both orthodox and alternative health assessment as well as therapeutic and educational strategies. Figures 4–11 and 4–12 represent the typical services available to adolescent and late adulthood women.

No matter what human development theories or therapies the nurse supports, it is wise to assess one's own developmental level and that of parents, younger brothers or sisters, clients, and friends. Physical and motor growth and development, cognitive, linguistic, psychological, spiritual, and moral levels are all important in an assessment. Understanding developmental levels helps the nurse expect and explain developmental crises, passages, or transitions. Sometimes the client or family member sees a behavior as inappropriate or abnormal when in fact it is an expected developmental task of a particular stage. Being able to predict certain high-risk transitional periods can help the nurse plan an individual or group learning program.

Certain human potential groups have been accused of capitalizing on developmental crises; they offer relief of symptoms and make false claims of short-term resolution of lifelong developmental problems. Every profession has a fringe of charlatanism or self-interest to contend with. Even with the techniques covered in this chapter, there have been false claims and fraud. Chapter 10 includes strategies for evaluating the competence of practitioners—both orthodox and alternative.

In the next section, broad recommendations for community action and social change will be proposed. On the interpersonal level, much can be said for some of the therapeutic approaches that support individual development which has either been hampered in the past or thwarted in the present. [34] Individual and group counseling and education are doing much to help professionals and clients view their problems in a developmental context.

COMMUNITY IMPLICATIONS
OF HUMAN DEVELOPMENT

The community implications of the human development process involve an attitude shift and an increasing awareness on the part of youth, middle-aged, and aged. This process should be seen as a gradual predictable unfolding of opportunity, not as hopeless predestination. The holistic health and human potential movement have done much to demonstrate the creative, positive aspects of growing, changing, and aging.

HEALTH ASSESSMENT

Annual physical examinations
School physical examinations
Vaginal examinations (gonorrhea
  culture, Pap smear)

Adolescence abuse
Rape
Wellness Inventory
Stress assessment

DIAGNOSES AND THERAPIES

Crisis and suicide intervention
Rape advocacy and counseling
Malnutrition, obesity
Minor accidents
Minor infections, illnesses

Family planning
Clairvoyant diagnosis
Psychic healing
Individual and group therapy.
Family therapy

Rap Sessions for Adolescents

Fears of violence
Who have been raped
Who have attempted suicide
Who are pregnant
Living with a chronic illness
Living with a disability

Living in a one-parent family
Living with an alcoholic parent
Loss of a parent, child, friend
Giving a baby up for adoption
Keeping a baby as a single
  parent

HEALTH EDUCATION

Anatomy and physiology of the
  female body
Growth and development
Reproduction: menstruation,
  conception, pregnancy, childbirth
  and child care
Contraception
Growing up female—sexual identity
Self-awareness
Alternate life styles
Man-woman relations
Common health problems, prevention
  and care

Nutrition
Addictions—drug, alcohol
Coping with stress
Community resources
Nonstereotyped care
  opportunities for women
Holistic health practices
Personal hygiene and grooming
Physical fitness and self-defense
Assertion training
Self help: Breast examination,
  vaginal inspection

HEALTH CARE OPTIONS FOR ADOLESCENTS

Creative movement
Rolfing
Massage

Yoga; tai chi
Relaxation
Meditation

FIGURE 4-11 Health care services for adolescent women

Reprinted from Loretta S. Bermosk and Sarah E. Porter, *Women's Health and Human Wholeness* (New York: Appleton-Century-Crofts, 1979), pp. 187–88.

HEALTH ASSESSMENT

Physical examination
Cancer screening
Following rape, abuse
Wellness Inventory

Stress assessment
Pre- and postoperative
Following injuries, accidents

DIAGNOSES AND THERAPIES

Crisis and suicide intervention
Rape advocacy and counseling
Anxiety, depression
Malnutrition, obesity
Postoperative care
Common infections and illnesses
Sexual therapy

Clairvoyant diagnosis
Psychic healing
Individual and group therapy
Couples therapy, family
 therapy
Feminist therapy

Therapeutic Rap Sessions—Self-help

Women who are divorced
Women who are widowed
Aging—handling the stress of caring
 for self, husband, parent with a
 debilitating illness, following
 surgery, or with cancer, who is
 dying

Dying and death
Women facing retirement
Weight loss
Nursing care of specific
 conditions
Management of pain

HEALTH EDUCATION

Anatomy and physiology of the
 female body, from age 60 onward
Physical, emotional, and spiritual
 needs of the aged
Aging process
Wellness Inventory
Reactions and management of stress
 and anxiety
Sex education: maintaining sensuality
 and sexual response, orgasm,
 masturbation, woman-man
 relationships, woman-woman
 relationships
Divorce, widowhood, living alone
Nutrition

Common health concerns of
 women: symptoms associated
 with aging, breast and uterine
 cancer, vaginal infections,
 cystitis
Addictions—drug, alcohol,
 tobacco
Living with retirement
Financial planning
Caring for the ill and aged in
 the home
Community resources
Healthing and holistic health
 practices

HEALTH CARE OPTIONS

Biofeedback
Hypnosis
Rolfing
Massage
Polarity Therapy
Creative Movement

Yoga
Tai chi
Relaxation, imagery
Meditation
REAL

FIGURE 4-12 Health care services for late adulthood women

Reprinted from Loretta S. Bermosk and Sarah E. Porter, *Women's Health and Human Wholeness* (New York: Appleton-Century-Crofts, 1979), pp. 200–01.

Infancy and Childhood

Federal, state, and locally funded programs of well baby immunization, family planning, abortion counseling, and genetic screening and counseling have been in operation for years. They operate through neighborhood or district health centers and through regional or city hospital outpatient clinics. The Department of Health and Human Services, Health Systems Agency, has a maternal child health division which administers these and other protectively oriented human development programs. Many states have special infant and early childhood assessment and stimulation programs. All public health departments provide neonatal and developmental assessments.

More recently, the federal government has established a Child Abuse Council to deal with preventive and therapeutic programs of referral and counseling. Adult education programs and community colleges offer parents a channel through which to learn more about childhood development and how to handle developmental problems through creative parenting, parent effectiveness training (see Chapter 7), and ages and stages classes and groups.

Adulthood and Aging

Various church groups offer premarital, creative divorce, and single parent groups to help facilitate each of these difficult transitions. Women's and men's consciousness-raising groups abound with (and without) official or voluntary agency support. Women's self-help group members span from child-bearing and parenting age to those experiencing menopause and aging.

The private enterprise system has stimulated entrepreneurs to offer many more human potential and transition counseling groups for every conceivable developmental problem and price range. The opportunities for self-help and group support are available for payment, barter, or at no cost. It is the role responsibility of the nurse as counselor and referral agent to become familiar with these support systems, to explain them to clients, and to encourage their decision-making processes. With practice, and in some cases, supervision, some of the methods can easily be incorporated into the nurse's own repertoire of skills. The human development process is stimulating some of the most exciting research and innovative theories and techniques. The nurse is responsible for examining and critiquing this body of information, and for applying appropriate facets of it to self and sharing it with clients.

Public policy should focus on the middle-middle- and late-middle-aged, now in good health, who, for the first time in history, are facing fifteen to thirty years of postparenthood and retirement. [34] Little provision has been made for the masses of people who are moving toward a well-aging stage of life. This group needs to be politicized and helped to feel that it is they who have to lobby for legislation and programs which do not sentence them to early withdrawal from society. The Lowenthal et al. study indicated that the preretirement group felt they had little impact on issues vital to their survival as participants in the community, and they also felt they had no role in the community and could not ever envision one. [36]

A life course orientation is needed in social, economic, and educational institutions. It must reach adolescents and young adults so that the postparental and preretirement stages do not present them with an empty future over which they have little control. Obviously, then, all helping professional schools should contain a life course program of instruction.

Another huge area of potential community response to the human development process in adulthood is the workplace. Enhancing the meaning of work and creating work organizations which promote development of the worker is a new way of looking at productivity and profit. Employers are beginning to recognize that a worker who feels cared for and who has incentives and resources within the work setting for self-improvement and for coping with stress, is much less expensive to maintain in the long run than one who requires disability, hospitalization, and alcohol rehabilitation. Therefore, stress reduction, transition counseling, and lifestyling programs are receiving a positive response from employers—especially in large corporations.

The middle-aged and elderly should be exposed to a life course orientation through well-publicized programs that are made easily accessible to them. The retirement age should not be mandatory; training facilities should be developed so that middle-aged people can prepare for a second career if desired; and the mass-media orientation of the youth culture should be modified. [36]

For the aging, community and church-sponsored preretirement groups, Senior Citizen Activity Centers and federally sponsored organizations such as the National Commission on the Aging are fighting to change society's stereotypical view of aging—one which the aging often have of themselves as well. The grant-funded SAGE Foundation will be described in Chapter 6 as a model in holistic self-care for the aging. SAGE (Senior Actualization and Growth Exploration) is comprised of four programs:

1. Core Group Programs, which are small intensive groups working toward self-care and leadership of other groups.
2. Institutional Programs in extended care facilities and convalescent centers.
3. Professional Training and Research Programs offering seminars, workshops, and programs for professionals.
4. National development and networking which instituted the National Association for Humanistic Gerontology in 1974. It held its first conference in the summer of 1979, which focused on positive views of old age and on an exchange of information related to healthy, successful aging. [14, 40]

Ken Dychtwald, the founder of the National Association for Humanistic Gerontology, quotes two of the SAGE participants who summarize some of the holistic philosophy and practices learned:

At SAGE I have been learning how to be alive and vital again. For example, I was recently at a party and ate some of the wrong things. When I went home, I suffered from a tachycardia [rapid heartbeat] attack. I immediately put myself into a state of deep relaxation and practiced yogic breathing and the attack quickly passed . . .In addition to becoming more aware of myself in a physical way, I have also been learning quite a bit about my mind and my feelings. In my SAGE group I had a chance to work through some of my long-repressed grief about losing six people including my brother within a short period of time. One day I was doing my deep breathing exercises when emotions started coming up and I began to cry . . . .I wept bitterly for two hours, and I wept away a score of sorrows. And, finally, I started to laugh, thinking of all the people who have loved me all my life and still love me . . . .

. . ."I've seen things go on here that are amazing . . .self-healing. Here we're learning to tap new personal power sources through our spiritual growth. I'm finding energy that I haven't had in years." [14]

If stages, critical periods, eras, and transitions are a necessary part of the developmental process, how can we better help individuals to cope with these changes without debilitating distress and crisis? Do we accept depression and illness as a normal part of growing, or are there alternatives? Holistic approaches and innovative research are demonstrating that incorporating, trying, and testing these theories and methods is a developmental task for holistic nursing.

REFERENCES FOR CHAPTER 4

[1] Heinz L. Ansbacher, "Rogers' 'Formative Tendency,' Smuts, and Adler: A Humanistic Consensus," *Journal of Humanistic Psychology*, 18, no. 3 (Summer 1978), 87–92.

[2] Roberto Assagioli, *Psychosynthesis* (Baltimore, Md.: Penguin Books, 1977).

[3] Roberto Assagioli, *The Act of Will* (Baltimore, Md.: Penguin Books, 1974).

[4] Loretta S. Bermosk and Sarah E. Porter, *Women's Health and Human Wholeness* (New York: Appleton-Century-Crofts, 1979).

[5] Eric Berne, *Games People Play* (New York: Grove Press, 1964), p. 25.

[6] Barbara Brennan and Joan Rattner Heilman, *The Complete Book of Midwifery* (New York: E. P. Dutton & Co., 1977), p. 103.

[7] Gail Bronson, "Aging Americans," *The Wall Street Journal*, October 29, 1979, p. 1.

[8] Marie Scott Brown, *Normal Development of Body Image* (New York: John Wiley & Sons, 1977).

[9] Irene M. Burnside, *Nursing and the Aged* (New York: McGraw-Hill Book Company, 1976).

[10] Joseph Campbell, ed., *The Portable Jung* (New York: Penguin Books, 1978), pp. 3–23.

[11] Victor Daniels and Lawrence Horowitz, *Being and Caring* (Palo Alto, Ca.: Mayfield Publishing Company, 1976).

[12] Sheila E. Dresen, "Autonomy: A Continuing Developmental Task," *AJN*, 78, no. 8 (August 1978), 1344–46.

[13] Rémy Droz and Maryvonne Rahmy, *Understanding Piaget* (New York: International Universities Press, 1976).

[14] Ken Dychtwald, "The SAGE Project: A New Image of Aging," *Journal of Humanistic Psychology*, 18, no. 2 (Spring 1978), 78–80.

[15] Jean Elder, *Transactional Analysis in Health Care* (Menlo Park, Ca.: Addison-Wesley Publishing Co., 1978).

[16] Erik Erikson, *Childhood and Society* (New York: W. W. Norton & Co., 1963), pp. 247–74.

[17] R. P. Esposito and others, "The Johari Window," *Journal of Humanistic Psychology*, 18, no. 1 (Winter 1978), 79–81.

[18] Selma Fraiberg, *The Magic Years* (New York: Charles Scribner's Sons, 1959), pp. 91–103.

[19] Arnold Gesell, *Youth* (New York: Harper & Row, 1956).

[20] Florence Goodenough and Leona E. Tyler, *Developmental Psychology*, 3rd ed. (New York: Appleton-Century-Crofts, 1959).

[21] Ezekial Green, "On Bonding and Babies," *San Francisco Sunday Examiner and Chronicle*, California Living Magazine, August 20, 1978, pp. 34–37.

[22] Mark Jonathon Harris, "How to Make It to 100," *New West,* January 3, 1977, pp. 16–28.

[23] Patricia Hess and Candra Day, *Understanding the Aging Patient* (Bowie, Md.: Robert J. Brady & Co., 1977).

[24] Jack Hofer, *Total Massage* (New York: Grosset and Dunlop, 1976), pp. 168–70.

[25] Dennis T. Jaffe, "The Holistic Family," *New Realities,* II, no. 1 (1978), 80–85.

[26] Muriel James and Dorothy Jongeward, *Born to Win* (Menlo Park, Ca.: Addison-Wesley Publishing Co., 1973), pp. 10–14.

[27] Margaret D. Jensen and others, *Maternity Care* (St. Louis: C. V. Mosby Co., 1976).

[28] George Kaluger and Meriem Fair Kaluger, *Human Development, The Span of Life* (St. Louis: C. V. Mosby Co., 1974).

[29] Marshall Klaus and John H. Kennell, *Maternal-Infant Bonding* (St. Louis: C. V. Mosby Co., 1976), p. 14.

[30] Lawrence Kohlberg, "The Cognitive-Developmental Approach to Moral Education," *Phi Delta Kappa* (January 1975), 670–77.

[31] Frederick LeBoyer, *Loving Hands* (New York: Alfred A. Knopf, 1976).

[32] Frederick LeBoyer, *Birth Without Violence* (New York: Alfred A. Knopf, 1975).

[33] Laurence LeShan, "Psychological States as Factors in the Development of Malignant Disease: A Critical Review," *Journal of the National Cancer Institute,* 22, no. 1 (January 1959), 1–11.

[34] Daniel J. Levinson and others, *The Seasons of a Man's Life* (New York: Ballantine Books, 1978).

[35] Alexander Lowen, *Bioenergetics* (Baltimore, Md.: Penguin Books, 1976).

[36] Marjorie Fiske Lowenthal, Majda Thurnher, David Chiriboga, and associates, *Four Stages of Life* (San Francisco: Jossey-Bass, 1975).

[37] Joann S. Lublin, "The Birthing Room," *The Wall Street Journal,* February 15, 1979, p. 1.

[38] Abraham Maslow, *Motivation and Personality* (New York: Harper & Row, 1954).

[39] Ruth B. Murray and Judith P. Zentner, *Nursing Assessment and Health Promotion Through the Lifespan,* 2nd ed. (Englewood Cliffs, N.J.: Prentice-Hall, Inc., 1979).

[40] *New Dimensions/Common Ground* (San Francisco: Baha-udin Alpine and Sherman Chickerings Copublishers) no. 20 (Summer 1979).

[41] Waldo E. Nelson and others, *Textbook of Pediatrics* (Philadelphia: W. B. Saunders Co., 1969).

[42] E. J. Phares, *Locus of Control in Personality* (Morristown, N.J.: General Learning Press, 1976), p. 250.

[43] Sharon L. Roberts, *Behavioral Concepts and Nursing Throughout the Life Span* (Englewood Cliffs, N.J.: Prentice-Hall, Inc., 1978), pp. 266–77.

[44] Mike Samuels and Nancy Samuels, *The Well Baby Book* (New York: Summit Books, 1979).

[45] Gail Sheehy, *Passages* (New York: Bantam Books, 1977), pp. 18–19.

[46] Sandra Sundeen and others, *Nurse-Client Interaction* (St. Louis: C. V. Mosby Co., 1976).

[47] Doris C. Sutterly and Gloria F. Donnelly, *Perspectives in Human Development* (Philadelphia: J. B. Lippincott, 1973).

Chapter 5
stress

CHAPTER OUTLINE

G. Stress and the Interpersonal Lifespace
   1. Crisis Theory—A Psychological Approach to Interpersonal Stress
   2. Crisis and the General Adaptation Syndrome
   3. Maturational and Situational Crises
   4. The Four Characteristic Phases of Crisis
   5. Factors Which Influence the Outcome of Crisis
   6. Crisis Prevention and Anticipation
   7. Families and Crisis
H. Society and Stress—The Community Lifespace
   1. Statistical Measurements of the Community's Health Status
   2. Social Network Index
   3. High-Risk Groups
   4. Occupational Health and Safety

CHAPTER OBJECTIVES

1. Trace the development of stress physiology from Cannon through Selyé's General Adaptation Syndrome.

2. Explain the three phases of stress, the concurrent physiological events, especially stress hormone levels, and appropriate nursing observations.

3. Describe the Local Adaptation Syndrome, listing the effects and the observations the nurse makes.

4. Differentiate primary, secondary, and tertiary prevention.

5. Explain the concept of risk and how the Health Hazard Appraisal utilizes this idea.

6. State five intrapersonal measurements used to assess stress levels.

7. Define crisis theory and compare it to Selyé's theory of stress.

8. Differentiate situational from maturational crises and describe three primary preventive activities that nurses can perform in crises evaluations.

9. Define and critique four statistical measurements of the community's health status. List three groups particularly at risk for stress and explain the rationale for the choices.

10. Describe the Social Network Index and the most recent research conclusions associated with it.

STRESSORS AND HOMEOSTATIC MECHANISMS

Hans Selyé's research and writings on stress have been selected as one of the most influential and all-encompassing theories of disease causation ever proposed, and as such, they will be emphasized here. Selyé's stress theory takes into consideration germ theory as well as host resistance and response mentioned in Chapter 1. More recently, Selyé has accepted any psychological, sociocultural, biological, and environmental stimuli as appropriate in eliciting a stress response. In short, stress has become a truly holistic pathophysiological theory with wellness and preventive health implications.

Hans Selyé was not the first physiologist to research stressful stimuli ("stressors") and their effects on the organism. Walter B. Cannon, a physician, published a paper in 1935 describing the "stresses and strains of Homeostasis." [11] Cannon adhered to the Hippocratic idea that disease was cured by a "vis medicatrix naturae," or natural power, and that the organism could maintain a steady state in the face of profound disturbances. [11]

These "homeostatic mechanisms" or adaptations, which automatically maintained equilibrium, included fluid and electrolyte balance, blood sugar, lipid, protein, and calcium regulation, acid-base balance, body-temperature control, nervous system regulation, sympathico-adrenal response, and immune system response. Modern physiology has elaborated on, specifically researched, and confirmed many of Cannon's original impressions about the "Wisdom of the Body." [11]

From Cannon's research some universal characteristics of homeostatic, regulatory, or adaptive mechanisms can be derived:

1. They are compensatory in nature.
   a. For example, *temperature control.* Extreme cold yields peripheral vasoconstriction, increased muscularity and shivering to return body temperature to normal.
   b. For example, *compensatory growth.* A slightly enlarged heart is often found in heavily stress-conditioned athletes to compensate for increased oxygen needs. (See Chapter 6 for more detail.)
2. They are self-regulatory and automatic in nature.
   a. For example, adrenocorticotrophic hormone (ACTH) is secreted from the pituitary automatically in stressful situations unless severe illness, accident, or surgery has damaged its ability to respond to stressors.
3. They tend to be negative feedback systems. Negative feedback redirects excesses or deficiencies *back to the norm.* (For example, the pituitary produces ACTH which drives the adrenal cortex to produce corticoids which inhibit further ACTH secretion of the pituitary.) Positive feedback constantly leads away from the norm and increases the deficiency or excess, eventually leading to exhaustion and death. (For example, during stress the regulatory negative feedback system is bypassed so that high corticoid levels do not inhibit further ACTH excretion and resulting higher corticoid levels, thus accounting for amazingly high blood levels of both.
4. The regulation of a single physiologic process may require the operation of multiple homeostatic negative feedback systems (for example, acid-base balance in the blood requires activation of the respiratory system and kidneys).

5. Some degree of deviation or error exists in all homeostatic mechanisms. (For example, the pancreas overresponds to a sugar load, secretes insulin, and produces hypoglycemia [low blood sugar] in a fasting subject.) [11, pp. 299-300]

THE GENERAL ADAPTATION SYNDROME (G.A.S.)

In 1936, Hans Selyé was experimentally injecting hormone extracts into rats and noticed a predictable response, that is, adrenocortical enlargement, atrophy of the thymus, spleen, and lymph nodes, and deep bleeding duodenal and stomach ulcers. Since he was searching for a new ovarian hormone, he was sorely disappointed. An intuitive thought motivated him to try injecting a variety of "nocuous" substances into the rats, which all yielded the same triad mentioned above. [50, pp. 22-24]

From this ill-fated experiment, Selyé developed the desire to pursue studying this nonspecific reaction of the body to any injury. Thus, the General Adaptation Syndrome (G.A.S.) was born. The last forty years have seen the growth of Selyé's theory to encompass the idea of any stressor, internal or external, positive or negative, activating some as yet unknown afferent system of one or more "mediators." These mediators carry the message to nocuous agents through neural or humoral pathways to the integrative centers which bring about the nonspecific triad, including stimulation of the pituitary adrenocortical system. Certainly, the theory has its critics, but none has been able to definitely disprove it.

The Neuroendocrine Physiology of Stress

The basic process of the General Adaptation Syndrome warrants description. A review of neuroendocrine anatomy and physiology is a prerequisite for tracing the psychophysiology of stress (Figure 5-1). Figure 5-2 summarizes the three basic stages of the stress response. Reference to both figures may assist you in the following explanation of a typical General Adaptation Syndrome response.

It is important to visualize the neurological and endocrine systems working harmoniously and sometimes overlapping their functions in response to a stressor or stressors. No matter how localized the original stress response is on one particular "target" organ (for example, the gastrointestinal tract: diarrhea), we must assume that the whole system can eventually become involved.

What structure in the brain is responsible for integrating the subcortical and cortical functions of the nervous system? Recent evidence seems to point to the *reticular activating* system (R.A.S.), a network of nerves located in part of the midbrain up into the thalamus. It serves as the master communicator between the cerebral cortex, hypothalamus, and brain stem. If this information is validated, it may "join" the historically disparate domains of mind and body.

The biggest gap in neurophysiological information appears to occur at this point in the communication of the stress signal from the reticular activating system to the hypothalamus. Pelletier suggests that the hypothalamus is particularly sensitive to both limbic system and cortical information about stress as well as to its

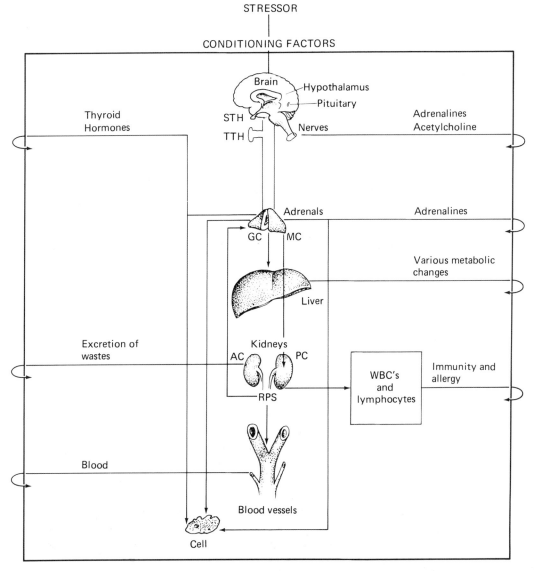

FIGURE 5-1 The fundamental pattern of all stress situations triggering the General Adaptation Syndrome

MC = Mineralcorticoids; PC = Pro-inflammatory corticoids
(Aldosterone and Deoxyxorticosterone [DOC])

GC = Glucocorticoids or AC = Anti-inflammatory corticoids
(Cortisol and Cortisone)

Adrenalines are epinephrine and norepinephrine

RPS = Renal pressor substances (renin and angiotensin)

STH = Somatotrophic hormone

Adapted from Hans Selyé, *The Stress of Life,* rev. ed. (New York: McGraw-Hill Book Company, 1978), p. 151.

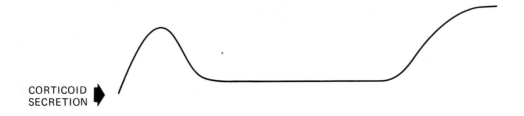

CORTICOID SECRETION ▶

Stage of Alarm
Auxiliary mechanisms are mobilized to maintain life so that the reaction spreads to large territories. No organ system is as yet specially developed to cope with the task at hand.

Stage of Resistance
Adaptation is acquired due to optimum development of the most appropriate specific channel of defense. Spatial concentration of the reaction makes corticoid production unnecessary.

Stage of Exhaustion
The reaction spreads again due to wear and tear in the most appropriate channel. Corticoid secretion rises, but can maintain life only until auxiliary channels are exhausted.

FIGURE 5-2 Summary of the three stages of the stress response

Adapted from Hans Selyé, *The Stress of Life,* rev. ed. (New York: McGraw-Hill Book Company, 1978), pp. 163–64.

long acknowledged function as the sleep-wakefulness, temperature, and hunger controller. [36, p. 53]

The hypothalamus has two functions, the second of which is essential in triggering the General Adaptation Syndrome. First, it triggers the autonomic nervous system to mutually excite and inhibit the sympathetic and the parasympathetic nervous systems. The effect is commonly identified as the fight or flight response and can be universally simulated by recalling or replaying an exciting or traumatic experience or accident. The second function of the hypothalamus is to stimulate the endocrine system by way of the pituitary, anteriorly causing it to secrete adrenocorticotrophic hormone (ACTH), thyrotrophic hormone (TTH), and somatotrophic (growth) hormone (STH), and posteriorly causing it to release vasopressin. Each of these hormones stimulates its own particular series of organs and responses.

Adrenocorticotrophic hormone stimulates the adrenal cortex (outer layer) to produce cortisone and cortisol, the antiinflammatory glucocorticoids (GC), so-called because they stimulate the liver to release glycogen stores and raise blood sugar levels. They are synthetically produced and used to reduce inflammation in various conditions. The adrenocorticotrophic hormone also causes a seemingly opposing set of proinflammatory mineralocorticoids (PC), called deoxycorticosterone and aldosterone, to be produced. Their function is to conserve fluid.

The adrenal medulla secretes epinephrine and norepinephine, which account for the "adrenalin rush" often associated with the first stage of a stress reaction. The adrenal medulla is stimulated by sympathetic nervous system filaments, *not* by the pituitary. Adrenalin increases carbohydrate metabolism, dilates arterials of the heart and skeletal muscles, accelerates heart rate and increases blood volume and respiration. Adrenaline also stimulates the fat tissue to release free fatty acids

(FFAs) which can be oxidized directly by the heart for more energy. The FFAs further suppress the liver's normal process of breaking down glucose, since the liver need not both synthesize and break down glucose simultaneously. [54, p. 47] Norepinephrine increases the blood pressure.

Other physiological functions that may be related to the G.A.S. trigger:

1. The thyrotrophic hormone which stimulates the thyroid to secrete thyroxine, thereby increasing the basic metabolic rate and causing the body to be more responsive to adrenalin.

2. The somatotrophic hormone whose function in stress is still in question. It definitely effects connective tissue cells and stimulates mineral corticoids and inflammation, but it is not certain that it works through the adrenal cortex.

3. The production of renal pressor substances (RPS) (for example, angiotensin) by the kidney during a stress reaction. It is easy to conclude that any of these "alarm" responses are lifesaving mechanisms and not desirable to any degree in a long-term stressful situation.

4. An individual response not connected to the G.A.S., but which can influence it at any point, is that of individual nerves to stressors. They react by producing adrenalines and acetylcholine (a substance which stimulates parasympathetic activity).

The typical progression of the stress response has been reviewed. More of Selyé's research regarding the General Adaptation Syndrome will follow. It is important to recognize that although his model is the most comprehensive to date and accounts for the entire gamut of psychosomatic diseases which are the result of long-term stress, it has some missing links. One gap is the previously mentioned hypothesized brain structure responsible for converting psychosocial stressors into neuroendocrine responses. Another may be the scientific rethinking of the nonspecificity of the General Adaptation Syndrome. For the present, acknowledgment of these critiques is sufficient for the holistic nurse to continue with the General Adaptation Syndrome as a basis for administering preventive holistic nursing care.

The Phases of the General Adaptation Syndrome

An early aspect of Selyé's research was the discovery of three distinct phases of the General Adaptation Syndrome, which he termed "alarm," "resistance," and "exhaustion." These stages seem to place the General Adaptation Syndrome in a time framework, but clinically it is difficult to assign specific durations to each stage. It is more difficult to predict such durations. The important point for practitioners is to support those defenses which come into play at the stage of resistance at which adrenocortical secretions have decreased and coping with the stressor has become the task of the specific organ system best fitted to deal with it. Another obvious intervention in the acute illness nursing care setting is to prevent the exhaustion stage at which the target organ breaks down and, if possible, to shift its function to another system in order to avoid total collapse and eventual death. A diagram in Figure 5–2 depicts the stages of the General Adaptation Syndrome and the subsequent adrenocortical blood levels.

Effects of the General Adaptation Syndrome

The General Adaptation Syndrome will cause:

1. an increase in cardiovascular output;
2. a decrease in blood flow to the skin, kidney, and other organs not essential for immediate survival, in order to ensure a ready supply to the more vital areas, such as the brain, skeletal, and heart muscles;
3. slowing of nonessential functions, such as digestion and excretion;
4. retention of salt and water by the kidneys to bolster the blood volume;
5. an increase in muscle tone;
6. increased acuteness of close vision and dilation of pupils so that maximum light can be used;
7. an increase in respiratory rate and depth to ensure adequate oxygenation of the blood;
8. an increase in metabolism to provide for immediate energy; and
9. activation of mechanisms to aid in heat dissipation since heat is a byproduct of metabolism. [10, pp. 81–82]

Nursing observations

The nurse makes the following behavioral observations:

Pupils: may be dilated; migraine headache may be present

Skin: may be pale or ashen color, cool to touch; palms "clammy" with perspiration

Nailbeds: may be pale, lacking usual pinkness

Mouth: may describe "Dry mouth"; lips may be pale in color, bruxism (grinding teeth)

Pulse: may be more rapid than usual; has feeling of full volume to touch; subjective complaint: client can feel/hear heart pounding

Blood pressure: may be elevated

Stomach: may have lack of, or excessive, appetite; diarrhea, indigestion, nausea

Intestinal tract: may be unable to defecate; may experience flatus, describe "gas pains" caused by retention of flatus (gas); abdomen may be distended

Genitourinary tract: premenstrual tension or missed menstrual cycles; may be unable to void or may indicate urge to urinate but have only small amount of urine

Skeletal muscles: hypermotility; pain in lower back or neck; activities may be very coordinated and precise or may be rigid or tremorous

Emotional: high-pitched, nervous laughter; stuttering, impulsive behavior, instability; subjective complaints including: feelings of unreality, weakness or dizziness, fatigue or being "keyed up," insomnia, hyperexcitation, irritability, depression, accident proneness

Respiration: depth and rate of respiration may increase; may note use of accessory neck and abdominal muscles in breathing

Temperature: may be elevated

Pain: reaction to pain may be reduced for a short time

Intellectual processes: ability to perceive relevant data and to problem solve may be increased

Clinical measurements of G.A.S. response

Clinical measurements that can assist the nurse in the assessment of a General Adaptation Syndrome response are:

1. increased blood levels of adrenalines, corticoids, ACTH, corticotropin-releasing factor (CRF) (disappears too quickly for accurate measurement);
2. blood creatine/creatinine ratio increases in alarm stage as urine concentrates;
3. increased cholesterol, triglyceride levels;
4. increased STH, glucagon, insulin, and prolactin levels (difficult to obtain with consistency and accuracy);
5. increased electroencephalograph (EEG) waves;
6. increased blood pressure; and
7. increased galvanic skin response (GSR) and increased electromyograph (EMG).

Effects of parasympathetic overstimulation

Should the *parasympathetic* division inadvertently stimulate *all* the organs it innervates at the same time as the sympathetic division is innervating its organs, massive behavioral disorganization would result. The nurse might observe effects opposite to those of sympathetic stimulation.

The Local Adaptation Syndrome (L.A.S.)

Another area of interest in Selyé's model of stress adaptation is the Local Adaptation Syndrome. As its name implies, it is a circumscribed specific reaction to injury that involves inflammation, swelling, redness, heat, and pain. The response involves adrenocorticotrophic hormone secretion and subsequent mobilization of antiinflammatory corticoids and proinflammatory corticoids, but response is restricted to the target, not to the entire system. An example of this response might be a bee sting in which a local reaction occurs in one person, but in another person who is sensitive or allergic to bee stings, the entire General Adaptation Syndrome might be triggered. In another situation, a person might be stung by a swarm of bees and be incapable of coping locally with the amount of antigen (toxin) in the system. Again, the entire G.A.S. is called into action. A Local Adaptation Syndrome may become a General Adaptation Syndrome, therefore, and certainly many of the same mechanisms operate in both.

Effects of the L.A.S.

The Local Adaptation Syndrome will cause:

1. dilation of blood vessels in the inflamed area to supply it with more red and white blood cells;
2. proliferation of fibrous connective tissue and its cells which encapsulate potential pathogens and prevent their spread into the blood stream;
3. connective tissue and cell proliferation, which also helps damaged or destroyed tissue to granulate or form new tissue to replace old; and

4. chemical substances to secrete from the blood and connective tissue which surround the irritant, neutralize its poisons and waste products, and kill any bacteria present. [50, pp. 131–34]

Nursing observations

The nurse observes the following manifestations of the L.A.S.:

1. *redness* and *heat* in a clearly circumscribed area around the injury (thus the term "localized" is often used to describe it);
2. *swelling* around the injury due to dilated blood vessels, leakage of fluid and cells from them, and the rapid increase of fibrous connective tissue;
3. *pain,* which is the response of the sensory nerve endings irritated by the injury and swelling;
4. *sero-sanguinous* (watery and bloody) *drainage* or pus, which may exude or be expressed from the wound. If the wound is closed, these exudates may give a hard, raised, smooth, and stretched appearance to the skin and may require heat or an incision; and
5. *restriction of movement* (splinting or guarding), which may occur in response to swelling and pain.

These cardinal signs of "rubor" (redness), "calor" (heat), "tumor" (swelling), and "dolor" (pain) have been used by health practitioners since Roman times to describe their observations.

FACTORS INFLUENCING STRESS RESPONSE

It should be noted that although the stress syndrome (General Adaptation Syndrome and Local Adaptation Syndrome) seems to be a universal response, it is mediated by many variables, which Selyé terms "conditioning factors." Some of these factors are briefly described in the next section. [50, p. 123] A few of the factors will be elaborated on in other chapters—for example, environment and lifestyle in Chapter 6.

Individual Make-up

Individual make-up includes unchangeable genetic and demographic characteristics, such as age, sex, race, and ethnic group. One of the most obvious and uncontrollable of these factors is heredity. Persons whose parents and grandparents have a family history of susceptibility of a particular organ (for example, the heart or the stomach) to stress, run an increased risk of that same organ's breaking down more quickly in themselves. They also have the advantage of having this knowledge as part of their conscious attempt to modify their lifestyle in order to reduce stress on that organ system. Other individual factors which can contribute to stress responses are immunity and innate resistance to stressors.

Another important element in individual make-up is *personality,* an overused term meaning the dynamic organization within an individual of those psychophysical systems that determine his unique adjustments to his environment. [26,

Gordon Allport as quoted therein, p. 39] Later in this chapter, the much publicized Type A and Type B Personality Assessment will be presented as a factor impinging on the stress response. Personality encompasses such concepts as self-image, self-esteem, body image, body type, personal attitudes and values, personality types, family and peer conditions, and educational development.

Cultural background contributes to the uniqueness of the individual—his or her attitudes and responses toward stress. Each culture has its own attitudes toward wellness and illness, health practices (diet, relaxation, exercise, etc.), coping, familial and community support systems, and healing rituals. Most cultural health belief systems support the holistic view of dynamic interaction of the human being with the environment. All aspects of the person (body, mind, spirit) are involved in illness and healing.

The more the holistic nurse learns about her own cultural background, the more able she will be to appreciate the cultural traditions of others. For an holistic overview of several major cultures and their health traditions, see Marie Branch and Phyllis Paxton, *Providing Safe Nursing Care for Ethnic People of Color*. [9]

Environment

Environment usually refers to those things outside oneself over which one has little control. For the purposes of this discussion, biological rhythms will be included as part of everyone's milieu. Some of these rhythms can be modified, and certainly, an awareness that rhythmic patterns exist and deeply influence our lives is prerequisite to learning how to use them. *Biological rhythms* are automatic, repetitive, rhythmic patterns found in plants, animals, and man. Endogenous rhythms come from within the organism, for example, sleep-wake and sleep-dream cycles. A *circadian rhythm* is an endogenous rhythm which reoccurs in a cyclic pattern within a twenty to twenty-eight hour period (about one day). Examples include body temperature, blood pressure, urine production, and hormone and blood sugar levels (see Figure 5–3). Exogenous rhythms are dependent on the rhythm of the external environment. The menstrual cycle, for example, is attuned to the lunar cycle. It is also an example of an infradian rhythm, that is, a rhythm longer than a circadian rhythm.

Data confirm a relationship between circadian rhythms and mental and physical illness. Births and deaths occur more frequently at night and in the early morning (1:00 a.m. is the peak hour for labor, for example); and the peak hours for suicides and accidents are also in the early morning hours. Adrenocortical (antiinflammatory) secretion is at its lowest level at midnight. Sensitivity to histamine peaks in the evening and at night. Breathing crises in asthma clients understandably increase in the evening.

Circadian rhythms are altered by certain drugs, especially barbiturates. Drug effects may be enhanced by administering the drugs when physiological functions are at desired maximal or minimal levels. For example, more pain medication may be needed at night than during the activity period of day. The rhythm of liver enzyme secretion will influence detoxification of certain drugs.

Persons from nine months of age through adulthood experience monocyclic—

RHYTHM	PEAK	LOW
Tidal volume	Afternoon	2 a.m.
Cardiac output	6 p.m.—midnight	4–6 a.m.
Blood pressure	3 p.m.	3 a.m.
Temperature	5 p.m.	5 a.m.
Growth hormone	Night	Day
Adrenocorticoid secretions	4–6 a.m.	Midnight
Adrenalin	6–8 a.m.	Late evening

FIGURE 5-3 Biological circadian rhythms in man

that is, one—major sleep period in twenty-four hours. Rapid eye movement (REM) or rejuvenating sleep occurs every 90 to 100 minutes. Nurses should realize that alterations in biological rhythms may occur and take several days to adapt to (1) during hospitalization or institutionalization; (2) anywhere new noise levels, lighting patterns, unfamiliar schedules for eating, sleeping, or hygiene occur; or (3) when persons cross time zones ("jet lag").

Nurses need to include information in the client history about the client's pre-illness patterns of sleep, rest, and food and fluid intake and output. It is important to control, when feasible, external factors to suit and support the client's normal routine, thereby lessening stress. Diagnostic tests procedures, surgery, and medications should be scheduled to suit the client's own biological clock when possible.

Research is currently being conducted on a method of contraception based on the lunar cycle, which attempts to regulate within a predictable period of time the menstrual cycle and ovulation. "Lunaception," as it is popularly called, is a method that has been used by African tribeswomen for thousands of years as an effective prognosticator of menstruation and ovulation. Light research with rats appears to confirm this use of biological rhythms, although more studies are needed to test the hypotheses. [44]

Other aspects of the environment include air, soil, water, noise and climatic conditions, esthetic amenities, and the quality of living and work surroundings. These variables can either contribute to high-level wellness or serve as risk factors for illness and/or disease.

The concept of environment can also include the socioeconomic, political, educational, recreational, and psychological climates people find themselves in from day to day. Accessible health care resources and facilities also contribute to people's feelings of environmental security.

Lifestyle

Lifestyle has been defined in an earlier section and it will be described in more detail in Chapter 6. It is often interpreted by the health community to refer to those personal habits which may or may not place an individual at risk for certain illnesses or conditions. Examples of lifestyle habits include time management, coping skills, eating, drinking and smoking habits, and so forth.

STRESS THEORY AND ILLNESS EXAMPLES

It is important to remember that no one stressor causes a General Adaptation Syndrome response. The nature of the stressors, their number, scope, and intensity, and the location of the target organ will all affect the individual's response.

Selyé likens the stress theory to the Gestalt School of Psychology which emphasizes wholeness and the interaction of the individual with the environment (see Chapter 9). The General Adaptation Syndrome can be viewed as a mosaic of organs, systems, and mechanisms or processes which act as a single unit, but are made up of an enormously complicated series of elements. Certainly, philosophical holism supports this point of view. Modern holistic practitioners see the stress process as a self-regulatory natural tendency to adapt to a fluctuating environment. The body-mind-spirit are interacting, interdependent elements of the stress response. Lifestyle elements, such as nutrition, exercise, and relaxation patterns, are supported by stress theory (they will be discussed in Chapter 6).

Simply summarized, then, the stress adaptation process is an elaborate neuroendocrine mechanism which helped prehistoric man to adapt to a physically hostile and threatening environment. All these primitive responses remain with us today despite the differences in the types of stressors.

The stress response can be viewed from two perspectives.

1. The first perspective includes real dangers to the body which require an emergency fight or flight and appropriate G.A.S. response. This response is often termed *primary fear.*
2. The second perspective is composed of acquired or conditioned fears, in which situation a previously neutral stimulus acquires the capacity to elicit the G.A.S. Sometimes this signal "anxiety" or secondary fear is appropriate—for example, a fire alarm can trigger anxiety in many people. When an acquired fear is inappropriate—such as in phobic fears of heights, elevators, etc.—it is often termed a psychosomatic or neurotic anxiety. [48, p. 402]

Chronic or inappropriate activation of the stress response is called dyponesis or faulty effort. [48, Whatmore and Kohli as quoted therein, p. 402]

In Western society today, exposure is not so much to physical threats such as predators, plagues, and famines as much as it is to tension, aggravation, anger, and guilt. Our environment today contains both physical and chemical pathogens and pollutants. Stress is frequently of a destructive rather than an exhilarating variety, and oftentimes it isn't even felt or diagnosed until years after its damage has been inflicted or become irreversible. Today's diseases are largely caused by the interaction of a susceptible individual with a destructive environment.

Stress has been directly linked with the following groups of diseases of adaptation:

1. heart attack, hypertension, angina, arrhythmia, migraine;
2. ulcers, colitis, constipation, diarrhea, diabetes;

3. infections, allergies, autoimmune diseases, cancer; and
4. backache, tension, arthritis. [2, pp. 21, 43, 61, 80]

Two commonly acknowledged conditions or precursors (high blood pressure and gastrointestinal ulcers) related to the diseases of stress will make use of some of the current information about the General Adaptation Syndrome which was presented earlier in this chapter. Figure 5-4 summarizes some health disruptions directly and indirectly related to stress. Some have only been theoretically linked to stress, while others have been shown to be strongly associated with it.

Acute Health Disruptions

LAS (e.g., protective response to injury—inflammation)
    Extrinsic (trauma, burns, etc.)
    Intrinsic (appendicitis, colitis, gastritis)
Shock (neuroendocrine response—GAS [decreased blood volume, cardiogenic shock, neurogenic shock])
Surgery (preoperative and postoperative GAS)

Chronic (Long-term health disruptions)

Aging can be defined as the cumulative effects of GAS:
    decreased ACTH
    adaptation energy reserves decrease
    increased risk of decreased response to stress
Immobility ("deconditioning" of body to stress)
Cancer (hormones, host resistance, and increased tumor growth)
Cardiovascular disorders (arteriosclerotic heart disease, hypertension, stroke)
Skin (rashes, hives, etc.)
Neuroendocrine problems (Hyper- and hypo-thyroidism, glycemia, adrenalism)
Gastrointestinal disorders (e.g., ulcers)

Other Health Disruptions

Immune disorders (asthma, allergies—major and minor autoimmune disorders)
    lupus erythematosis
    arthritis
    rheumatic fever
    multiple sclerosis
    hepatitis
Psychosomatic disorders (migraine, ulcers, allergies, asthma, etc.)

FIGURE 5-4 Stress: a summary of potential applications for nursing

High Blood Pressure

Blood pressure is related to the stress response via the adrenal glands and the kidneys. The kidneys help to control blood pressure by regulating the salt concentration in the blood and by secreting substances (pressors) that cause the blood vessels to constrict. Constriction of the blood vessels decreases the total volume and raises blood pressure in much the same way as running water passing through narrow pipes raises water pressure.

The adrenal glands secrete aldosterone, which increases blood sodium content, which in turn acts as a signal to the kidneys to secrete pressors. Constriction of the vessels is also stimulated by the pituitary gland. All these actions serve to cause an elevated blood pressure. [54, p. 48] If a stress reaction is prolonged and the blood pressure is elevated for an extended period of time, severe hypertension and kidney damage can ensue, thereby perpetuating a vicious feedback cycle.

It appears that in long-term stress, the glucocorticoids may play a dominant role. Glucocorticoids are also a causative factor in the next stress disorder to be discussed.

Gastrointestinal Ulcers

When the brain responds to stress, it automatically sends a signal to the vagus nerve in the stomach, which stimulates gastric acid secretion. While the acids in the digestive tract are capable of dissolving tissue, the lining of the stomach and intestines is normally protected from being dissolved in its own fluid. Steroids, which are released during stress, somehow decrease the ability of the intestinal lining to withstand the stomach acidity. In chronic stress, this can lead to ulceration of the lining.

The proinflammatory hormones can wreak their own havoc with the cardiovascular system in long-term stress. Not only do they constrict arterial walls, but they can also cause tears in them which are repaired and replaced with plaques or callouses of cholesterol. Cholesterol is readily available due to the high circulating blood levels during stress. This eventually causes atherosclerosis, the precursor to heart attacks, strokes, and a host of other cardiovascular diseases. In summary, extraordinary or continually unwanted stress costs its victims energy, deprives them of tranquility, facilitates the occurrence of some diseases, and even outrightly causes others.

PREVENTION OF STRESS-RELATED DISORDERS

In dealing with the broad spectrum of stress-related disorders, the objective of holistic nursing is to prevent their occurrence. Preventive health has been commonly divided into primary, secondary, and tertiary prevention. [51]

Primary, Secondary, and Tertiary Prevention

Primary prevention involves developing an awareness of overt and covert clues to potential areas of risk to the client's well-being. This is also termed prospective medicine, wellness medicine, or health promotion. This area is of particular concern to holistic nurses. It is conservatively estimated that 90 percent of the population falls into this preventive health category. [23, p. 105] The preventive aspects of nursing are particularly evident in the area of specific protection for a communicable disease for which there is artificial active immunity available. Preventive nursing also encompasses detecting an early sign of a correctable disability or developmental lag, for example.

Secondary prevention occurs after a condition or disease is diagnosed. The goal here is prevention of secondary complications. A classic example is arteriosclerotic heart disease (hardening of the arteries), in which the goal is to prevent a coronary (heart attack) or cerebral vascular accident (stroke).

Tertiary prevention involves the rehabilitation and prevention of further disability following an effect of a disease process. An example is the paralysis resulting from a stroke which can cause the further complications of immobility. These complications can be anticipated, and in many cases, prevented.

Since this book focuses on wellness, primary prevention and protection will be emphasized. Primary protective holistic nursing care is generally not something a nurse can do for a client. Rather, the objective is to help the person help himself to stay healthy. Immunization is an example of something the health care provider can do to accomplish this goal. With the advent of vaccines and antibiotics, many of the leading causes of death have changed from communicable diseases to diseases or accidents that are self-induced. In these instances, the responsibility for preventing stress disorders lies squarely with the individual.

Risk Factors and Prevention

Many of the leading causes of death have precursors (forerunners) that can be identified. Some of these precursors cannot be eliminated (that is, family history), but others, such as cigarette smoking or alcohol consumption, are self-induced and can, if the client is aware of them and is willing to change his lifestyle, be eliminated. Thus, the client's risk for specific illnesses or even death can be reduced.

The various factors involved in causing diseases such as heart disease are called *risk factors*. Risk is defined as the probability that an individual will develop an illness or disability. Since risk is a statistical term expressed in percentages or odds, it is not a pronouncement of life or death on a particular individual. Risk predicts the likelihood that an event will occur in a clearly defined population. LaLonde has outlined the typical analytical process for defining a population at risk for coronary artery disease:

> *Mortality from coronary artery disease:*
> *Predisposing morbid condition:* atherosclerosis

Contributing factors: serum lipids, hypertension, diabetes, obesity, high fat diet, lack of exercise, stress, relative absence of estrogens, cigarette smoking

Population at risk: males over forty years of age with foregoing conditions or habits [24, p. 39]

The American Heart Association has outlined certain risk factors for coronary artery disease (Figure 5-5) in a similar but more specific manner.

One way to determine the risk factors of a disease process is to study large populations of people both with and without the disease to see in what ways the two groups resemble and differ from one another. The presence of a risk factor does not imply that the disease always follows. Other factors, such as heredity, environment, and lifestyle, may play a significant part.

OVERT PROBLEMS AND PERSONAL ATTRIBUTES

Familial occurrence of coronary disease at an early age
Hypertension
Electrocardiographic abnormalities
Diabetes mellitus
Lipid abnormalities involving serum cholesterol and triglycerides and their lipoprotein vehicles
Obesity
Gout (hyperuricemia)
Certain personality-behavior patterns

ENVIRONMENTAL FACTORS

Cigarette smoking
Lack of physical activity
Emotionally stressful situations
Diet

RISK FACTORS

1. Serum cholesterol of more than 260 mg percent, a fasting triglyceride of more than 250 mg percent, or a prominent electrophoretic pre-beta lipoprotein band
2. Sustained blood pressure over 160/95 mm HG
3. Body weights 30 percent or more above standards listed in tables of desirable weight
4. Fasting blood sugar of more than 120 mg percent, or a casual blood sugar of 180 mg percent, decreased glucose tolerance or significant glycosuria
5. History of gout or a uric acid level over 7.5 mg percent
6. Electrocardiographic abnormalities
7. Habitual cigarette smoking

FIGURE 5-5 Coronary heart disease: contributing factors

Source: American Heart Association, "Heart Facts, 1978 and 1980," (Dallas: American Heart Association Communication Division, 1978 and 1980).

From an epidemiological standpoint, a risk factor should satisfy four criteria in order for it to be associated with disease causation:

1. The incidence (frequency with which disorders arise) of the disease in a population must be proportional to the population's exposure to the factor.
2. The distribution of the disease—in geography, time, by sex, and among various population groups—should be consistent with the distribution of the suspected factor.
3. The factor should produce the same disease, or one corresponding to it, in experimental animals in the laboratory.
4. The removal of the factor or the reduction of exposure to it by the human population should reduce the incidence of the disease in the population. [53, p. 36]

Epidemiological data have formed the basis for the table of high-risk groups for cancer shown in Figure 5-6. Not all risk factors mentioned in this chapter have met this criteria due to the research logistics and restrictions. One such factor is the emotional component of stress. The most well-documented risk factors for cardiovascular disease are cigarette smoking, hypertension (often an effect of stress),

---

The following table, based on epidemiological studies, lists major factors for common cancers.*

LUNG

+ Heavy smoker, over age 50
+ Smoked pack a day for 20 years
+ Cigarette cough
+ Started smoking at age 15 or before
+ Smoker working with or near asbestos, arsenic, nickel compounds, coal

BREAST

+ Lump or nipple discharge
+ History of breast cancer
+ Close relatives with history of breast cancer
+ Over age 35; especially over 50
+ Never had children; first child after age 40

* *Age-adjusted:* a method used to make valid statistical comparisons by assuming the same age distribution among different groups being compared.

COLON-RECTUM

+ History of rectal polyps
+ Rectal polyps run in family
+ History of ulcerative colitis
+ Blood in stool
+ Over age 40
+ Foods high in animal fat, sugar, and highly refined foods, foods low in fiber

SKIN

+ Excessive exposure to sun/radiation
+ Fair complexion
+ Work with coal tar, pitch, or creosote

UTERINE-CERVICAL

+ Unusual bleeding or discharge
+ Frequent sex in early teens or with many partners
+ Low income background
+ Poor care during or following pregnancy
+ Aged 40–49
+ Took synthetic estrogens (oral contraceptives, DES, Fertility pills)

UTERINE-ENDOMETRIAL

+ Unusual bleeding or discharge
+ Late menopause (after age 55)
+ Diabetes, high blood pressure, and overweight
+ Aged 50–64

ORAL

+ Heavy smoker and drinker
+ Poor oral hygiene

OVARY

+ History of ovarian cancer among close relatives
+ Aged 50–59

PROSTATE

+ Over age 65
+ Difficulty in urinating

STOMACH

+ History of stomach cancer among close relatives
+ Diet heavy in smoked, pickled, or salted foods
+ Some link with blood group "A"

FIGURE 5-6 Cancer: early detection—high-risk groups

Sources: American Cancer Society Facts, 1978; Anna Eng, Betty Jean Carter and Christine Williams, "Personalizing Primary Cancer Prevention Education for Students," *Health Values: Achieving High-Level Wellness,* 3, no. 6 (November/December 1979), 304–8.

diabetes, and hyperlipidemia (a possible effect of stress). Others *may* include heredity, obesity, and physical inactivity. Yet altogether, these risk factors account for less than half of the cardiovascular mortality.

It was the consensus of the First National Conference on Emotional Stress and Heart Disease that "emotional stress should be considered a risk factor equal to other recognized risk factors." [35, p. 266] As the nurse moves into the intrapersonal lifespace and begins to look at her own level of stress, the emotional component of the stress adaptation life process will take on more meaning. Experimental research is now being conducted to evaluate the influence of emotion on health risk status.

The area of preventive wellness-oriented health will be explored. The basis for the questions on inventories and assessments (found in the appendices) will often be statistical data compiled about certain risk factors in relation to predicting health or illness—in some cases with relative accuracy. But, projecting health and hazards is a new science and art; it still has a long way to go, although the initial attempts are encouraging.

Health Hazard Appraisal

Dr. Lewis Robbins and Dr. Jack Hall, two Indianapolis physicians, developed the Health Hazard Appraisal. [41] Their appraisal is preceded by the usual medical history and physical exam, and is followed by a thorough discussion with the client of certain lifestyle elements which will yield total assessment of his/her health (risk status).

Robbins and Hall's model merits some study. It is based on the idea that health and illness can be placed on a continuum (as mentioned in Chapter 1) and indicated in the chart below. The type of health care needed can be identified by knowing which level the person is at on the health side. A person can be at one of the following three levels:

1. At no risk for a specific illness/accident—the person is at no risk now; but this is a good time to reinforce lifestyle patterns that will, if continued, prevent possible risks in the future. This is an important time to begin general health education.

2. The person is not at risk yet, but he is now more vulnerable to risk because of age, occupation, race, sex, or other reasons. Continuing to reinforce positive lifestyles and to provide health education is imperative. Anticipatory teaching can be directed toward preventing diseases or accidents to which the person has become or may become vulnerable.

3. Precursors are present, and although no illness signs or symptoms are present, the person is at greater risk for a specific illness or accident. His risk is higher than the average person's risk. Patient education can be specific to help identify how his lifestyle, if continued as it is, will lead to illness. Intervention is imperative at this point to prevent the patient from reaching stage 4.

On the illness side of the continuum, a person can be at any one of the following levels:

4-5. Signs and symptoms of a specific disease are present; the person is in the early stages of an illness.

6. The disease is now present; a crisis has occurred. [41]

1	2	3	4	5	6
NO RISK	VULNERABLE TO RISK	PRECURSOR(S) PRESENT	SIGNS PRESENT	SYMPTOMS PRESENT	CRISIS

In steps 4–6, diagnoses can be made and specific medical treatments instituted. Health maintenance care must not be focused on prevention of disease progression or on reversing the client's precrisis state. The primary objective of health care has now changed; it is no longer prevention but rather curing the illness that is present.

The Health Hazard Appraisal is being utilized and has now been taken by more than 200,000 people across the country; it is also being used by a few health departments, the San Francisco Health Department among them. [45] The information is processed by computer and yields:

	Sample Person	Recommendations
Chronological Age	51	Exercise program
Appraisal Age	65	Quit smoking
		Lose sixty pounds
Attainable Age	52	Make out will
(with recommended lifestyle modifications)		

The computer has calculated the risk of dying from certain risk factors for an average American population. It is understandable that such an appraisal can serve as a powerful motivator.

A Health Risk Index is shown in the appendix. Basically, if the nurse can view the various risk factors for certain major prevalent illnesses, turn them around, and look at the positive side, then a risk factor becomes a potential lifestyle modification element. Thus, if a risk factor for coronary artery disease is a body weight 30 percent over the life tables standards, the appropriate lifestyle modifications will be nutrition and exercise. A popular version of a risk factor analysis and its effect on longevity is shown in Figure 5–7.

STRESS AND THE INTRAPERSONAL LIFESPACE

From the preceding material, it becomes clear that certain information based on relevant risk factor analyses can be obtained about self and clients which can prevent certain illnesses and optimize health. In the following section, several health inventories, questionnaires, and self-tests will be presented and critiqued. It is intended that the holistic nurse evaluate her own lifestyle in terms of health, and then apply those knowledges and tools to her interactions with clients.

Stress Symptom Checklist

John Friedrich and others have suggested a symptom checklist self-evaluation tool for monitoring stress in self and/or a client. This checklist is presented in Figure 5–8. Although the checklist does not have research to support its use, it can still serve as a sensitive self-test.

Wellness Inventory

The Health Hazard Appraisal has already been mentioned. A more wellness-oriented test that can be easily self-administered is John Travis' Wellness Inventory. In fifteen minutes, a student or client can self-assess his health habits. The inventory is an educational tool which refers the person to interesting facts about certain risks to health and suggests appropriate references. The Wellness Inventory goes beyond conventional risk factors to some more untested assumptions at times. If

Can You Pass the Test of Time?

The following test, though *not* validated, is based on the best scientific evidence available today. While scientists still don't know all of the variables causing long life, they are aware of some of the phenomena that seem to be correlated with longevity. The test is based on that data. The life expectancy tables are taken from the latest census figures; they reflect average life expectancy for the entire United States population. Racial differences do exist: At birth life expectancy for most non-whites averages over six years lower, although by 65 it's less than one year lower.

Life Expectancy Table

AGE	MALE	FEMALE	AGE	MALE	FEMALE	AGE	MALE	FEMALE	AGE	MALE	FEMALE	AGE	MALE	FEMALE
26	70.5	77.3	35	71.3	77.7	44	72.3	78.4	53	74.1	79.6	62	76.9	81.4
27	70.6	77.3	36	71.4	77.8	45	72.5	78.5	54	74.3	79.7	63	77.3	81.6
28	70.7	77.4	37	71.5	77.8	46	72.6	78.6	55	74.6	79.9	64	77.7	81.9
29	70.8	77.4	38	71.6	77.9	47	72.8	78.7	56	74.9	80.1	65	78.1	82.2
30	70.9	77.5	39	71.7	78.0	48	73.0	78.9	57	75.2	80.3	66	78.6	82.4
31	70.9	77.5	40	71.8	78.0	49	73.2	79.0	58	75.5	80.5	67	79.0	82.7
32	71.0	77.5	41	71.9	78.1	50	73.4	79.1	59	75.8	80.7	68	79.5	83.0
33	71.1	77.6	42	72.0	78.2	51	73.6	79.3	60	76.2	80.9	69	79.9	83.3
34	71.2	77.6	43	72.2	78.3	52	73.8	79.4	61	76.5	81.2	70	80.4	83.6

Find your life expectancy on the table above, as based on your age and sex. Keep a running score by adding and sub-tracting years as you answer each of the following questions. The final number is your personalized life expectancy.

Heredity

1. Longevity of parents or grandparents
Add 2 years if 2 of your grandparents lived to age 80 or beyond. If your mother lived to 80 or beyond add 1.5 more; if your father reached 80 add another 2.
+ _____

2. Relatives and cardiovascular disease
Subtract 4 if any parent, grandparent, sister or brother died of a heart attack or stroke before 50. If anyone died of any of the above before 60, subtract 2.
+ _____

3. Other heritable diseases
Subtract 3 for each incident of diabetes, thyroid disorder, breast cancer (for women), cancer of the digestive system, asthma, emphysema or chronic bronchitis among parents or grandparents.
+ _____

Health and Diet

4. Weight
Subtract 1 per 10 pounds overweight.
+ _____   − _____

5. Smoking
Under a cigarette pack a day, subtract 2; 1 to 2 a day, subtract 4 to 7; 2 or more, subtract 8 to 12.
+ _____   − _____

6. Drinking
For light to moderate drinkers—up to 2 drinks per day—add 3. For heavy drinkers—over 3 drinks per day—subtract 8. Teetotalers subtract 1. Moderate drinking reduces stress and is a digestive aid. Heavy drinking, however, produces all kinds of physiological damage. The negative correlation between teetotaling and life expectancy may reflect that teetotalers have rather rigid value systems, and they may undergo stress in maintaining those systems.
+ _____   − _____

7. Exercise
If you exercise moderately—jog, bike,
ride, take long walks or swim 2 or 3 times weekly—add 3. Just exercising on weekends isn't enough.
+ _____   − _____

8. Sleep
If you sleep 9 hours a day, subtract 4. For more than 10 hours, subtract 6. Adults who sleep that much use too many hours in non-physical activity. Also, people who sleep a lot may be unhappy and sleep as an escape, or they may be ill. Depressed people have shorter life expectancies.
+ _____

9. Regular physical examinations
Women over 30 who give monthly breast self-examinations and have at least an annual breast examination and pap smear add 2. Men over 40 who have an annual physical with a proctoscopic examination every year add 2. If cancer is detected early enough, it can be treated and controlled.
+ _____   − _____

Education and Occupation

10. Years of education
Less than high school, subtract 2; 4 years beyond high school, add 1; 5 or more years beyond high school, add 3. School does not make you live longer, but higher education correlates with increased income and opportunity and access to better health care.
+ _____

11. Type of occupation
If your occupation is in the professional category, add 2—except if you're a musician, architect or pharmacist, subtract 1. (Why the negative correlation between longevity and these occupations exists is uncertain. Perhaps musicians, architects and pharmacists will know.) If you work in rugged heavy labor, you risk accidents; subtract 2. Occupations associated with overeating, such as being a chef or a baker, subtract 2.
+ _____

12. Annual income
If it's over $40,000 per year, subtract 2. People in higher income brackets probably experience more stress earning that much and consume more rich food.
+ _____

13. Activity on the job
If your job is active—housework, construction work, etc.—add 3. If it's sedentary—office work—subtract 3.
+ _____

14. Age and work
If you are over 60 and you are still working, add 2.
+ _____

Lifestyle

15. Rural vs. urban dwelling
If you live in an urban area, subtract 1. If you live in a rural area, add 1. City dwellers experience more stress.
+ _____   − _____

16. Marital status
If you are married or living with someone permanently, add 3. If you're single, subtract 1 for each unwedded decade past age 25. Married people live longer.
+ _____   − _____

17. Personality type
If you are a calm, passive person, add 1 to 3. If you're aggressive, intense and competitive, subtract 1 to 5—you are prone to cardiovascular disease.
+ _____

18. Risk-taking—auto accidents
If you use your car's seat belts regularly and follow speed limits, add 1. Auto accidents are among the top 10 killers.
+ _____

19. Happiness
If you are basically content with life, add 1 to 2. If you're unhappy—worried, tense and guilty—subtract 1 to 3.
+ _____

Test designed by Dr. Diana S. Woodruff of Temple University, as adapted from "Will You Live to Be 100," by Judith Bentley, *Family Health*, January, 1975.

FIGURE 5-7   A popular version of a risk factor analysis

Reprinted with permission of Mark Jonathan Harris, "How to Make it to 100," *New West*, 2, no. 1 (January 3, 1977), 28.

There are many symptoms of tension which imply a need for relaxation. In order to be able to cope with tension, it is helpful to become aware of some of these symptoms. By completing the following check list, you can gain further insight into your status regarding relaxation.

	Frequently (1)	Quite Often (2)	Seldom (3)	Never (–1)
1. Do you feel insecure?				
2. Do you often feel over-excited?				
3. Do you feel anxious?				
4. Do you worry when you go to bed at night?				
5. Is it difficult for you to fall asleep at night?				
6. Do you find it difficult to relax when you want to?				
7. Do you wake up in the morning feeling tired and loggy?				
8. Do you find it difficult to concentrate on a problem?				
9. Do you often feel tired during the day?				
10. When playing a sport, do you find it hard to concentrate on it?				
11. Is it hard for you to stay awake at work or in class?				
12. Do you feel upset and ill-at-ease?				
13. Do you lack self confidence?				
14. Do you often worry during the day over possible misfortunes?				
15. Do you frequently feel bored?				
16. Do you often feel discouraged?				
17. Do you have nervous feelings?				
18. Do you feel depressed?				
19. Do you have any type of twitch?				
20. Do you have frequent headaches?				
21. Do you have frequent colds, earaches, or sore throats?				
22. Do you have any persistent pains in joints or feet?				
23. If you feel yourself becoming tense, do you find it difficult to relax?				
24. Do you notice that you seldom find time to relax or stretch during the day?				
25. Do you exercise regularly?				
26. Do you often find that you exhibit tension by scowling, clenching fists, tightening jaws, hunching shoulders or pursing lips?				
27. Do your shoes, belt or other items of clothing fit too tightly?				
28. When you notice any of the tension symptoms, do you find it difficult to stop or minimize them?				
29. Are you unable to "let go" easily when you feel tense?				

The foregoing was merely designed to bring attention to areas which may reflect tension in your daily life. If you wish to rate yourself, the following scale will reflect, to a degree, your tension potential. Score: Frequently (1), Quite Often (2), Seldom (3), Never (–1).

Score	Rating
0–19	Above Average Tension Control
20–39	Average Tension Control
40–55	Low Tension Control
56–84	Poor Tension Control

FIGURE 5-8 Stress symptom checklist

Reprinted with permission from John A. Friedrich, "Tension Control Techniques," in Roger Harris and Lawrence W. Frankel, eds., *Guide to Fitness After Fifty* (New York: Plenum Press, 1977), pp. 337–38.

some of the inherent biases (such as sex) can be overlooked, the Wellness Inventory can be used as a helpful self-motivating aid.

Nutrition, Health, and Activity Profile

The nutrition, health, and activity profile helps the student/client determine his/her dietary intake of protein, carbohydrates, fats, vitamins, minerals, fiber, and calories, and compares it to recommended norms. This is also done for each of the other lifestyle elements, namely, exercise, stress, environment, and self-responsibility. Current research is cited, as well as issues over which there is still considerable controversy—vitamin-mineral supplementation, for example. The self-administered profile suggests recommended reading for those eager to do further study. An example of the profile format and a sample analysis is contained in the Appendices.

The profile is mailed to Pacific Research Systems, where it is computer analyzed and returned with personalized recommendations. This individualized profile is a potent motivator. Seemingly "healthy" students and clients are often shocked by their low levels of wellness. This state of readiness to learn lifestyle modifications can be utilized by holistic nurses to counsel and teach themselves and their clients.

Body Print

The Institute of Health Research, one of the Institutes of Medical Sciences at Pacific Medical Center in San Francisco, has devised an individually referenced blood chemistry profile composed of two dozen lab tests, which, along with an extensive medical history, physical exam, and stress EKG, forms a "Body Print." This "Body Print" is likened to a fingerprint in that it is unique and is not compared to what has customarily been considered "normal" range for a healthy population.

This distinctive range of normal for each individual is a relatively new idea. It is now being shown that what is considered a "normal" serum cholesterol, for example, is really an average based on a typically obese, out of shape, stressed American population. In other words, our norms are not synonymous with healthy.

The Health Research group is discovering that there is a huge "grey" area between optimum health and obvious disease. Certain biochemical changes occur which indicate trends toward disease long before it actually occurs. The mapping out of this trend can serve as a warning which allows time for lifestyle modification techniques which are much less costly and distressing than treatment after the onset of disease.

Refer once again to Drs. Robbins and Hall's list of the stages of the health-illness continuum on page 152. It serves as a reminder that degenerative disease takes a long time to develop. Likewise, signs and symptoms occur long before a disease manifests itself clinically. Restyling life habits can alter unhealthy trends toward disease.

Neurophysiological Stress Profile

Dr. Kenneth Pelletier has developed a neurophysiological stress profile to detect which target organ is at risk of being adversely affected by chronic stress. This profile monitors brain wave activity through an EEG, muscle activity through an electromyograph, peripheral hand and foot temperature, galvanic skin response, blood pressure, electrocardiogram, and respiration rate and pattern. [36, pp. 79–80] After five years of research, Pelletier has recommended the extension of monitoring methods to include biochemical measurements, blood analysis reflective of tissue fatigue, respiration-gas analysis, immunological reactivity, and a host of other subtle variables. [36, p. 81]

Social Readjustment Rating Scale— Life Events and Illness Index

Pelletier and other authorities on stress acknowledge the role of psychosocial life events in the causation of disease. The most noted and popularized researchers in this area are Dr. Thomas Holmes and Dr. Richard Rahe, who developed the Social Readjustment Rating Scale in 1967. [22; see Figure 5-9] The scale assigns numerical values to stressful life events. After adding up the number of points attached to events which have happened to the nurse or client in the last year, the score is compared against the following table:

0–150	30 percent chance of becoming ill
150–299	50–50 percent chance of developing illness or change in health status
300 or over	80 percent chance of developing a serious illness or change in health status

Once the nurse or client has evaluated himself or herself in terms of recent stressful events, he or she can apply some preventive measures as suggested by Dr. Holmes:

1. Become familiar with the life events and the amount of change they require.
2. Put the scale where family members can see it easily several times a day.
3. With practice, recognize a life event when it happens.
4. Think about the meaning of an event and identify some of the feelings experienced with the event.
5. Think about different ways to adjust to a particular event.

Rank	Life event	Mean value
1	Death of spouse	100
2	Divorce	73
3	Marital separation	65
4	Jail term	63
5	Death of close family member	63
6	Personal injury or illness	53
7	Marriage	50
8	Fired at work	47
9	Marital reconciliation	45
10	Retirement	45
11	Change in health of family member	44
12	Pregnancy	40
13	Sex difficulties	39
14	Gain of new family member	39
15	Business readjustment	39
16	Change in financial state	38
17	Death of close friend	37
18	Change to different line of work	36
19	Change in number of arguments with spouse	35
20	Mortgage over $10,000	31
21	Foreclosure of mortgage or loan	30
22	Change in responsibilities at work	29
23	Son or daughter leaving home	29
24	Trouble with in-laws	29
25	Outstanding personal achievement	28
26	Wife begin or stop work	26
27	Begin or end school	26
28	Change in living conditions	25
29	Revision of personal habits	24
30	Trouble with boss	23
31	Change in work hours or conditions	20
32	Change in residence	20
33	Change in schools	20
34	Change in recreation	19
35	Change in church activities	19
36	Change in social activities	18
37	Mortgage or loan less than $10,000	17
38	Change in sleeping habits	16
39	Change in number of family get-togethers	15
40	Change in eating habits	15
41	Vacation	13
42	Christmas	12
43	Minor violations of the law	11

6. Take time to arrive at important decisions.

7. Try to anticipate life changes when possible and plan for them in advance.

8. Try to set a steady pace without last minute hurrying.

9. When a task is accomplished, it should not be looked at as a time to stop all preventive measures. [14, Holmes as quoted therein, p. 11]

Nurses and clients can compile their own individual stressful events hierarchy. The goal is to think of twenty frequently occurring stressful events and to arrange them in order from the lowest level of stress to the highest. Each item is assigned a rank from 1 through 20, with a point value assigned to each. Total relaxation equals zero Subjective Units of Distress (SUDs), while the most stressful situation on the hierarchy is rated at 100 SUDs. [14, pp. 120–22] An example follows:

1. Doctor's appointment   10
2. Having friends over for dinner   15
3. Coming home tired at 6 o'clock, and then having to shop, cook, and do homework   30
4. Going to bed late and getting up early, unprepared for clinical experience   40
5. Taking an unprepared for exam   50
6. Leaving child home sick while having to go to school and work   75

Type A and Type B Personality

The most well-known study connecting personality with illness (cardiovascular disease) is the Type A and Type B behavior study conducted by Meyer Friedman and R. H. Rosenman in the late 1960s in San Francisco. The result, in 1971, was a personality profile of the "Type A personality," predisposed to coronary artery disease. The "Type B personality" ran a relatively low risk of incurring the disease.

To determine the personality for self or client, administer the Type A and B questionnaire (located in the appendices). Basically, the Type A person suffers from what the researchers call "Hurry Sickness." A preoccupation with time, goals (which are usually stated in numerical terms), and achievement characterizes the Type A person. The qualities and behaviors are numerous and complex and bear a striking resemblance to the left-brain yang-dominated syndrome detailed in Chapter 1.

FIGURE 5-9   (Opposite page) Social readjustment rating scale

Reprinted with permission from Thomas H. Holmes and Richard H. Rahe, "The Social Readjustment Rating Scale," *The Journal of Psychosomatic Research*, 11, no. 2 (August 1967), 216.

Stress Awareness Diary

A Stress Awareness Diary has been suggested by Davis, McKay, and Eshelman. [14, pp. 19–20] The nurse or client is asked to record the time that a stressful event occurs, to give a very brief description of the event and of the symptom(s) that could be related to the stress. An example follows:

Time	Stressful Event	Symptom
6:30 A.M.	No breakfast, rushing, late for a clinical experience	Headache, nausea, tightness in stomach

In Chapter 6, stress diary information can be used to recognize characteristic stress responses to particular events or interactions. Appropriate stress management techniques can then be incorporated.

If the nurse has self-administered and scored each of the questionnaires, inventories, and appraisals mentioned, a profile of certain health promotive lifestyle habits begins to emerge. The elements of nutrition, stress reduction, fitness and conditioning, environmental awareness and action, and above all, self-awareness and responsibility, keep reoccurring. They all can be viewed as lifestyle themes or modifications which will be part of every preventive and therapeutic regimen mentioned in this book. These are not revolutionary ideas; in essence, they are endorsed by all sectors of the wellness-illness, holistic-allopathic health care community.

It is important for the student to self-experience as much of the preceding material as possible before proceeding to the Interpersonal Lifespace and Stress section.

STRESS AND THE INTERPERSONAL LIFESPACE

Much of the intrapersonal experience with stress can be brought into the interpersonal setting. The role of nurse/client was reviewed in Chapters 2 and 3, and certain differences have been explained. Expectations exist on both sides of the nurse-client relationship. The client is probably motivated by some stress or desire to prevent its harmful effects. With all the nurse's knowledge about the stress concept and its behavioral manifestations, one or more stress assessments may be indicated and administered.

Once the nurse has ascertained that stress is indeed present at some level, the next step is to determine how able the client is to handle it. Obviously, in a wellness setting the physiological adaptive mechanisms are still functioning, but what about the psychological coping abilities and mechanisms? How much social support is the individual or family able to mobilize?

Crisis Theory—A Psychological Approach
To Interpersonal Stress

One of the most practical, time-tested frameworks for predicting and handling the psychological aspects of stress was proposed by Gerald Caplan in 1964. [12] Selyé had been formulating his useful biological construct (G.A.S.) when an entire set of similar ideas expressed in psychological terms appeared at about the same time in a different discipline, namely, psychiatry and mental health. Given the old duality problem of mind-body separation, it is not surprising that two such different yet similar analyses of the stress problem should develop.

Crisis and the General Adaptation Syndrome

An attempt will be made to compare the two concepts of stress and crisis. The student may have to make some creative leaps at times, but Caplan's ideas about Crisis Theory (anticipation and management) are often more applicable to interpersonal nursing situations which require immediate analysis and action than are Selye's neuroendocrine formulations and rationales. The strong parallels between the two theories are shown in Figure 5–10.

Rather than using the word *stressor,* Caplan prefers the more all-encompassing word, *crisis,* which he defined as

> . . . any transient situation that necessitates reorganization of one's psychological structure and behavior, that causes a sudden alteration in the person's expectation of themselves, and that cannot be handled with the person's usual coping mechanisms. [13, p. 35]

CRISIS THEORY (Caplan)	STRESS THEORY (Selyé)
Phase 1: Initial impact or shock phase	Alarm
Phase 2: Defensive retreat	Resistance
Phase 3: Recoil or Acknowledgment	
Phase 4: Adaptation, Change, or Resolution	Exhaustion

FIGURE 5-10 A comparison of Selyé's stages of stress and Caplan's phases of crisis

Maturational and Situational Crises

Crises can be divided into two types—*maturational* and *situational. Maturational* or *developmental crises* are transition points, the periods that every person experiences in the process of biopsychosocial growth and development that are accompanied by changes in thoughts, feelings, and abilities. Erikson and other developmental psychologists have identified these major transition states as:

Prenatal to Infancy
Infancy to Childhood
Childhood to Puberty and Adolescence
Adolescence to Adulthood
Maturity to Middle Age
Middle Age to Old Age
Old Age to Death

With appropriate support, a person is normally able to meet the challenge of growth from one stage of life to another. It is in this sense that developmental crises are considered normal. It is possible to prepare for them; they need not be nightmares, and people can enjoy a sense of self-mastery and achievement from successful completion of developmental tasks. However, these periods can become a period of turmoil and stress if there is a lack of the normal social supports. The challenge in each phase is to move on. Sometimes, however, various situational factors make this a seemingly impossible task.

Situational or *accidental* ("life accident") *crises* are external events or situations, not necessarily a part of normal living—often sudden, unexpected, and unfortunate—which loom larger than the person's immediate resources or ability to cope and which demand a change in behavior. Some common situational crises are loss of a parent or spouse through death or divorce, loss of job or status, urban dislocation, fire, natural disaster, and the diagnosis of a chronic or fatal illness. It should be remembered that an individual in a major transition state is already vulnerable. Add to that the stress of a traumatic event and the person is even more likely to experience a crisis.

The essential factor influencing the occurrence of crisis is an imbalance between the difficulty and importance of the problem and the resources immediately available to deal with it. The usual homeostatic, direct problem-solving mechanisms don't work. The individual is "upset"—usually associated with such subjective feelings of displeasure as anxiety, fear, guilt, or shame. There is a feeling of helplessness and ineffectuality in the face of an insoluble problem, which feeling is associated with some disorganization of functioning. The person is less effective than he or she usually is.

The Four Characteristic Phases of Crisis

Phase 1: Shock. The initial rise in tension from the impact of the stimulus calls for the habitual problem-solving responses of homeostasis.

Phase 2: Defensive Retreat. The person's usual problem-solving ability fails. The stimulus continues and is associated with a rise in tension and upset.

Phase 3: Recoil. The individual's anxiety level rises even further. The increased tension moves the person to use every resource available—including unusual or new means—to solve the problem and reduce the increasingly painful state of anxiety. There may be active resignation and giving up of certain aspects of goals as unattainable. Complementarity between the person and others which was disturbed is now reestablished.

Phase 4: Adaptation or Resolution. If the problem continues and can neither be solved with need satisfaction nor avoided by need resignation or perceptual distortion (adaptation), the tension mounts beyond a further threshold or its burden increases over time to a breaking point (resolution). Major disorganization of the individual with drastic results can then occur.

Factors Which Influence the Outcome of Crisis

Some variables which can alter the response to a crisis, as well as to stress, include the person's age, genetic endowment, cultural background, state of physical and emotional health, and level of energy to deal with the crisis. The objective facts of the crisis situation, the person's previous experiences with similar situations, and the person's own perception of the event are also important considerations. Finally, the individual's own coping mechanisms, the availability and response of family, friends, and other resources will effect the outcome of a crisis.

The duration and outcomes of crisis—acute emotional upset—can last from a few days to a few weeks. The person can return to his or her precrisis state and can grow from the crisis experience through discovery of new resources and ways of solving problems, or the person can reduce tension by moving into adaptive or maladaptive neurotic or psychotic patterns of behavior.

Crisis Prevention and Anticipation

Helping people in crisis through primary prevention includes:

1. identifying the people at risk through crisis assessment. (Developmental crises are predictable; situational crises are not as easy to predict.) This involves asking: What is the probability that a hazardous event will occur? What is the probability that the individual will be exposed to the hazard? What is the vulnerability of the individual?
2. assessing whether a particular person is or is not in crisis. This is characterized by difficulty in managing one's feelings, for example, anxiety—which includes a sense of dread, fear of losing control, an inability to focus on one thing, physical symptoms of G.A.S. response, alcohol or drug abuse, trouble with the law, and inability to effectively use available help.

Secondary and tertiary prevention imply that some form of psychoemotional disability has already occurred because of the absence of primary prevention. The intent is to shorten the rehabilitation time and long-term disability. These levels of prevention will not be considered in this text.

A strategy for helping people in stress or crisis will be included in the next chapter. The current goal is to assess the individual and/or family in crisis to determine either their risk for experiencing a crisis or whether they have already entered the active crisis phases mentioned.

Families and Crisis

If a family or group is thrown into crisis through one or more of its members, the nurse should assess the members of the family or group as well as the client seeking help. The nurse should be able to answer the following questions:

1. Is the family's communication network open?
2. Are the roles of the family or group members complementing one another?
3. Does the group provide warmth, reassurance, absolution, and consolidation?
4. Does the family or group allow the client to verbalize anxiety, hostility, depression, and other feelings?
5. Does the family or group support the client's own decision-making power?

Caplan acknowledges the validity of the "organismic tension" the individual or family in crisis is experiencing. He, like Selye, does not see stress only as a negative wearing force. They both admit to the conditioning, maturing effects of effectively resolving a stressful (crisis) situation.

SOCIETY AND STRESS—THE COMMUNITY LIFESPACE

Health and illness have been related to stressful intrapersonal and interpersonal environments. In the community, national and international context, health, illness, and social stress can be directly correlated. The Holmes Scale has been examined from a personal standpoint. It reflects the types of societal events that have value to most people and can cause them considerable stress.

Another element which profoundly influences stress response is the quality of the social support system. An assessment of this community system has been termed the Social Network Index (SNI) by Dr. Lisa Berkman, and she has tested it with some success. The SNI will be described later in this section.

Environmental stress has been correlated with an increase in mammary cancer, hypertension, and even in the lymphocytic immune response to antigens. [48] Levi suggests that societal stressors such as high population density produce discontent, aggressive behavior, alienation, and mental and psychosomatic illnesses. [28, p. iii] Other areas of community concern are environmental pollution, energy conservation, poverty, unemployment, famine, nuclear, chemical, and bacteriological warfare (not to mention more conventional methods), loneliness, and rapid social change. Even the threat of these stressors occurring—if they are not already doing so—produces ongoing stress in the population.

The community is recognizing these social problems on an international level.

The WHO 27th World Health Assembly Technical Discussions indicated that high-level social and health planners are considering these questions by agreeing to focus on:

1. the importance of all aspects of the human environment, including the psychosocial and socioeconomical factors, for human health and man's well being;
2. the increasing awareness that psychosocial factors can precipitate or counteract physical and mental ill health, profoundly modify the outcome of health action, and influence the quality of life; and
3. the resulting need for a holistic and ecological approach in social and health action and for the corresponding reorientation of medical and paramedical education and training. [28, p. xiv]

Statistical Measurements of the Community's Health Status

An overview of the level of health or disease of the community is best obtained by looking at statistical measurements of positive and negative tendency. The positive measurements of a population's health status are the birth and fertility rates and the life expectancy, such as the popularly adapted one used in the "Can You Pass the Test of Time?" quiz in Figure 5-7.

Unfortunately, the measurement of community health is largely gauged in terms of negative statistics, that is:

Mortality Data: general, infant and maternal, disease specific, stillbirth and abortion mortality

Morbidity Data: certain communicable diseases, certain congenital defects and birth injuries, hospital admissions, health and disability insurance claims data from special national health surveys, special disease registries, for example, crippled children, cancer, or special research programs [41]

Other negative data sources including divorce, alcoholism, drug addiction, and crime rates. Failure of community organizations are reflected in unemployment rates, illiteracy rates, and lack of vital community services

This data can then be cross-correlated with demographic data (age, sex, and cultural group information) to provide a means for discovering possible causal relationships and for predicting future trends in illness.

Social Network Index

One of the most fascinating large sample studies to date regarding stressful life events, health practices, and utilization of health services will be discussed in Chapter 6. The same stratified representative population of 6,928 people was used for a study by Dr. Lisa Berkman and Dr. Leonard Syme in which social networks were correlated to host resistance and mortality. Four sources of social contact were examined—marriage, contacts with close friends and relatives, church membership, and informal and formal group associations. This social network index not only measured the number of social ties but also the type and extent of involvement.

People who belonged to a church or temple had lower mortality rates than those who did not. Mortality was predicted independently of other known risk factors, for example, serum cholesterol levels, physical activity, alcohol intake, obesity, health practices, and socioeconomic status.

Included in the discussion by the researchers was the hypothesis that although stressful social circumstances may play a role in the causation of disease (depending on the strength of other pathogenic variables, for example, a virulent microorganism), when disease agents are less pathogenic, social factors may play a decisive role in health status. Although the study was measuring mortality, it is suggested that social circumstances such as social isolation may influence host resistance and affect vulnerability to disease in general. [7, p. 201]

A nursing assessment of the social network or support system is often critical, especially when persons are undergoing significant and stressful life changes. It is important for holistic nurses to remember that even positive life changes, such as a wanted pregnancy, have been shown to be negatively affected by lack of social supports. It is clear that many "nonhealth" variables affect health. These factors must be included in the nursing health assessment.

High-Risk Groups

Ignoring individual psychobiological programming, three very broad high-risk groups for community stress problems are infants and children, old people, and the physically, mentally, financially, and socially handicapped—that is, drug and alcohol abusers, prisoners, and the educationally handicapped. The special proneness to stress is evident in each of these populations.

Of particular interest, however, are the aging in our society. Although several major theories of aging have been proposed, recent excitement seems to center around some theory-related research on stress by Paola Timiras of the University of California, Berkeley. [57] Figure 5–11 summarizes this complex and fascinating idea of a brain-endocrine-regulated biological clock.

Alex B. Comfort, the gerontologist and physiologist, describes aging as an increase in the number and variety of homeostatic faults. Selyé views aging as the result of all the stresses to which the body has been exposed during a lifetime and corresponds to the stage of exhaustion in the General Adaptation Syndrome. [49, p. 93]

Medicine will certainly be interested in the applications of this research, but what does it mean for society? It is already calculated that by 1985 the population of persons in the United States over seventy years of age will rise 11 percent for men and 14 percent for women. As life is extended in communities, are senior citizens being sentenced to the complications of the degenerative diseases of adaptation and to a high probability of long-term institutionalization? How can the aging prevent the negative effects of aging and cope with the effects that have occurred? What methods of coping have been developed? These questions will be addressed in Chapter 6.

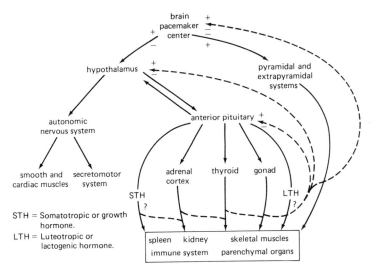

The brain-endocrine theory of programmed aging postulates that neurons in the higher brain centers are the "pacemakers" that regulate the biologic clock controlling growth, development, aging, and death. These neurons in the pacemaker center stimulate (+) or inhibit (−) the neurosecretory cells of the hypothalamus, which controls anterior pituitary secretions of tropic hormones. These, in turn, regulate other endocrine secretions or act directly on the target tissues or organs. Hormones determine metabolic activity and function of responsive tissues and organs in addition to modulating neuroendocrine interactions by positive or negative feedback (*dashed lines*) on the pituitary, hypothalamus, and other brain structures. The hypothalamus, through the autonomic nervous system, also regulates secretomotor functions and smooth and cardiac muscles, an action shared by the hormones as well. Finally, the pacemaker neurons influence the rate of stimulation of the pyramidal and extrapyramidal systems, which control skeletal tone and movement.

FIGURE 5-11 A brain-endocrine theory of aging

Reprinted from Paola S. Timiras, "Biological Perspectives on Aging," *American Scientist*, 66, no. 5 (September/October 1978), 605–13. Reprinted with permission of *American Scientist, Journal of Sigma Xi*, The Scientific Research Society.

Occupational Health and Safety

In discovering the community implications of stress, the occupational community cannot be overlooked. In 1970, the Occupational Safety and Health Act was enacted and provided:

> . . . that every man and woman is entitled to a workplace free from recognized hazards and that employers have the obligation of providing such a workplace. A purpose of OSHA is to assure insofar as practicable that no employee shall suffer diminished health, functional capacity, or life expectancy as a result of his or her work experience. [54, p. 184]

Since that time, OSHA enforcers have been uncovering a shocking number of work-related diseases. Some of the more publicized of these long-term disabling conditions have been "black lung" and "asbestosis." Chronic degenerative diseases are particularly difficult to document and diagnose because of their slow, silent, insidious onset. Occupational health is becoming particularly sensitive to precursors of ill health and risk factors. The results are programs that emphasize prevention and health promotion.

Physical and chemical hazards can occur in any work environment. In the health care work setting, the responsibility for the welfare and supervision of human beings is an added stressor. If, in addition, health workers are faced with working conditions or job requirements that do not allow them to perform as efficiently as possible, then they suffer the added burden of knowing that their inefficiency can directly affect the health of human beings. Administrative rules, lack of facilities, and the staff's preventing the workers from giving clients optimum care constitutes an even greater source of stress to them. Health-care workers must also deal regularly with sickness and death. All these stresses can add up to what is often termed "burn out" syndrome, which will be discussed in Chapter 10.

The direct relationship between stress on the job and disease is complex, but it is clear that job stress and demands can lead to increases in disease risk factors, such as increased cholesterol levels and hypertension. Even if stress does not cause physical ailments and disabilities, it still can lead to mental suffering and ill health—a sufficiently exorbitant price to pay for earning a living.

Some innovative occupational preventive health programs will be mentioned in later chapters. Industry is finding that an investment in a stress reduction program, for example, can save thousands of dollars in illness and compensation payments.

In summary, divorce, unemployment, poverty, delinquency, and crime rates are powerful testimony to the inability of our society to cope with its many social needs and social stresses. Stellman emphasizes the need for social supports:

> The isolated nuclear family . . . too often keeps children from their grandparents, aunts, and uncles, and dissolves the familial support system that had been a part of human existence until urbanization and industrialization disrupted it. Each nuclear family is now forced to provide for itself all its survival needs, as well as housekeeping and child-care duties. The lack of success that this arrangement has had is evident from the 29 percent of all females who are divorced and from the fact that 13 percent of all families are headed by single women. The young are alienated; the middle aged are striving and struggling toward heart disease, cancer, and the restlessness and uselessness of retirement; and the old are impoverished and lonely. [54, pp. 207–08]

Surely, we face some challenging stressors, which are having their predictable effect on us in the form of the diseases of civilization that have been alluded to in this chapter. We cannot escape stress; we couldn't survive without some of it. However, can we limit its effects and condition ourselves to withstand its impact? Chapter 6 explores the processes of creatively adapting, coping, and living optimally with stress.

REFERENCES FOR CHAPTER 5

[1] Donna C. Aguilera and Janice M. Messick, *Crisis Intervention,* 3rd ed. (St. Louis: C. V. Mosby Co., 1978).

[2] Ann Aikman and Walter McQuade, *Stress* (New York: Bantam Books, 1974).

[3] Donald B. Ardell, *High Level Wellness* (Emmaus, Pa.: Rodale Press, 1977).

[4] Nedra Belloc, "Relationship of Health Practices and Mortality," *Preventive Medicine,* 2, no. 1 (March 1973), 67–81.

[5] Nedra Belloc and Lester Breslow, "Relationship of Physical Health Status and Health Practices," *Preventive Medicine,* 2, no. 1 (March 1972), 409–21.

[6] Herbert Benson, *The Mind/Body Effect* (New York: Simon and Schuster, 1979).

[7] Lisa F. Berkman and S. Leonard Syme, "Social Networks, Host Resistance, and Mortality: A Nine Year Follow-up Study of Alameda County Residents," *American Journal of Epidemiology,* 109, no. X (October 1979), 186–204.

[8] Jerry E. Bishop, "Age of Anxiety: Stress of American Life Is Increasingly Blamed for Emotional Turmoil," *The Wall Street Journal,* vol. C, no. 64, April 2, 1979, pp. 1 and 26.

[9] Marie F. Branch and Phyllis Paxton, *Providing Safe Nursing Care for Ethnic People of Color* (New York: Appleton-Century-Crofts, 1976).

[10] Marjorie L. Byrne and Lida F. Thompson, *Key Concepts for the Study and Practice of Nursing,* 2nd ed. (St. Louis: C. V. Mosby Co., 1978).

[11] Walter B. Cannon, *The Wisdom of the Body* (New York: W. W. Norton & Co., 1932).

[12] Gerald Caplan, *An Approach to Community Mental Health* (New York: Grune and Stratton, 1961).

[13] Gerald Caplan, *Support Systems and Community Mental Health* (New York: Behavioral Publications, 1974).

[14] Martha Davis, Matthew McKay, and Elizabeth Eshelman, *The Relaxation and Stress Reduction Workbook* (Richmond, Ca.: New Harbinger Publications, 1980).

[15] G. E. Alan Dever, *Community Health Analysis—A Holistic Approach* (Germantown, Md.: Aspen Systems Corporation, 1980).

[16] René Dubos, *Man Adapting* (New Haven, Conn.: Yale University Press, 1965).

[17] Erik P. Eckholm, *The Picture of Health* (New York: W. W. Norton & Co., 1977).

[18] Daniel Girdano and George Everly, *Controlling Stress and Tension: A Holistic Approach* (Englewood Cliffs, N.J.: Prentice-Hall, Inc., 1979).

[19] Mark Jonathan Harris, "How to Make It to 100," *New West,* 2, no. 1 (January 3, 1977), 28.

[20] Roger Harris and Lawrence W. Frankel, eds., *Guide to Fitness After Fifty* (New York: Plenum Press, 1977).

[21] Lee Ann Hoff, *People in Crisis: Understanding and Helping* (Menlo Park, Ca.: Addison-Wesley Publishing Co., 1978).

[22] Thomas H. Holmes and Richard H. Rahe, "The Social Readjustment Rating Scale," *The Journal of Psychosomatic Research,* 11, no. 2 (August 1967), 213–18.

[23] John H. Knowles, ed., *Doing Better, Feeling Worse* (New York: W. W. Norton & Co., 1977).

[24] Marc LaLonde, "A New Perspective on the Health of the Canadians," a working paper, (Ottawa: Minister of National Health and Welfare Information, 1975).

[25] Richard S. Lazarus, "Psychological Stress and Coping in Adaptation and Illness," *International Journal of Psychiatry in Medicine,* 5, no. 4 (Fall 1974), 321–33.

[26] Richard S. Lazarus, *Patterns of Adjustment,* 3rd ed. (New York: McGraw-Hill Book Company, 1976).

[27] Lennart Levi, *Society, Stress, and Disease* (New York: Oxford University Press, 1971).

[28] Lennart Levi, *Psychosocial Stress: Population, Environment, and Quality of Life* (New York: John Wiley & Sons, 1975).

[29] Gay Luce, *Body Time* (New York: Bantam Books, 1973).

[30] John C. McCamy and James Presley, *Human Life Styling* (New York: Harper & Row, 1975), p. 324.

[31] Alan McLean, ed., *Occupational Stress* (Springfield, Ill.: Charles C Thomas, 1974).

[32] David Mechanic, "Stress, Illness and Illness Behavior," *Journal of Human Stress,* 2, no. 2 (June 1976), 2–6.

[33] Carolyn L. Morris, "Relaxation," *AJN,* 79, no. 11 (November 1979), 1958–59.

[34] Alice I. O'Flynn-Comiskey, "The Type-A Individual," *AJN,* 79, no. 11 (November 1979), 1956–58.

[35] Dean Ornish, "Mind-Heart Interactions: For Better and For Worse," *Health Values: Achieving High Level Wellness,* 2, no. 5 (September/October 1978), 266.

[36] Kenneth Pelletier, *Mind as Healer, Mind as Slayer* (New York: Dell Publishing Co., 1977).

[37] Kenneth Pelletier, *Toward a Science of Consciousness* (New York: Dell Publishing Co., 1978).

[38] Kenneth Pelletier, *Holistic Medicine from Stress to Optimum Health* (New York: Delacorte Press, 1979).

[39] Richard H. Rahe and Ransom J. Arthur, "Life Change and Illness Studies: Past History and Future Directions," *Journal of Human Stress,* 4, no. 1 (March 1978), 3–15.

[40] Judith M. Richter and Rebecca Sloan, "A Relaxation Technique," *AJN,* 79, no. 11 (November 1979), 1960–64.

[41] Lewis C. Robbins and Jack H. Hall, *How to Practice Prospective Medicine* (Indianapolis, Ind.: Methodist Hospital of Indiana, 1970).

[42] Judith Rodin and Ellen J. Langer, "Long-Term Effects of a Control-Relevant Intervention with the Institutionalized Aged," *Journal of Personality and Social Psychology,* 35, no. 12 (December 1977), 897–902.

[43] Edward S. Rogers, *Human Ecology and Health* (New York: Macmillan, 1960).

[44] Art Rosenblum, ed., *The Natural Birth Control Book* (Philadelphia: The Aquarian Research Foundation, 1976).

[45] Davis Ross, "Computing the Odds on Dying," *San Francisco Sunday Examiner and Chronicle,* February 17, 1980, p. 6.

[46] Sister Callista Roy and Sharon Roberts, *Theory Construction in Nursing and an Adaptation Model* (Englewood Cliffs, N.J.: Prentice-Hall, Inc., 1979).

[47] Gary Schwartz and David Shapiro, *Consciousness and Self-Regulation,* vol. 1 (New York: Plenum Press, 1976).

[48] Gary Schwartz and David Shapiro, *Consciousness and Self-Regulation,* vol. 2 (New York: Plenum Press, 1978).

[49] Hans Selyé, *Stress Without Distress* (New York: The New American Library, 1974).

[50] Hans Selyé, *The Stress of Life* (New York: McGraw-Hill Book Company, 1976).

[51] Sherry L. Shamansky and Cherie L. Clausen, "Levels of Prevention: Examination of the Concept," *Nursing Outlook* (February 1980), 104–08.

[52] Marcy J. T. Smith and Hans Selyé, "Reducing the Negative Effects of Stress," *AJN,* 79, no. 11 (November 1979), 1954–55.

[53] David M. Spain, "Atteroschlerosis," *Scientific American,* 215, no. 2 (August 1966), 48–56.

[54] Jean Stellman, *Women's Work, Women's Health: Myths and Realities* (New York: Pantheon Books, 1977).

[55] "Stress," *Blue Print for Health,* published by The Blue Cross Association, XXV, no. 1 (1974).

[56] Ogden Tanner, *Stress* (New York: Time-Life Books, 1977).

[57] Paola S. Timiras, "Biological Perspectives on Aging," *American Scientist,* 66, no. 5 (September-October 1978), 605–13.

[58] Arthur Vander, *Human Physiology and the Environment in Health and Disease* (San Francisco: W. H. Freeman & Co., 1976), p. 36.

[59] Ingrid Waldron and others, "The Coronary-Prone Behavior in Employed Men and Women," *Journal of Human Stress,* 3, no. 4 (December 1977), 2–18.

[60] Jean Watson, *Nursing: The Philosophy and Science of Caring* (Boston: Little Brown, 1979).

[61] Kerr L. White, "Prevention as a National Health Goal," *Preventive Medicine,* 4, no. 3 (September 1975), 247–51.

Chapter 6
lifestyling

CHAPTER OUTLINE

A. Self-Responsibility
  1. The Intensive Journal: The Period That is Now
  2. Rational Emotive Therapy
  3. Assertiveness Training
  4. Time Management
B. Nutrition: Background and Research
  1. Intrapersonal Nutrition
  2. Community Nutrition: U.S. Dietary Goals
  3. Orthomolecular Chemistry
  4. Overnutrition and Obesity
  5. Food Additives
  6. Herbs
  7. Controversial Topics
C. Fitness and Conditioning
  1. Aerobic Conditioning
    a. Training Effect
    b. Positive Effects
    c. Physiologic Effects of Running
    d. Caloric Expenditure and Lean Body Mass
  2. Fitness Tests
    a. The Harvard Step Test
    b. 12-Minute or One-and-a-Half-Mile Test
    c. Treadmill Test
    d. Contraindications
  3. Community Fitness and Conditioning Programs
    a. Beginners
    b. Senior Citizens
  4. Other Aspects of Exercise
    a. Overuse—Athletic Syndrome
    b. Disuse; Immobility; Aging
    c. Misuse: Storing Tension in Target Muscles

D. Stress Reduction and Management
  1. Nonmovement
    a. Biofeedback
    b. Autogenic Training
    c. Jacobson's Progressive Relaxation
    d. The Feeling Pause
    e. Palming
    f. Visualization
  2. Movement
    a. Yoga
    b. Tai-Chi Ch'uan
    c. Massage
    d. Zone Therapy, Reflexology, and Foot·Massage
    e. Acupuncture and Acupressure
    f. Touch for Health
    g. Rolfing
  3. Stress Reduction Programs
    a. Coping Skills Training
    b. Coping and Crisis Intervention
    c. Support Systems and Groups
    d. Clinical Applications of Stress Management and Lifestyle Modification
E. Community Coping: Environmental and Political Awareness
  1. Governmental Policies and Programs
  2. Private and Cooperative Programs
    a. Senior Actualization and Growth Exploration (SAGE)
    b. Aerobic Dance
    c. The Northern California Conference on Occupational Stress
    d. The Self-Care Movement
    e. The Women's Self-Help Movement

CHAPTER OBJECTIVES

1. Define the terminology related to the five lifestyle elements of self-responsibility, nutrition, fitness and conditioning, stress reduction, and environmental awareness.

2. Differentiate aggressive, passive, and assertive style behavior. Choose a nonassertive situation you would like to "rescript" and apply the five steps for change to it.

3. Choose a stressful event or an irrational idea you have experienced and apply Ellis' Rational Emotive approach to it.

4. List three time management techniques and state their importance for nursing.

5. Explain the nutritional topics of fasting, protein, and fiber to another person, presenting a positive and a negative aspect of each.

6. Describe the potential risks evident in a diet high in refined carbohydrates and cholesterol.

7. Discuss the benefits and possible risks inherent in megavitamin therapy.

8. Differentiate organic and dynamic fitness, flexibility, strength, endurance, and cardiovascular conditioning.

9. Identify the positive physiological and psychological effects attributed to aerobic conditioning.

10. Describe one fitness test, its strengths, and its shortcomings.

11. Differentiate disuse, misuse, and overuse in relation to fitness and conditioning.

12. Describe the relaxation response and contrast it to the stress response.

13. Contrast two movement and two nonmovement stress-reduction techniques.

14. Assess your own level of self-responsibility, nutrition, stress reduction, fitness and conditioning, and environmental awareness, using the tools supplied in this chapter and in the appendices.

15. Design a plan to modify areas assessed as needful of change in your lifestyle on the basis of your self-assessment.

16. Describe one intrapersonal, interpersonal, and community coping strategy for each of the five human lifestyle elements used in a simulated stressful situation.

17. Outline six steps which the lay and professional helper can use to help relieve a stressful crisis situation with a client.

18. Identify the major objectives of the self-care movement. List one example of a group that is working toward the self-care ideal and how it is achieving its goals.

For years, nurses have been writing "reduce stress," "refer for nutritional counseling," "plan exercise program," in their care plans in response to client health problems. Given the present level of knowledge about the stress-adaptation process, how do these lifestyle goals fit into a preventive health program? Furthermore, what kinds of information and skills will be demanded of holistic nurses from clients and colleagues as the stress response becomes more a part of daily life in an increasingly complicated urban environment?

The body's stress response has been examined. Adaptation has been defined as those processes—biological, psychological, social, or cultural—which aid the human organism in its attempt to return to homeostasis. [25, p. 261] The General Adaptation Syndrome adaptive response has been explored in some depth, largely from a physiological perspective. The potential for acute and long-term illness as a result of *prolonged* G.A.S. and fight or flight responses has been projected.

A psychological approach to stress has been proposed using Caplan's theory of crisis. Lazarus [50] and others are adding to this ever-expanding body of knowledge. More comprehensive theories of stress-adaptation encompassing sociocultural factors are the focus of much ongoing research. It should be remembered that stress-adaptation in itself is not a pathological concept, although it has been applied largely in medical and psychiatric areas. The fields of psychosomatic and behavioral medicine have developed to meet the needs of the 50 to 70 percent of all clients seen in medical practices whose complaints are reportedly stress initiated, mediated, or exacerbated. [83, p. 401] More nurses are becoming stress management consultants and teachers to help clients solve these stress-related problems.

To clarify the considerable blurring of the meaning of coping, the term *lifestyling* will be used to mean all the knowledges and skills of health promotion and disease prevention *consciously* applied to manage stress and its related effects, specifically in the areas of self-responsibility, nutrition, fitness and conditioning, stress reduction, and environmental awareness. Coping methods and support systems will be included in the word lifestyling. Traditional psychological defense mechanisms such as denial, repression, and so forth, will not be discussed.

Adaptation refers to those biological, psychological, social, and spiritual responses *automatically* called into play in response to a stressor. The process of adaptation depends not only on the number, scope, intensity, and type of stress with which an individual, group, or community is faced, but also with their skills, capacities, and support systems which can be summoned up to deal with that challenge. [60, p. 2]

This chapter will outline some lifestyle modifications for dealing with stress and will suggest some techniques that are within most people's grasp. The first area of focus—self-responsibility—has been discussed in detail. However, it is such a pivotal concept with regard to any stress-management practice that a few more comments are in order. The other four areas yet to be covered are: (1) nutrition, (2) fitness and conditioning, (3) stress reduction and management, and (4) environmental awareness and action.

The chapter will conclude with selected clinical applications and examples of the lifestyling practices which individuals, groups, and communities are using to promote high-level wellness.

Within the wellness continuum, there are many generative, innovative strategies for nurses and clients to condition themselves to better withstand stress. Conditioning implies learning a planned, increasing series of adaptations in preparation for coping with stress. Numerous productive intrapersonal and interpersonal mind/body/spirit coping mechanisms exist to help clients and nurses deal with daily unpreventable stresses or acute crisis situations during or after their occurrence. The first step, covered in Chapter 5, is to become aware of stress and its protective as well as psychosomatic outcomes.

The next task is to look at all the techniques nurses and clients have at their disposal to modify the effects of stress appropriately. All the exercises and methods contained in this chapter require openness, commitment, flexibility, and practice. Results are often not dramatic, but very subtle, and require patience and evaluation criteria that measure qualitative and minute changes.

Lifestyle patterns and resulting health problems are often the most difficult to change because the results seem unsubstantial and often can't be measured for many years. If nurses and clients can readjust their criteria of success and redefine their unrealistic expectations of overnight changes, especially in areas such as smoking cessation or weight loss, change will occur and be more lasting. Readiness to change is a key factor in all the lifestyle elements. An anonymous Italian Proverb summarizes the problem nicely:

> "Between saying and doing
> there lies the ocean" *

SELF-RESPONSIBILITY

Self-responsibility as defined in Chapter 2 is the reflective response of the self to choose freely from a variety of alternatives. Self-responsibility is based on self-awareness.

Self-awareness occurs when nurses or clients assess their own levels of stress, fitness, nutrition, self-responsibility, and environmental awareness. Once nurses or clients perceive and then internalize this information, they may indicate a desire to make some lifestyle changes. Until these steps occur, the nurse's role is really that of an advocate and teacher who explains and clarifies information related to the mind-body response to stress. The nurse also supports current productive methods of coping, noting nonproductive habits as well as those which are not working for clients or for themselves.

It is important to note that both the nurse and the client have within themselves the knowledge, tools, materials, and energy to maintain health. What clients may lack in factual or technical expertise, they make up for in "inside" information about themselves. This contribution is respected and encouraged by the nurse, for without it and the clients' participation, none of the lifestyle changes will occur or be maintained for any length of time.

Self-responsibility begins when clients grasp the fact that the body is innately wise and striving toward optimal health in the face of a continuing series of stressful interactions with the environment.

Samuels and Bennett, in their self-health manual, *The Well Body Book,* have coined the phrase "the three-million-year-old-healer"; they refer to the body, which has evolved its own unique way to protect and heal itself in over three million years of adaptation to stress. [79] Sometimes the mind fools the body into perceiving a

* Quoted in Paul Watzlawick, *The Language of Change* (New York: Basic Books, 1978), p. 138.

situation as stressful, thereby triggering a full-scale stress response that is inappropriate to the situation or to the long-term welfare of the entire system.

It is easy to demonstrate the effect sad or tension-filled thoughts can have on the physical performance of the individual (via heart rate, blood pressure monitoring, muscle testing, and other biofeedback methods). Once clients recognize the autonomic control they can learn, they have achieved another step toward accepting responsibility for their own health. Voluntary "control" over involuntary somatic functions was at one time an heretical idea. Science now acknowledges that when the mind creates fear and worry, the body manifests muscle tension and vasoconstriction. This reaction is termed negative arousal. Chronic muscle tension and vasoconstriction have their predictable long-term effects (see Chapter 5). When the mind experiences love, peace, and harmony, the body responds with decreased muscle tension, vasodilation, and increased subjective body feelings of warmth and well-being.

If the first adaptation is the stress which includes the "fight or flight" response, then the second is the relaxation response. Eliciting the relaxation response can have more powerful effects, in some cases, than drugs or surgery. Relaxation will be examined in the stress reduction section of this chapter. The role of self as healer is one that many clients have difficulty accepting. It is actually simpler for some clients to abrogate their power to heal themselves to someone who may not even know them. It is easier to blame someone else for illness. Most nurses and clients will need to experience this self-healing or self-destructive ability before proceeding to change.

Albert Schweitzer neatly summarized the self-help concept and role of the supportive professional in an interview over twenty years ago with Norman Cousins:

> The witch doctor succeeds for the same reasons all the rest of us succeed. Each patient carries his own doctor inside him. They come to us not knowing the truth. We are at our best when we give the doctor, who resides within each patient, a chance to go to work. [17]

A recent bestseller contains twenty-five questions to help people assess their mastery of the self-responsibility concept. [26, p. 15] This self-inventory has not been scientifically tested, but it may serve as an initial step toward evaluating one's willingness to assume responsibility for health and life (see Figure 6–1).

The self-responsibility concept, then, begins with a self-examination and a determination of what one can do for a health problem or practice making use of one's own inner healing resources. If this assessment yields a medical problem that requires specialized medical expertise, then those services are sought.

Most of the time, however, the real or potential stressors can be defined and the body–mind adaptation examined either by the client or with the assistance of a professional helper. Clients can then contract with themselves to work toward certain clearly delineated health goals within a specific time period. The nurse supports these efforts at predetermined intervals until the long-term goal of self-care is reached.

Chapter 2 suggested some brief self-awareness, self-responsibility exercises. The self-responsibility assessment mentioned at the beginning of this section may be

1. Do you believe that your mind is your own?
2. Are you capable of controlling your own feelings?
3. Are you motivated from within rather than from without?
4. Are you free from the need for approval?
5. Do you set up your own rules of conduct for yourself?
6. Are you free from the desire for justice and fairness?
7. Can you accept yourself and avoid complaining?
8. Are you free from hero worship?
9. Are you a doer rather than a critic?
10. Do you welcome the mysterious and the unknown?
11. Can you avoid describing yourself in absolute terms?
12. Can you love yourself at all times?
13. Can you grow your own roots?
14. Have you eliminated all dependency relationships?
15. Have you eliminated all blame and fault-finding in your life?
16. Are you free from ever feeling guilty?
17. Are you able to avoid worrying about the future?
18. Can you give and receive love?
19. Can you avoid immobilizing anger in your life?
20. Have you eliminated procrastination as a lifestyle?
21. Have you learned to fail effectively?
22. Can you enjoy spontaneously, without having a plan?
23. Can you appreciate and create humor?
24. Are you treated by others the way you want to be?
25. Are you motivated by your potential for growth rather than by a need to repair your deficiencies?

Total: Yes __ No __

If you score 8 or more in the No column, read some of the references cited at the end of Chapter 2. (Also try some of the exercises by Dyer recommended in his book.)

FIGURE 6-1 25 questions designed to measure capacity to choose happiness and fulfillment

Adapted by permission from Dr. Wayne W. Dyer, *Your Erroneous Zones* (New York: Avon Books, 1976), p. 15–16.

simplistic and prepackaged, but it serves as the beginning of an arduous, and at times exhilarating, path to self-discovery and enlightenment.

The Intensive Journal: The Period That is Now

One of the most promising tools for stimulating the process of self-responsibility and self-growth is seen in the Intensive Journal developed by Ira Progoff, a noted depth psychologist and student of Jung and D. T. Suzuki. Progoff spent years developing, testing, and experimenting with the journal with his clients. In his Intensive Journal Workshops, Progoff encourages people to work through each of the questions below and to record their responses. [73] Sometimes, the insights gained can be dramatic. Often the messages are unclear and unfamiliar because they may come from the right hemisphere of the brain which focuses on visual, intuitive, and nonlinear, nonanalytic thought.

The beginning exercise summarized here is loosely adapted from The Period Log. It clearly focuses on the period that is here and now. The Period Log is only one in a series of self-awareness exercises which, through extensive self-exploration, open the door to the Intensive Journal, a lifetime self-discovery and development process.

One of the elements that makes the Intensive Journal different from other journals used throughout history is that it is not set up as a chronology of events, but rather as an inner dialogue with the self—yielding a kind of self-wisdom. Progoff's achievement lies in the format for the Intensive Journal which is constructed so as to allow self-direction and self-integration of learning rather than reliance on outside feedback.

The Period Log addresses a highly individual point in a person's life that is not set apart as a specific time sequence—it could be days, weeks, or even years. The present moment can only be distinguished from the past or future by the fact that we are still involved in the results, consequences, thoughts, or decisions raised by that period. The present period may be a significant life change, transition, or definable life accident (for example, ''It started the day my father died'', etc.). Discovering this period, Progoff suggests, is best begun by switching off the conscious mind—perhaps through a relaxation exercise.

The question, ''Where am I now in my life?'' is presented to the relaxed person. Like any indirect question that the right hemisphere is asked to consider, it is placed ''out there'' without any judgment or analysis. The answers to the questions, ''What is this period? where did it begin? what events surround it?'' should flow—not cause intense concentration. Different kinds of images present themselves; some are auditory, some visual, some merely feelings. Again, no judgment is placed on the kind of image. If some descriptive word or phrase comes to mind, this can be written in the log.

Returning to the conscious level, we begin to answer specific questions in the Period Log having to do with *now:*

1. What memories are there of the time?
2. Do dissension or disharmony characterize the period?
3. Have there been times of love or friendship?
4. Are there any family or work relationships or social events that are particularly significant?
5. Have any religious, spiritual, psychic, or inner experiences occurred?
6. Are these considered important?
7. Can any dreams be remembered?
8. Do any dreams persist or recur? Are these important to remember for later recall?

9. Have any creative insights or ideas been brought up?

10. Do any illnesses characterize this period?

11. What persons are important to you during this time? List them and describe their significance very briefly.

12. What outside activities or work have been of particular value?

13. What have been the positive aspects of this work? What have been the negative aspects of this work?

14. Have any major lifestyle changes occurred during this time? If so, what?

15. Have you had any community or political involvement at this time?

16. Are any artforms particularly attractive to you at this time (for example, music, theatre, etc.)?

17. Have any dramatic life events occurred during this time?

18. Has any thing or event or inner experience changed the course of your life? If so, describe it *very* briefly. [73, pp. 64–78]

Many of the responses to these questions are examined and analyzed in more detail later in the Intensive Journal. The Period Log is the beginning of putting our life experiences and our lives in focus.

Rational Emotive Therapy

In Chapter 2, Rational Emotive Therapy was briefly discussed. Its originator, Albert Ellis, believed that inappropriate response to stress, or negative arousal, was the result of irrational ideas or beliefs which could be replaced by realistic self-talk. Ellis puts forth the idea that self-controlled thoughts are what create anxiety, fear, depression, and so on.

Ellis believes that ten basic irrational ideas can perpetuate a negative cycle which results in anxiety, feelings of worthlessness, fear, and physiological symptoms of stress. The ten ideas and their rational explanations are listed in Figure 6–2. Check off those which approximate your own beliefs.

It takes a certain level of self-awareness to admit indulgence in some of the beliefs mentioned. Once a belief is admitted, however, some rules for rational thinking can be applied:

1. It doesn't do anything to me. It doesn't make me anxious or afraid.

2. Everything is exactly the way it should be, having been caused by a long series of causative events.

3. All humans are fallible creatures. Setting unreasonable expectations merely increases the chances for disappointment and unhappiness.

4. It takes two to have conflict.

5. The original cause is lost in antiquity and searching for it is difficult, painful, and a waste of time.

6. We feel the way we think. Our interpretations of events cause emotions. [20, Goodman as quoted therein, pp. 109–10]

Some of the rules have an autosuggestive quality about them. In a later sec-

1. **It is an absolute necessity for an adult to have love and approval from peers, family and friends.**
   In fact, it is impossible to please all the people in your life. Even those who basically like and approve of you will be turned off by some behaviors and qualities. This irrational belief is probably the single greatest cause of unhappiness.
2. **You must be unfailingly competent and almost perfect in all you undertake.**
   The results of believing you must behave perfectly are self blame for inevitable failure, lowered self esteem, perfectionistic standards applied to mate and friends, and paralysis and fear at attempting anything.
3. **Certain people are evil, wicked and villainous, and should be punished.**
   A more realistic position is that they are behaving in ways which are antisocial or inappropriate. They are perhaps stupid, ignorant or neurotic, and it would be well if their behavior could be changed.
4. **It is horrible when people and things are not the way you would like them to be.**
   This might be described as the spoiled child syndrome. As soon as the tire goes flat the self-talk starts: "Why does this happen to me? Damn, I can't take this. It's awful, I'll get all filthy." Any inconvenience, problem or failure to get your way is likely to be met with such awfulizing self statements. The result is intense irritation and stress.
5. **External events cause most human misery—people simply react as events trigger their emotions.**
   A logical extension of this belief is that you must control the external events in order to create happiness or avoid sorrow. Since such control has limitations and we are at a loss to completely manipulate the wills of others, there results a sense of helplessness and chronic anxiety. Ascribing unhappiness to events is a way of avoiding reality. Self statements *interpreting* the event caused the unhappiness. While you may have only limited control over others, you have enormous control over your emotions.
6. **You should feel fear or anxiety about anything that is unknown, uncertain or potentially dangerous.**
   Many describe this as, "a little bell that goes off and I think I ought to start worrying." They begin to rehearse their scenarios of catastrophy. Increasing the fear or anxiety in the face of uncertainty makes coping more difficult and adds to stress. Saving the fear response for actual, perceived danger allows you to enjoy uncertainty as a novel and exciting experience.
7. **It is easier to avoid than to face life difficulties and responsibilities.**
   There are many ways of ducking responsibilities: "I should tell him/her I'm no longer interested—but not tonight . . . I'd like to get another job, but I'm just too tired on my days off to look . . . A leaky faucet won't hurt

anything . . . We could shop today, but the car is making a sort of funny sound.''

If you have checked this idea, please add your standard excuses to avoid responsibility here:

Area of Responsibility   **_Method of Avoidance_**

_____   _____

_____   _____

_____   _____

_____   _____

_____   _____

_____   _____

8. **You need something other or stronger or greater than yourself to rely on.** This belief becomes a psychological trap in which your independent judgement, and the awareness of your particular needs are undermined by a reliance on higher authority.

9. **The past has a lot to do with determining the present.** Just because you were once strongly affected by something, that does not mean that you must continue the habits you formed to cope with the original situation. Those old patterns and ways of responding are just decisions made so many times they have become nearly automatic. You can identify those old decisions and start changing them *right now.* You can learn from past experience, but you don't have to be overly attached to it.

10. **Happiness can be achieved by inaction, passivity and endless leisure.** This is called the Elysian Fields syndrome. There is more to happiness than perfect relaxation.

FIGURE 6-2 Albert Ellis' ten basic irrational ideas

Reprinted with permission from Martha Davis, Elizabeth Eshelman, and Matthew McKay, *The Relaxation and Stress Reduction Workbook* (Richmond, Ca.: New Harbinger Publications, 1980), pp. 106–07.

tion of this chapter (page 262), autohypnotic suggestions will be described. Suggesting to the unconscious, through the right hemisphere, a positive or rational view of the world can have the effect of changing that chaotic world or the individual's response to it.

Refuting irrational ideas, like any of the lifestyle modifications mentioned in this chapter, requires openness, a willingness to change, and a commitment to a certain amount of homework. In the case of refuting irrational beliefs, approximately twenty minutes is recommended to work through each stressful event that occurs. The suggested format follows:

1. *The stressful event:* an abbreviated *objective* description.
2. *Rational ideas:* reasons why the event occurred and what you plan to think or do about it.
3. *Irrational ideas:* all the negative, self-deprecating thoughts, beliefs, and assumptions that enter your mind.
4. *Emotional response:* label the emotion in one or two words, for example, I'm angry, etc.
5. Select an irrational idea from (3) and challenge it by using the rules for refuting irrational ideas mentioned earlier.
   a. Does any evidence exist for the falseness of the idea; if so, what?
   b. Does any evidence exist for the truth of the idea; if so, what?
6. What is the worst that could happen?
7. What good things might occur?
8. What alternative thoughts, emotions, and actions can be generated? [20]

This simple technique can be practiced and shared with clients. Since there is no research data either to support or to dismiss the technique, it falls into the category of helpful hints which work for some people. The nurse needs to evaluate its efficacy with self and at least to keep anecdotal records with clients. Chapter 8 will suggest a problem-solving technique to encourage and spell out such evaluation.

Assertiveness Training

Directly related to coping with stress and developing self-awareness and responsibility is cultivating assertiveness, that is, the ability to express personal rights and feelings. Several sets of personal and professional rights have been articulated in the Appendices. Nurses and clients don't express their feelings or defend their rights because they have been conditioned to accept certain mistaken assumptions. Davis, Eshelman, and McKay have listed some of these assumptions and the respective rights they tend to oppress (see Figure 6–3).

Differentiating one's own habitual style of interpersonal behavior is one of the first steps in assertiveness training. Reading about the following three behavior styles, and then evaluating one's own style from them, can be helpful.

1. *Aggressive style behavior* includes fighting, accusing, threatening, and overwhelming others. This type of person is often confused with an assertive one when in fact they bear little resemblance to one another. An aggressive person creates fear and hostility.
2. *Passive style behavior* encourages oppression of real feelings and allows others to do as they please at personal cost. The passive style person may not have any enemies, but he is often harboring anger and resentment—which takes its toll in the long run.
3. *Assertive style behavior* encourages expression of feelings, consideration of others, and direct action toward clearly stated goals. An assertive person realizes that the other two methods are ineffective and cause more stress than they alleviate.

FIGURE 6-3 Some common mistaken assumptions vs. legitimate rights

Reprinted with permission from Martha Davis, Elizabeth Eshelman, and Matthew McKay, *The Relaxation and Stress Reduction Workbook* (Richmond, Ca.: New Harbinger Publications, 1980), pp. 133–34.

Mistaken Traditional Assumptions	Your Legitimate Rights
1. It is selfish to put your needs before others' needs.	You have a right to put yourself first, sometimes.
2. It is shameful to make mistakes. You should have an appropriate response for every occasion.	You have a right to make mistakes.
3. If you can't convince others that your feelings are reasonable, then they must be wrong, or maybe you are going crazy.	You have a right to be the final judge of your feelings and accept them as legitimate.
4. You should respect the views of others, especially if they are in a position of authority. Keep your differences of opinion to yourself. Listen and learn.	You have a right to have your own opinions and convictions.
5. You should always try to be logical and consistent.	You have a right to change your mind or decide on a different course of action.
6. You should be flexible and adjust. Others have good reasons for their actions and it's not polite to question them.	You have a right to protest unfair treatment or criticism.
7. You should never interrupt people. Asking questions reveals your stupidity to others.	You have a right to interrupt in order to ask for clarification.
8. Things could get even worse, don't rock the boat.	You have a right to negotiate for change.
9. You shouldn't take up others' valuable time with your problems.	You have a right to *ask* for help or emotional support.
10. People don't want to hear that you feel bad, so keep it to yourself.	You have a right to feel and express pain.
11. When someone takes the time to give you advice, you should take it very seriously. They are often right.	You have a right to ignore the advice of others.
12. Knowing that you did something well is its own reward. People don't like show-offs. Successful people are secretly disliked and	You have a right to receive formal recognition for your work and achievements.

(continued)

envied. Be modest when complimented.	
13. You should always try to accommodate others. If you don't, they won't be there when you need them.	You have a right to say "no."
14. Don't be anti-social. People are going to think you don't like them if you say you'd rather be alone instead of with them.	You have a right to be alone, even if others would prefer your company.
15. You should always have a good reason for what you feel and do.	You have a right not to have to justify yourself to others.
16. When someone is in trouble, you should help them.	You have a right not to take responsibility for someone else's problem.
17. You should be sensitive to the needs and wishes of others, even when they are unable to tell you what they want.	You have a right not to have to anticipate others' needs and wishes.
18. It's always a good policy to stay on people's good side.	You have a right not to always worry about the goodwill of others.
19. It's not nice to put people off. If questioned, give an answer.	You have a right to choose not to respond to a situation.

FIGURE 6-3 (continued)

Sharon and Gordon Bowers have developed an Assertiveness Questionnaire (see Figure 6–4) in which the respondent categorizes each item according to applicability and degree of comfort: (1) comfortable; (2) mildly uncomfortable; (3) moderately uncomfortable; (4) very uncomfortable; and (5) unbearably threatening. [20, pp. 140–42]

After responding to the questionnaire, the Bowers suggest looking at items in the (2) to (3) range rather than tackling the most threatening situations. They suggest choosing a specific situation to be rewritten, and describing that situation being careful to include specifics—such as who, when, what, how—regarding your fear of the outcome should you act assertively, and what your personal goal is, in specific terms. Once the situation is recorded accurately, a "script" for change can be planned:

1. Define your goals, needs, wants, rights.
2. Choose a time and place to discuss the problem, if possible.

FIGURE 6-4 Assertiveness questionnaire

Reprinted with permission from Martha Davis, Elizabeth Eshelman, and Matthew McKay, *The Relaxation and Stress Reduction Workbook* (Richmond, Ca.: New Harbinger Publications, 1980), pp. 140–41.

A *Check here if the item applies to you*	B *Rate from 1–5 for discomfort*	
		WHEN do you behave non-assertively?
_____	_____	asking for help
_____	_____	stating a difference of opinion
_____	_____	receiving and expressing negative feelings
_____	_____	receiving and expressing positive feelings
_____	_____	dealing with someone who refuses to cooperate
_____	_____	speaking up about something that annoys you
_____	_____	talking when all eyes are on you
_____	_____	protesting a rip-off
_____	_____	saying "no"
_____	_____	responding to undeserved criticism
_____	_____	making requests of authority figures
_____	_____	negotiating for something you want
_____	_____	having to take charge
_____	_____	asking for cooperation
_____	_____	proposing an idea
_____	_____	taking charge
_____	_____	asking questions
_____	_____	dealing with attempts to make you feel guilty
_____	_____	asking for service
_____	_____	asking for a date or appointment
_____	_____	asking for favors
_____	_____	other _____
		WHO are the people with whom you are non-assertive?
_____	_____	parents
_____	_____	fellow workers, classmates
_____	_____	strangers
_____	_____	old friends
_____	_____	spouse or mate
_____	_____	employer
_____	_____	relatives
_____	_____	children
_____	_____	acquaintances
_____	_____	sales people, clerks, hired help
_____	_____	more that two or three people in a group
_____	_____	other _____

(continued)

```
A
Check
here if
the item
applies
to you
                        WHAT do you want that you have been unable to
                             achieve with non-assertive styles?
_____              approval for things you have done well
_____              to get help with certain tasks
_____              more attention, or time with your mate
_____              to be listened to and understood
_____              to make boring or frustrating situations more
                             satisfying
_____              to not have to be nice all the time
_____              confidence in speaking up when something is im-
                             portant to you
_____              greater comfort with strangers, store clerks, me-
                             chanics, etc.
_____              confidence in asking for contact with people you
                             find attractive
_____              getting a new job, asking for interviews, raises,
                             etc.
_____              comfort with people who supervise you, or work
                             under you
_____              to not feel angry and bitter a lot of the time
_____              overcome a feeling of helplessness and the sense
                             that nothing ever really changes
_____              initiating satisfying sexual experiences
_____              do something totally different and novel
_____              getting time by yourself
_____              doing things that are fun or relaxing for you
_____              other _____
```

FIGURE 6-4 (continued)

3. Define the particular problem as clearly and simply as possible.
4. Describe feelings which indicate assuming of responsibility for "I messages," such as "I feel."
5. State the request as briefly and understandably as possible.
6. Reinforce the positive reasons and benefits for the person's cooperating with the request. [20]

It is important that body language (described in Chapter 7) be consistent with assertive behavior, that is, communicate directness, self-confidence, etc. Other techniques for facilitation of assertiveness and prevention of blocking and manipulation by the other person will be mentioned in Chapter 10.

Time Management

Finally, a more mundane aspect of self-responsibility is time management. As the nurse becomes more and more involved in her professional role, the value of time becomes crucial. Poor personal time managers may be able to avoid temporarily the stress that comes from procrastination or chronic rushing to meet deadlines, but most health care situations cannot tolerate poor and inefficient decision making.

Symptoms of poor time management have been outlined as:

rushing

chronic vacillation between unpleasant alternatives

fatigue or listlessness, with many slack hours of nonproductive activity

constantly missed deadlines

insufficient time for rest or personal relationships

the sense of being overwhelmed by demands and details, and of having to do alot that you don't want to do most of the time. [20, McKay as quoted therein, p. 150]

All time management techniques suggest:

establishing priorities that indicate most important goals and that allow decision making based on those priorities

creating new time by realistic scheduling and elimination of low priority tasks

learning to make basic decisions using a systematic approach

Chapter 8 will suggest such a method for problem solving.

The self-responsibility exercises and suggestions mentioned are merely the beginning for the self-aware, practicing holistic nurse. The chapter references offer a further start. More in-depth courses and trainings are offered, often for continuing education in nursing credit for relicensure. Application of these techniques to nursing practice is now under way. Scientific evaluation of the effectiveness of these approaches is the responsibility of every holistic nurse, for it is through this research that a clearly defined, workable body of holistic nursing knowledge will develop.

NUTRITION: BACKGROUND AND RESEARCH

Nowhere in the risk factor human lifestyle elements is there more controversy than in the burgeoning area of nutrition. *Nutrition* includes all the processes by which food is ingested, assimilated, and utilized to promote health and prevent disease.

Nurses have traditionally involved themselves with therapeutic nutrition or diet therapy which focuses on the illness-specific dietary requirements of the client. Nutrition courses in nursing and medical education focus on therapeutic illness-oriented nutritional interventions rather than on those values, principles, and practices which optimize and enhance wellness.

Once again, the content in this chapter will center around nutritional approaches which directly relate to certain prevalent risks to wellness. Certain issues which are believed by a growing group of recognized researchers to influence the overall internal environment of the cell and the complex biochemical balance thereof will be explored briefly.

Some special nutrient deficiency-prone groups will be pinpointed, and the position that even the average American diet is vitamin and mineral deficient will be advocated. The following reasons support the stand that many Americans are subclinically undernourished:

1. increased environmental pollution;
2. increased stressful lifestyles;
3. persistently unhealthy habit patterns—for example, alcohol and cigarette intake; and
4. increased food refining and processing, and the use of additives which bleach or cancel out many of the nutrients formerly present in foods.

Even when undernutrition is not directly lethal, it raises the odds of early death from other causes; at the very least, it impairs health and infringes upon the right to a full life. Those at risk for particular problems resulting from malnutrition or undernutrition should be mentioned. Groups particularly plagued by serious undernutrition are the American Indians living on reservations, migrant workers, the urban and rural poor and their unborn children, and the aged.

The general term "protein-calorie" malnutrition is commonly used to describe the undernutrition of the poor. Early and severe malnutrition is an important factor in later intellectual development above and beyond the effects of social-familial influences.

A particularly crucial attribute of the brain's growth spurt, which probably lasts from about the twentieth week of fetal life to two years after birth, is its apparent chronological inflexibility. If certain kinds of growth do not occur within a specified period, the opportunity for that growth may be lost forever. This period presents a once in a lifetime opportunity for normal development, which is why undernutrition is profoundly more serious for this group than for any other.

Undernutrition accentuates and even creates a lack of stimulation and experience that hinders personal development. Often apathetic and socially withdrawn, the poorly nourished tend to be less sociable than the well-fed. Physical and mental fatigue, the inability to concentrate, and low motivation doom them to poor performance at school. Frequent illness means frequent absence from the classroom. Thus, poorly nourished children fall behind in a critical learning period and suffer irreversible losses of opportunity. [48] Some supplemental nutrition and food programs have been federally initiated to help combat this massive problem. They will be discussed in the community coping section of this chapter.

Before the nurse becomes immersed in a sea of conflicting documents regarding the latest advances in nutrition, two points regarding any of its research need to be made. First, there exists a tremendous variation in individual requirements for nutrients. Nonetheless, some attempts to universalize these demands have been made by the United States Department of Agriculture and the Food and Nutrition Board, National Academy of Science National Research Council. At best, Recommended Daily Allowances (RDA's) constitute a reference point from which to embark on a personal nutrition plan.

Second, nutritional research is conducted largely on animal populations with short lifespans—for example, fruitflies—and as evidence becomes more admissible, the experiment involves more expensive animals with longer lifespans. It is unrealistic to expect human subjects to submit to a carefully controlled experiment under laboratory conditions for any extended length of time exceeding 1 percent of their total lifespans. An exception would be the now contested practice of experimenting on prisoners, mental hospital clients, and other captive populations.

The result is that much of the data obtained from such trials does not have the clarity or precision of a physics or chemistry experiment. Conclusions are often extrapolated from lower-level life forms and are mistakenly applied to humans when the mechanism being studied is often different or absent in man.

Material presented in this section will be classified as clinically proven in controlled animal or human trials, the opinion of recognized authorities on the subject, or the testimony of large numbers of people to a reputable nutritional source. Conflicting or opposing information about various topics will also be covered and noted as such.

Intrapersonal Nutrition

Perhaps the best way to begin sorting out a nutritional plan consistent with current findings, but comfortable for the individual, is to look at exactly which foods clients are eating and how they feel about them—before, during, and after eating. A long recommended method is to conduct a twenty-four-hour recall of exactly which foods are ingested and in what quantities and then converting that data into caloric, protein, fat, carbohydrate, vitamin, and mineral values. These values are then compared to the hypothetical norms or standards referred to earlier. Recommendations for dietary changes are then made. More often than not, habits, cultural food values, psychological and social needs, geographic location, and financial status have not been considered. Thus, the recommendations will quickly be ignored or abandoned.

If the client is oriented to the purpose of a seven-day "Diet, Exercise, Relaxation and Feeling Diary" which asks not only for the food ingested, but for the feelings and circumstances surrounding that intake, as well as for the other lifestyle elements of exercise and relaxation, a bigger picture of the relationship of food to total health begins to emerge (see Figure 6-5).

The nurses and clients will soon see for themselves certain eating, exercise, and stress patterns. They may even sense a cyclical pattern to their food cravings and responses. Certain stimuli will trigger certain food responses. Some will become aware of eating as coping, loving, etc.

When clients submit the completed diary, they will already have reached some conclusions about their eating, exercising, and relaxing habits. The nurse encourages clients to draw more conclusions, answering questions about nutrition and other areas that inevitably ensue. Nurses and clients also have their own mixed bag of beliefs, facts, and faddish ideas about food. The nurse explores these at this time, clarifying and discussing incorrect information.

Holistic practitioners advocate listening to the body's internal messages about food. Much attention is paid to the way food is prepared, its freshness, how it blends with other foods, how it feels to eat it (taste, smell, tactile sensations), the mood surrounding eating, and finally, what it does to aid the body. All this may sound like a simplistic approach, but it implies that clients have a certain prerequisite level of nutritional knowledge and an awareness of healthful food preparation techniques.

Given all this information, what does the client feel like doing about his current nutritional status? Answers or goals—such as gain weight, lose weight, eat more vitamins and minerals, consume less fat and refined carbohydrates, gain more energy, etc.—appear.

The client may have some very specific needs and desires or he may shift the responsibility to the nurse. The client may wish a review of the current medical position on certain topics before continuing the plan. A summary of some of the major issues in nutrition follows. It is not meant to be exhaustive or as a substitute for requisite nutrition courses.

Community Nutrition: U.S. Dietary Goals

Despite the protests of conservative nutritionists who felt few changes were necessary in dietary goals for the United States, the Senate Select Committee on Nutrition and Human Needs has advocated some ambitious recommendations and its goals are tied directly to the major killers—coronary heart disease, stroke, hypertension, cancer, and diabetes. Dental caries are another major health problem cited. (Figure 6-6 illustrates these goals, as published in 1977.) The Committee has a history of progressive stances in the face of enormous pressure from the Food and Drug Administration, special interest groups, and the medical establishment.

Orthomolecular Chemistry

Orthomolecular medicine is one of the more controversial issues debated among nutritionists, chemists, and medical professionals. It has been defined by Linus Pauling as the system for the preservation of good health and the treatment of

SEVEN DAY DIET, EXERCISE, RELAXATION AND FEELING DIARY

All foods, drinks, sauces, sweeteners, kinds of bread, and times are recorded. The time, kind, and amount of exercise is recorded, as is the type and amount of exercise. Any feeling experienced before, during, or after any of the above are recorded. Observations can include physical signs, experiences, or conclusions.

Day	Breakfast	Lunch	Dinner	Snacks	Exercise	Relaxation	Feelings	Observations
1								
2								
3								
4								
5								
6								
7								

FIGURE 6-5 Seven day diet, exercise, relaxation, and feeling diary

Dietary Goals for the United States*

1. To avoid overweight, consume only as much energy (calories) as is expended; if overweight, decrease energy intake and increase energy expenditure.
2. Increase the consumption of complex carbohydrate and "naturally occurring" sugars from about 28 per cent of energy intake to about 48 per cent of energy intake.
3. Reduce the consumption of refined and processed sugars by about 45 per cent so that it accounts for about 10 per cent of total energy intake.
4. Reduce overall fat consumption from approximately 40 per cent to about 30 per cent of energy intake.
5. Reduce saturated fat consumption to about 10 per cent of total energy intake: balance that with polyunsaturated and monounsaturated fats, which should account for about 10 per cent of energy intake each.
6. Reduce cholesterol consumption to about 300 mg. a day.
7. Limit the intake of sodium by reducing the intake of salt to about 5 Gm. a day.

    * Goals recommend that current protein intake (12 per cent of calories) should be continued.

Changes in Food Selection and Preparation Suggested by U.S. Dietary Goals

1. Increase consumption of fruits and vegetables and whole grains.
2. Decrease consumption of refined and other processed sugars and foods high in such sugars.
3. Decrease consumption of foods high in total fat, and partially replace saturated fats, whether obtained from animal or vegetable sources, with polyunsaturated fats.
4. Decrease consumption of animal fat, and choose meats, poultry, and fish, which will reduce saturated fat intake.
5. Except for young children, substitute low-fat and nonfat milk for whole milk, and low-fat dairy products for high-fat dairy products.
6. Decrease consumption of butterfat, eggs, and other high-cholesterol sources. Some consideration should be given to easing the cholesterol goal for premenopausal women, young children, and the elderly in order to obtain the nutritional benefits of eggs in the diet.
7. Decrease consumption of salt and foods high in salt content.

FIGURE 6-6 U.S. dietary goals, and changes in food selection and preparation suggested by U.S. dietary goals

From the Select Committee on Nutrition and Human Needs, United States Senate: Dietary Goals for the United States, second ed. (Washington, D.C.: United States Government Printing Office, December, 1977).

disease by varying the concentrations in the human body of substances that are normally present there and that are required for health. [68, p. 208]

Orthomolecular medicine uses nutrition and nutrients as they have rarely been used before in the belief that vitamins, essential amino acids, minerals, proteins, and carbohydrates are native to the body and can possibly do a great deal of good when administered properly. It is also felt by advocates of this "new medicine" that the powerful plant and chemical substances now used to heal are alien to the human organism and have only been used and evaluated for a relatively short period of time, whereas the basic nutrients are as old as life itself.

A position traditionally held by the medical establishment is that deficiency and starvation states, such as scurvy, beriberi, or marasmus, can be averted and treated by providing adequate or supplemental amounts of appropriate body nutrients. When deficiency states are not evident, however, no supplementation is considered necessary. This position is opposed by proponents of orthomolecular medicine.

Vitamins

A *vitamin* is defined as an organic chemical present in food in extremely small amounts. It is essential for normal health, and a deficiency disease will result without it. A vitamin cannot be made by the body. [61] The most publicized of nutrients is ascorbic acid or Vitamin C.

Vitamin C

This vitamin was discovered fifty years ago by Albert Szent-Gyorgyi, and has been popularized as a cure for the common cold and the flu by Linus Pauling, the Nobel-prize-winning biochemist. Dr. Pauling's research has led him to the conclusion that this water-soluble antioxidant is indispensable for the formation of collagen tissue and serves as the "intracellular cement" in tissues. It is essential for cell metabolism, wound healing, any bodily stress response (L.A.S. or G.A.S.), and growth.

Every cigarette smoked expends ten milligrams of the body's Vitamin C. This requires replacement, if not increased intake, of Vitamin C. Vitamin C's antioxidative properties block the oxidative transformation of nitrate additives into carcinogenic nitrosamines. [2] In combination with another potent antioxidant, Vitamin E, it can be added to nitrate-preserved meats to prevent some of the harmful oxidative effects.

The polarization of the scientific community regarding Vitamin C centers around Linus Pauling's claim that 1,000 mgm. of Vitamin C per day will cause 45 percent fewer colds and 60 percent fewer days of sickness in normal populations. [2]

Pauling's background, grounded in theoretical biochemistry, not in practice-based medicine, was one reason for the large number of clinical trials organized to test and refute his theory.

It was already well-known that large doses of Vitamin C are less completely absorbed with greater amounts excreted. A brief increase in blood levels does occur for from 1 to 2 hours, but then the background body store levels of Vitamin C adjust back to their previous levels. In a few cases, it has been noted that tissue Vitamin C levels may also reach a similar plateau. This state is termed "saturation," which appears to occur at approximately 4 grams in most adults (see Figure 6–7). It would take approximately 120 mgm. of Vitamin C per day to maintain this level. In 1976 the recommended daily requirement was reduced from 60 to 45 mgm. per day of Vitamin C. Despite this information, other theorists have supported Pauling's claims, for example, Irwin Stone in his findings published in 1972 in the popular book, *The Healing Factor: Vitamin C Against Disease.* [92] Some factors that have been found to contribute to an additional need for Vitamin C are exposure to the acute stresses of illness, accident, surgery, or the chronic stress of smoking and pollution. There is a desperate need, however, for clinically controlled studies on humans. Many are in progress, but their results will not be published for several years.

Vitamin C appears to be important in collagen formation and is in some way involved in the growth of fibroblasts, osteoblasts, and rodontoblasts, as well as in the hydroxylation of proline and lysine. It contributes to wound healing and to the formation of some neurotransmitters. It enhances iron absorption and inhibits copper absorption.

A few studies have documented the antioxidative properties of Vitamin C in the prevention of nitrosamine formation from the nitrates used to cure bacon.

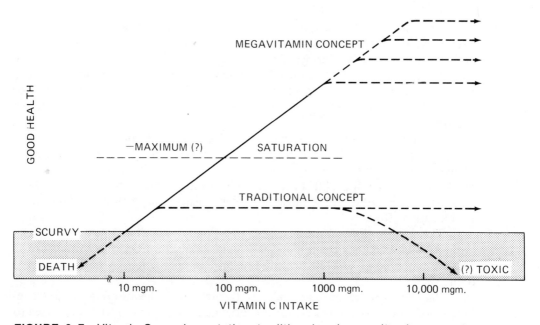

FIGURE 6-7 Vitamin C supplementation: traditional and megavitamin concepts

Serum cholesterol levels have been shown to decrease, which helps retard the development of arteriosclerotic heart disease.

Ewan Cameron, a Scottish surgeon, startled the scientific community with his hypothesis and limited clinical studies using Vitamin C in massive doses (10, 20, and 30 thousand mg. per day) as an anticancer drug. In Cameron's studies, terminal cancer patients have claimed pain relief and extended survival rates. In cases such as these, the risks of massive vitamin C intake are outweighed by the possibility of health for the individual.

In response to Pauling's and others' demands for a governmentally sponsored study replicating Cameron's work, the National Institute of Health partially supported Dr. Edward Creagen and his colleagues at the Mayo Clinic. Dr. Creagan's study was composed of 123 terminal cancer patients, evenly matched for all variables except the megadoses of Vitamin C given to the experimental group. The conclusion of the study was that no therapeutic benefit was demonstrated from high dose Vitamin C treatment. [18]

Linus Pauling countered these results with one important variable that was entirely different from the Scottish study—previous experiences with chemotherapy and/or radiation. Only 4 percent of Cameron's study had received such therapy, whereas all but eight in the Mayo Clinic study had such prior treatment. Since Pauling's theory is based on the idea that Vitamin C potentiates the body's protective mechanisms and cytotoxic drugs damage the immune system, the clients in Creagan's study should not have been eligible. In summary, the replicative Mayo Clinic study was not replicative. The trial did show a 33 percent increase in median survival time for Vitamin C-treated clients as well as significant pain controlling effects, improved appetite, and increased strength.

Two potential problems have been uncovered in the studies on Vitamin C. One problem surfaced in an Australian experiment, in which one of the participants experienced an increase in urinary oxalic acid, which, in prone individuals, could lead to oxalic acid kidney stones. Another problem arises when, after having been on high doses of the vitamin for one or two weeks, the body adapts to it, and, should a person wish to discontinue its use, must then be slowly "weaned" off in order to prevent a rebound fall in blood level and the onset of scurvy-like symptoms.

Vitamin B Complex

Vitamin B was discovered in 1886 by the Dutch physician, Eijkman, who went to Java to study beriberi, a peripheral nerve disease. His discovery was not recognized by the scientific community until thirty years later. This water-soluble vitamin was thought to be a single vitamin, but it is now known that the B-complex contains almost a dozen vitamins or vitamin-related factors. [106, p. 68] The B-complex should be treated as a whole rather than as supplementing certain vitamins within the complex for maximum benefit to occur. Its functions include coenzyme in carbohydrate, protein, and energy production. It is essential in red blood cell formation, nerve function, and growth.

Numerous studies have linked pyridoxime (B_6) deficiency with atherosclerosis.

High intakes of saturated fat and animal protein make demands for B_6; therefore, many American diets are deficient in this nutrient. [105, p. 282]

It has been hypothesized that nicotinic acid (niacin) inhibits the mobilization of FFA's (free fatty acids—recall stress response in Chapter 5) from the fat tissue which reduce the production of very low density lipoproteins (VLDL) in the blood which lower the plasma cholesterol. [105, p. 287]

Oral contraceptives have been shown to cause pyridoxine (B_6) deficiency in some women. The major symptom—depression—may be dispelled with 20 mg. of pyridoxine daily.

Vitamin A

Vitamin A has long been associated with vision and skin. The recommended daily requirements are: men—5,000 IU daily; women—4,000 IU; pregnant women—5,000 IU; and lactating women—6,000 IU. A recent study at Penn State University found that 99 percent of those eating fast foods at the cafeteria services were receiving less than 1/4 of their recommended daily allowance of Vitamin A. [34] Such deficiencies were formerly thought to occur primarily in underdeveloped nations, where Vitamin A deficiencies rank as the leading cause of childhood blindness. But such studies as the one conducted at Penn State are proving that assumption false.

Xerophthalmia (dry eye) is the general term for ocular disorders that range from an ability to see in dim light to total blindness. One-tenth of India's children are said to suffer "night-blindness" from lack of Vitamin A. [27, p. 43]

Animal studies indicate that Vitamin A-supplemented animals were protected from chemically-induced bladder cancer. Over the counter ointments containing Vitamins A and D have long been used by informed consumers for their wound-healing properties. Other claims of Vitamin A include control of menorrhagia [55] and its essential role in the development of mature sperm. [97]

From such well-substantiated initial findings stem some sensationalized unproven exaggerations of the mythical powers of Vitamin A. Well-founded theories and facts thus become transformed by the food faddist media into incredible allegations, and because of such reporting that the credibility of the entire nutrition field comes into question.

Vitamin E D-alpha Tocopherol

Vitamin E was discovered at the University of California at Berkeley in 1923 and was immediately promoted by faddists as the youthful elixir. In 1968 the Food and Nutrition Board included it in the RDAs, setting the amount at 20 to 30 units for adults. It is believed that very few, if any, Vitamin E deficiencies exist, since it is found in nearly every food.

Vitamin E is completely fat soluble, occurs in the fatty portions of our food, and is stored in the adipose tissues. It stabilizes the lipid portions of the cell's membranous parts. Vitamin E is stored for long periods of time in the body. Approximately 10 times the Recommended Daily Allowance is required to double the tissue concentrations of Vitamin E.

One of the most noted of Vitamin E's reactions is with the notorious, destructive "free radicals," which are suspected by some theorists to be the perpetrators of old age. A major source of these substances is the polyunsaturated fats the public has converted to in its fight against high cholesterol. Vitamin E not only converts the free radicals into nonreactive, nonharmful forms, but it also frees the fats from further oxidative deterioration.

Another interesting property of Vitamin E is its ability to inhibit the oxidative production of prostoglandins which control many cellular and physiologic processes, including inflammation. The antiinflammatory effects of Vitamin E are yet to be reported in controlled studies.

Vitamin E has been shown to provide protection against lung damage by the oxidant photochemicals of smog and air pollution, ionizing radiation (sun or x-rays), and smoking.

Another interesting observation reported in the *American Journal of Clinical Nutrition* in March 1978, is the low levels of Vitamin E and selenium (another antioxidant mineral) found in tumor clients. [4] Vitamin E has already been theoretically linked with bolstering the immune system.

Vitamin K

Vitamin K is a fat-soluble vitamin stored in small amounts in the liver. Vitamin K controls the synthesis of prothrombin needed to initiate the blood-clotting mechanism. There is no requirement stated for it since clinical disease or treatment states would be the only cases for replacement therapy.

Vitamin D

Vitamin D is a fat-soluble vitamin which acts almost in a hormone-like fashion. It regulates and controls calcium and phosphorous absorption from the small intestine and their deposition in the bones. Although the RDA is 400 IU, it is believed that most of this requirement is received from sunlight. Toxicity can occur and presents itself in the form of calcification in the kidneys (stones), lungs, and bones.

Minerals

A *mineral* is defined as any naturally occurring nonorganic homogeneous solid substance. There are nineteen or more minerals that form the mineral composition of the body. These minerals must be supplied in the diet; a varied diet of vegetable and animal products will accomplish this. [61, p. 632]

Calcium

Calcium is essential to bone and teeth development and muscle contractibility. The average American diet contains 700 to 1,200 mg. of calcium. The RDA is 1,000 mg. in modest servings. [105, p. 24] Milk products and most dark green vegetables provide 300 mgs. Certain groups of people are at risk of calcium deficiency. They include people with milk allergies, pregnant clients, clients who are immobile, people under stress, postmenopausal clients, those on cortisone therapy, and clients who suffer from malabsorption.

For these clients bone meal seems to be a good supplement because it contains phosphorous as well as calcium, which must be balanced in what is termed the Ca-PO_4 ratio. Severe calcium deficiency symptoms are dramatic—muscle spasms, tetany, and eventually, cardiac arrest.

Iron

The most widespread deficiency disease of vitamin or mineral is anemia, resulting from inadequate intake of iron or other vitamins or from iron losses to blood parasites (for example, hookworm) in underdeveloped countries and in certain risk populations in developed nations.

Iron is a key component of hemoglobin as well as a constituent of muscle protein and of several enzymes that allow cells to convert nutrients into energy. The RDA is 10 milligrams per day; the average American diet supplies 10 to 20 mgms.

Certain groups fall into high risk categories. They are: children from six months to five years old, a period of rapid growth and expanding blood volumes; pregnant women; those adolescent girls who indulge primarily in junk foods and/or crash diets; and those infected with blood parasites.

Foods rich in iron include meats, fish, green leafy vegetables, beans, dried fruits, and whole grain wheat. The body absorbs heme iron (contained in meat, fish) more readily than nonheme foods (contained in whole wheat, nuts, dried fruit, legumes).

Iron overdosage can be signaled by constipation, diarrhea, upset stomach, or dizziness. In 1976, the accidental iron poisoning of children requiring hospitalization was reported 82 times. [23]

Zinc

The mineral zinc was discovered a few decades ago and it is fast becoming a widely acclaimed substance in the treatment of everything from taste deficiencies to Crohn's disease (a chronic intestinal inflammatory condition). The RDA established in 1974 is 15 mgms., and it is thought that the American diet provides 10 to 15 mgms.

Certain groups of people do not get enough zinc, however; for example, clients who drink alcohol or consume significant amounts of sugar; those with a wound; those suffering from anemia; and severely burned clients. The aging appear to be particularly susceptible to decreases in taste sensations and to corresponding low zinc levels. More research is needed to confirm their need for zinc supplements.

Nausea, vomiting, and loss of appetite can indicate zinc overdosage symptoms. Supplementing normally occurring zinc in meat, liver, seafood, milk, and whole grain products is a hotly debated issue.

Selenium

Selenium is one mineral whose function is unknown, and it is thought that too much could be harmful. However, it is known as a major antioxidant, and one study observes significantly lower cancer death rates in areas with naturally high soil levels of selenium. Other studies indicate correspondingly similar inverse relationships in which low levels of soil selenium occur in areas with higher levels of fatal breast cancer. [30, p. 65]

Selenium-rich food sources include seafood, whole grain cereal, bread products, and organ meats. In light of what promising information is known thus far, more extensive research on this mineral is indeed warranted.

Sodium and Potassium

Both sodium and potassium are electrolytes essential to the maintenance of body fluid balance and life. They play a large part in illness-oriented replacement therapy, especially intravenous therapy in acute-care situations.

The wellness aspects of sodium center around the recommendation that all Americans should restrict their sodium intake whether their cardiovascular status is compromised or not. The average person in an industrial country consumes at least ten times more salt than is needed for efficient cardiovascular functioning. The sodium, in turn, causes more fluid to be retained than the body actually requires. Many feel that stress and high salt intake work together insidiously to promote hypertension.

Special problems arise for those who self-medicate with substances which stimulate urination and excretion, diuretic-like medications for "premenstrual stress" or excess fluid retention. Potassium replacement, in a natural food form such as bananas, must be taken concurrently in order to maintain body fluid electrolyte balance. Tea, especially certain herbal teas, performs similar diuretic functions without the potentially harmful side effects of diuretics.

Overnutrition and Obesity

The American diet is not one of "overnutrition" so much as it is one of imbalanced nutrients. It is usually excessive in lipids, calories, cholesterol, salt, and "empty calories."

The term "empty calories" was coined in 1955 to describe foods essentially devoid of "protein, essential minerals, and vitamins." [105, p. 282] A high consumption of empty calories—carbohydrate foods heavily sweetened with white sugar—is, no doubt, a major causative factor in the disease cluster of obesity, diabetes, and atherosclerosis. [105, p. 320]

In the United States, 10 to 20 percent of all children and 35 to 50 percent of the middle-aged are overweight. Obesity is often defined as the condition of being 20 percent or more over a desirable weight determined mainly on the basis of morbidity and mortality statistics. Obesity interests the medical profession because obese people run a higher risk of premature death than other people do. Men who are 10 percent overweight have a one-third higher mortality rate in any given year than those of average weight, primarily because of their exceptional susceptibility to high blood pressure, diabetes, and coronary artery disease. Death rates for men who are more than 20 percent overweight are even higher. A person who is 20 percent overweight is at least twice as likely to develop diabetes than a person of normal weight. [27, p. 68]

Sugar

Excess sugar is statistically associated with atherosclerosis and heart attacks. [110] Yudkin stated that a person assessed by their study as taking more than 110 grams (4 ounces) of sugar a day was perhaps five or more times as likely to develop myocardial infarction as one taking less than 60 grams a day. [110]

Americans consume about 140 grams of sugar a day. Per capita sugar consumption globally has doubled since 1950. The average person in the world now eats forty-four pounds of sugar a year. [27] In addition to all the aforementioned dangers sugar presents, in solid form it is particularly conducive to tooth decay and plaque formation.

Simple and Complex Carbohydrates

It is important to distinguish simple from complex carbohydrates because so many fad diets condemn all forms of this valuable energy source. In fact, carbohydrates spare protein so that it can continue to build tissue. Carbohydrates also prevent essential reserve fatty stores from being broken down as they are in the ketosis which occurs with starvation, the acidosis of diabetes, and in a few popular "fad" diets.

The simple carbohydrates are monosaccharides (glucose, fructose, and galactose) and disaccharides (sucrose, lactose, and maltose). These sugars are highly refined, contain few vitamins, and require very little mastication or digestion before being absorbed and carried into the circulation via the intestinal villi. Carbohydrate metabolism requires cofactors, such as the B vitamins and magnesium, in order to convert glucose into energy. If these cofactors are not supplied, as they are in the complex carbohydrates, the body stores must supply them.

The complex carbohydrates include starch (grain, potatoes, beans, roots), dextrins, cellulose (fiber), stems, leaves, seeds and grain hulls, pectins, and glycogen. The starches are the most important carbohydrate sources.

Hyperglycemia and Hypoglycemia

It is hypothesized that an overuse of refined carbohydrates contributes to the high incidence of hyperglycemia (high blood sugar) and hypoglycemia (low blood sugar) in the United States. The basis for this stems from a common effect observed in glucose tolerance tests in which the fasting subject is loaded with a glucose preparation and then proceeds to secrete insulin to lower the blood sugar level. In a significant number of people, oversecretion of insulin occurs causing the sweating, headache, tremors, flushing, increased heart rate, thready pulse, and sometimes, fainting, characteristic of low blood sugar. This condition can frequently be induced in a normal hungry nonhypoglycemic person by performing a coffee and refined carbohydrate (for example, a sweet doughnut) load, and then waiting ninety minutes to two hours for the same results mentioned above to occur.

The crux of the nutritional lifestyle change advocated in this text is to move toward the complex carbohydrates—whole grains, vegetables, natural fruits—and away from the refined sugars. This, coupled with the other changes touched upon in this book, will open the door to a complete and balanced healthful nutritional lifestyle.

Food Additives

Other nonnutritional food substances to be considered are additives. Intestinal additives are antioxidants, stabilizers, emulsifiers, flavors, and colors. Our complex food distribution system necessitates their use to replace lost nutrients and to prevent spoilage.

In the 1950s, Dr. Benjamin Feingold, an allergist, discovered a connection between certain low molecular compound food substances and allergy, as well as with behavioral and psychological problems. He has spent the last twenty years observing, researching, and developing what has been popularly termed the Feingold Diet. From his studies, it appears that many minimal brain dysfunctional (MBD) and hyperkinetic children are highly sensitive to certain food additives, colorings, and flavorings. Rigid adherence to the Feingold Diet, which eliminates all artificially dyed and flavored foods and drugs and/or those foods containing salicylates (for example, aspirin), seems to alleviate symptoms. [32]

Dr. Feingold's work has been disputed, but it has given thousands of parents and children hope for normal lives without a reliance upon central nervous system stimulant, antianxiety, antipsychotic, antidepressant, and anticonvulsant medications.

Since the time of Dr. Feingold's studies, certain colorings have been taken off the market and the entire procedure for responsible labeling of food products has come into question. The federal agency responsible for insuring the safety of such substances is the Food and Drug Administration, an agency in the Department of Health and Human Services.

In 1960, the Food Additive Amendment to the Food, Drug and Cosmetic Act of 1938 was enacted. Any additive was to have substantial test data to prove its safety in order first to be used in food. Since the research time and costs involved would have been staggering, the GRAS (Generally Regarded as Safe) list was established. Additives could be used if no ill effects had been observed in humans to date; however, any new additives would have to go through a rigorous testing and evaluation process. There is no clear estimate on exactly how many additives exist, but figures range upwards of several thousand.

That many clients with dismal-sounding medical and psychiatric diagnoses could be cases of additive sensitivity does not require a far stretch of the imagination. Merely as a preventive measure, then, many parents have begun limiting preprocessed, prepackaged, additive-laden "junk foods."

Herbs

Although herbs are not commonly acknowledged as nutrients, some of them not only contain valuable vitamins and minerals, in addition to serving as roughage, but they have also been used for centuries for their preventive and curative properties.

The responsible practice of herbology, herbalism, and herbal medicine requires knowledge of normal and pathologic states, of botany, and of pharmacology. Health is seen holistically as a positive homeostatic state, and disease as a disturbance of that balance by an external or internal cause. Treatment is a highly individual matter and is assessed, monitored, and tailored to fit the person. Herbs are not always harmless, but they appear to have fewer side and cumulative effects than do drugs.

Recently, Gupta and colleagues studied the effect of onion on fibrinolytic activity. They reported that it prevented the rise in serum cholesterol known to be brought about by high fat diets. [36]

Another common member of the allium family, garlic, was studied for its hypocholesteremic and fibrinolytic effects on a very small sample. The fibrinolytic properties were commensurate with those in the Gupta study, but the hypocholesteremic effects were not as striking. [36]

Cooking with natural herbs and spices is a practice that is reviving in this country, and clinical investigation on the healing properties of herbs is on the increase. Traditional "wives' tales" regarding certain herbs and teas may prove to be more fact than fiction.

Controversial Topics

Fasting

Fasting is an old practice that is also enjoying a renaissance. Some groups advocate purifying the system before entering into a new, healing lifestyle or culture. Recall the fluid and electrolyte needs of the body. If these are satisfied along with vitamin and mineral supplementation, limited fasting, *with qualified supervision,* can be accomplished.

Acute-care, institutionalized clients frequently find themselves in fasting situations. The major difference is that in the hospital the clients' basic fluid, electrolyte, vitamin, and mineral needs are artificially (intravenously) compensated for because other more pressing needs supersede those for oral intake of food. Medical nursing supervision is continuous in an in-patient setting.

Vegetarianism and Protein

Another popular dietary practice is varying degrees of vegetarianism. Lactovegans (consumers of milk products, vegetables, and fruits), ovovegans (consumers of eggs, vegetables, and fruits), and vegovegans are the three types of vegetarianism in practice. The major critique of vegetarianism in this country has always been, "But how do they get their protein?"

A simple, clear explanation has been offered by Frances Moore Lappé in *Diet for a Small Planet.* [28] In the book she explains the necessity of completely filling out the Essential Amino Acid Pattern in order for the body to make protein. If even one amino acid (the limiting amino acid) is partially missing, the use of the others in protein synthesis is proportionately reduced.

Ewald describes the NPU (Net Protein Utilization) for every food and recipe that Lappé has mentioned in order that combinations of foods will maximize NPUs. Recipes encourage eating beans and wheat together to more than double the NPUs, for example. [28]

Several years ago the macrobiotic diet was severely criticized for this type of protein deficiency. The original diet called for certain amounts of soy and sesame seeds, along with brown rice. This, in fact, was a high protein combination, but it lacked other essential vitamins and minerals.

The macrobiotic diet attempts to balance the yin and yang—initially through the use of whole grains, fish, carrots, corn, and tea. According to proponents of the macrobiotic diet, a person can eventually subsist on the rice, soy, and sesame combination.

Fiber

Over the past sixty-five years, the ratio of animal to vegetable protein in our diets has doubled, the amount of sugar has increased 66 percent, while at the same time starch consumption has decreased 22 percent. With the adoption of processed foods in the American diet, therefore, the intake of fiber and trace minerals has decreased.

Fiber is divided into two types—*crude* and *dietary*. Crude fiber is the material remaining after food has been digested with dilute acid and alkali. Dietary fiber is any material remaining undigested after food's passage through the small intestine. It is composed of cellulose, hemicellulose, liguan, pectin, vegetable gums, and other indigestible substances. Its function is to take up water, increase stool bulk, absorb organic materials, and carry them out of the intestinal tract. Crude fiber is only one-fifth to one-half of dietary fiber.

Fiber or roughage is usually thought of as the indigestible part of plant cell-walls. Dietary fiber exists mainly in the outer layers of grain kernels and in raw or lightly cooked fruits and vegetables. It adds bulk to the diet and it also absorbs water and swells in the stomach and intestines. The stools of those with high-fiber diets are softer and larger than the stools often associated with those whose diets are low fiber, and, as such, they tend to pass through the body more quickly. The consumption to elimination process often lasts three or more days for Westerners, whose diet contains less fiber than it once did, whereas it averages only a day or two for traditional African villagers, whose diet is high in fiber and among whom bowel cancer is rare. The relatively dense low-fiber stool may expose the colon wall to higher concentrations of certain carcinogens.

Fats

Fats are divided into three groups—simple, compound, and derived. Of the compound lipids, the lipoproteins are most important because they contain cholesterol, triglycerides, and fatty acids.

Almost all tissues in the human body synthesize cholesterol. The newly synthesized cholesterol appears immediately in the plasma. The amount of cholesterol synthesized by the liver far exceeds that of any other contributor and is known as endogenous cholesterol. The liver also synthesizes phospholipids and maintains them in a balanced ratio. If this balance is maintained, the feared arterial fatty deposits or plaques are presumably prevented from forming. It is still not clear to what extent dietary restriction of cholesterol affects the most common types of lipid disorders associated with atherosclerosis.

Studies indicate a correlation between a high-fat diet and cancer. Clients with cancer of the colon have an above normal output of bile acids. The combination of high-bile acids and a high-fat diet has produced colon cancer in animals. Increased fat diets influence hormone production and alter the prolactin/estrogen ratio toward levels that increase the risk of breast cancer.

Lecithin

Lecithin is a phospholipid found in the membrane lining of all cells. It is another supplement that has been gaining popularity since the publishing of a limited, but positive, report in the *Australian and New Zealand Journal of Medicine* in June 1977. [87] In a very small sample of patients with high cholesterol levels, three out of seven clients experienced up to an 18 percent drop in cholesterol, particularly the LDL (low-density lipoprotein). Some replicative studies are being conducted to confirm this study and the initially positive reports of selected physicians regarding lecithin.

Twenty-one hypercholesterolemic patients were treated with two tablespoons of soybean lecithin three times daily for three months. Six clients discontinued the large dosage due to intolerance. Of the fifteen remaining clients, twelve showed a reduction of 41 percent in serum cholesterol levels. This had not occurred following regimens of low-fat diets lasting from one month to ten years. The clients were placed on a maintenance dose of one to two tablespoons of lecithin daily, which had been shown to be as effective in maintaining normal cholesterol levels once they were attained. [63]

Lecithin assists in the absorption of fat from the food we consume and aids in transporting it through the bloodstream. It has been compared to the "unsticking" commercial products—for example, "Pam"—containing lecithin.

Smoking

It is redundant to quote the familiar statistics from the original Surgeon General's report on the risk of smoking and its effect on lung cancer and cardiovascular disease, morbidity, and mortality.

The updated 1980 Surgeon General's Report on smoking reemphasizes the original risks, and in addition, stresses the negative effects on:

1. women, particularly those on birth-control pills;
2. infants, who can suffer low birth weights if their mothers smoke;
3. teenagers, particularly young women; and
4. workers in industrially risky areas who face increased risk of cancer of the lung, mesothelioma, and other occupation-specific cancers.

Some more recent data add to the overwhelming proof against smoking. Seventy-five percent of the cancers of the oral cavity and pharynx can be attributed to the association of alcohol and tobacco. One study indicated that 39 percent of the urinary bladder cancer in males may be due to tobacco. And 85 percent of cases of lung cancer in the United States, and 95 percent of those in the United Kingdom, are due to tobacco. [86]

Health Foods, Natural Foods, and Organic Foods

The President's Office of Consumer Affairs makes the following distinction in an attempt to protect the public from the fallacy, fraud, and misrepresentation often associated with the following terms:

Organic Foods are foods that have been produced without the use of pesticides and/or fertilizers.

Natural Foods are those foods that have no added preservatives, emulsifiers, or artificial ingredients.

Health Foods is a misnomer, unless taken to include all foods containing nutrients essential for growth, development, and body maintenance.

Estrogens

Estrogens play a role in keeping the phospholipids (lecithin) high, as well as having a protective value in atherosclerosis and heart disease, which helps prove that the *ratio* of circulating phospholipids to cholesterol in the blood is most important—*not the amount* of circulating cholesterol per se. [106, p. 26]

In summary, we do not know what an optimum diet is. The dietary goals presented by the Senate Select Committee on Nutrition and Human Needs say specifically that we eat too much, too much fat, too much cholesterol, too much sugar, and too much salt. We should eat more raw fruits and vegetables and use more unsaturated oils.

As nurses evaluate their own and clients' nutritional lifestyles, it is important to assess the rationale behind the dietary practice. What needs does the diet fulfill? (Possible answers are: discipline, cultural demands, religious devotion, punishment, reward, purification, self-esteem, etc.)

Personal lifestyles constitute one of the strategic frontiers of preventive medicine in developed countries today. Three prominent U.S. medical researchers recently wrote: "It can be said unequivocally that a significant reduction in sedentary living and overnutrition, alcoholism, hypertension, and excessive cigarette smoking would save more lives in the age range forty to sixty-four than the best current medical practice." [44]

By studying the lives of 7,000 men and women in California, Dr. Nedra B. Belloc and Dr. Lester Breslow have assembled eye-opening evidence of the health importance of personal habits. They correlated both physical well-being and lifespans to adherence to seven basic practices:

1. sleeping seven to eight hours each night
2. eating three meals a day at regular times with little snacking

3. eating breakfast every day
4. maintaining desirable body weight
5. avoiding excessive alcohol consumption
6. getting regular exercise
7. not smoking

They wrote that "the physical health status of those reported following all seven good health practices as consistently about the same as those thirty years younger who followed few or none of these practices." Men at age forty-five who follow three or fewer of these practices can expect to live to sixty-seven, while those following six or seven of the practices can expect to live to seventy-eight. Similarly, they found that forty-five-year-old women who follow six or seven of the health practices push their average age of death to eighty-one, while women who abide by three or fewer of the practices can expect to die at seventy-four. [5, 27]

FITNESS AND CONDITIONING

Fitness has been categorized as *organic,* that is, a state in which the body is free of disease or infirmity and is well-nourished. The type of fitness described in this section is referred to as *dynamic fitness,* which involves the resources to move vigorously, to do, to live energetically. Dynamic fitness can be divided into four major aspects—strength, endurance, flexibility, and cardiovascular conditioning. All the aspects of fitness are subject to the "overload principle" in order to be truly effective.

It is the overload principle which ties dynamic fitness to the theory of stress described in Chapter 4. *Overload* is a physical demand or physiologic stress imposed upon the body which exceeds that normally endured. Physical capacity is developed by the expenditure of varying amounts of energy that impose such extra stresses on the body. This causes the body to make more specific adaptations to these stresses, thereby allowing more effective performance of future tasks. Slowly but progressively, imposition of more work on the body *after* it adjusts to current workloads causes greater adaptation and increased fitness.

Another principle—the Specific Adaptation to Imposed Demands, or SAID— as coined by Wallis and Logan in 1964 explains how individuals could improve physical fitness with the least effort and in the shortest amount of time. [35] This could be done for each of the aspects of fitness by imposing a specific set of demands for that area. The area of cardiovascular conditioning could be improved by an increasing program of aerobic exercise, for example. Since no one exercise can satisfy the requirements of all four areas, a total fitness program needs to be designed for each person. Thus, although a yoga program might satisfy flexibility requirements, strength, endurance, and conditioning would require another form of exercise.

Strength is defined as the amount of force or power a muscle or group of muscles can exert and use to overcome resistance. Weight lifting and some forms of calisthenics, such as push-ups, can develop this aspect of fitness. *Endurance* is the ability to persevere and to continue with a workload. This quality allows a person to withstand a certain amount of fatigue, distress, or pain and can be achieved by an activity such as jogging. *Flexibility* describes the elasticity of the muscles and the ability to put each muscle group through its maximum range of motion. Flexibility can be accomplished through any stretching or warm-up series of exercises.

Fitness and conditioning are lifestyle modification factors that are no strangers to clinical research investigations and epidemiological studies. Fitness has been correlated with prevention of coronary heart disease since 1953 when a sample of sedentary London bus drivers were compared to their more active conductor counterparts. The bus drivers were found to have a higher evidence of coronary heart disease and myocardial infarctions (heart attacks). [98, Morris as quoted therein, p. 90] Later studies conducted in the United States, such as the Framingham Study, substantiated the idea that exercise provided some type of protection from cardiovascular diseases. [98] The exact mechanism by which physical activity provides its preservative effects is still in question, and this is partially the reason for the nonadmissibility of lack of exercise as a direct causative factor in heart disease. (Some research strengthening the case for fitness is presented later in this section.) Desire for health and fear of death are only two of many reasons people choose to exercise. The health professional is left having to make a decision whether to recommend it as a valid health intervention or not. In the face of highly suggestive evidence supporting exercise not only as a legitimate health risk reducer but as an enhancer of self-esteem, decreaser of anxiety, and contributor to the overall quality of life, it will be encouraged and promoted here.

In the late fifties, Dr. Hans Kraus coined the term "hypokinetic disease" to mean the product of overstress and underexercise. [35] The otherwise healthy forty- or fifty-year-old who was physically inactive was observed to show signs of aging earlier in life, functioned at an overall lower level, and was less able to maintain homeostasis when faced with the daily stresses of life. This low level of function combined with forced suppression of the "fight or flight response" was shown by Kraus to enhance the incidence of disease. [35, Kraus as quoted therein]

Other studies substantiated the idea of hypokinetic disease as any disease or symptom group produced by lack of exercise and "overstress," such as:

Myocardial infarction [Kraus, 1959; Morris and Crawford, 1959, as quoted in Kraus 1973]

Hypertension and overweight [Johnson et al., 1956]

Nervous tension [Sainsbury and Gibson, 1954]

Musculoskeletal pains and headache [Appleton, 1956; Kraus and Hirschlaid, 1953; Kraus, 1959, as quoted in Kraus, 1977]

[35, Kraus as quoted therein]

Today we describe hypokinetic disease as diseases or symptoms of lifestyle patterns. The prescriptions being offered do not include overnight panaceas such as diet pills and tranquilizers. Physicians are finding themselves issuing exercise, relaxation, and dietary "prescriptions." Clients are so accustomed to returning from health care agencies with a piece of paper that legitimizes what is often common sense, that they seek and receive such "orders."

Aerobic Conditioning

We recognize that strength, endurance, and flexibility are important and inseparable aspects of fitness, but here we will, of necessity, focus on cardiovascular conditioning. Cardiovascular conditioning is here termed *aerobic conditioning,* which is based on the principle that the body—particularly the heart and lungs—is subject to a planned series of stresses (exercise) to which the whole body naturally adapts to produce long-term beneficial body-mind changes. Although many activities classify as aerobic, the prototype of running will be investigated in depth because the bulk of the exercise physiology research available has been conducted on runners. Much of the data appear valid and applicable to certain other exercise areas.

Dr. George Sheehan, a sports physician, likes to translate training into Selyé's stress model: Applying increasing amounts of work (Stage 1) with a resultant improvement in performance (Stage 2), but stopping before exhaustion (Stage 3—"peaking too soon"). [85] Stage 3 applied to exercise or "overuse syndrome" will be examined later in this section. Its obverse effect, "disuse," will be studied in order to contrast the various aspects of the conditioning versus deconditioning adaptations the body makes when faced with planned stressors or their complete absence.

Dr. Ken Cooper was the first to gather data on a significant captive sample (the U.S. Air Force) on which he tested his aerobic conditioning program. The goal of the program was to increase the maximum amount of oxygen that the body could process at a given time. The body subjected to exercise was required to rapidly breathe large amounts of air, termed venous/oxygen consumption, or VO^2, and forcefully deliver large volumes of blood and oxygen to all parts of the body—an excellent indicator of the status of the cardiopulmonary vascular system.

Training Effect

The changes over time caused by aerobic exercise were termed the "training effect." Whether this effect had occurred or not was measured via a treadmill device attached to respiratory, electrocardiographic, blood pressure, and pulse monitoring equipment, respectively.

The training effect achieved the following in the test subjects:

1. It strengthened the muscles of respiration and tended to reduce the resistance to air flow, ultimately facilitating the rapid flow of air in and out of the lungs.
2. It improved the strength and pumping efficiency of the heart, enabling more blood to be pumped with each stroke. This improves the ability to more rapidly transport life-sustaining oxygen from the lungs to the heart and ultimately to all parts of the body.
3. It toned up muscles throughout the body, thereby improving the general circulation, at times lowering blood pressure and reducing the work on the heart.
4. It caused an increase in the total amount of blood circulating through the body and increased the number of red blood cells and the amount of hemoglobin, making the blood a more efficient oxygen carrier. [15, pp. 16–17]

Positive Effects

People who engage in aerobic exercise for 20 to 30 minutes, 3 to 4 times per week also claim that it fulfills some basic psychological needs for them:

1. The need for movement
2. The need for self-assertion
3. The need for alternation of stress and relaxation
4. The need for mastery over themselves
5. The need to indulge themselves
6. The need to play
7. The need to lose themselves in something greater than themselves ("Feeling one with the universe")
8. The need to meditate
9. The need to live their own rhythms [31]

Along with these feelings comes the revelation that self-control and self-creation are within the grasp of the ordinary person. The body responds to stimulation and calculated stress in the perfect way that it was designed to. Recognition of and participation in this growth process brings with it a true discovery experience for some.

Physiologic Effects of Running

A brief review of the physiologic effects of running illuminates the following interrelated effects:

1. Nerves become more efficient at transmitting impulses and at activating muscle fibers.
2. Muscle contractions become more efficient. The number of mitochondria (which produce an energy-producing substance, a subunit of RNA, adenosine triphosphate—ATP) increase.
3. Arteries develop collateral circulation and capillaries become more dense. It is hypothesized that this also occurs with the coronary arteries, but no studies have yet established this as a fact.
4. Fibrinolysin (a substance that breaks up small clots) appears in greater quantities.
5. Cholesterol and triglycerides become less concentrated.
6. Very high-density lipoproteins increase; very low-density lipoproteins decrease.
7. The catecholamines—epinephrine and nonepinephrine—which potentially cause pathogenic effects of chronic stress, usually released during the alarm stage of the stress response, decrease in fit clients.
8. The heart's muscle fibers lengthen and the coronary arteries enlarge. Blood flow to the heart may increase to five times resting levels. A trained heart at rest may pump twice as much as an untrained one (the stroke volume is larger). Resting heart rates can decrease 10 to 20 beats per minute in trained persons. Bradycardia is not uncommon.
9. Resting diastolic blood pressure is decreased.

10. The breathing muscles become stronger and more efficient, and the volume of oxygen inspired per minute triples.

11. The thermoregulatory mechanism becomes more efficient, that is, the body sweats and cools more quickly.

Since the manner in which cholesterol is distributed among the lipoproteins may be associated with the risk of developing coronary artery disease, the high concentration of high-density lipoproteins is important. The overall cholesterol level decreases only slightly with conditioning. This may be due to changes in the body weight and mass.

Cholesterol is a vital part of the cell wall and is the basis of bile acids and sex hormone formation. Triglycerides are an energy source stored in fat tissue. Cholesterol and triglycerides exist together with protein in the form of lipoproteins. There are three types of lipoproteins, classified according to density:

VLDL   Largest and least dense; carry most of the triglycerides (or TGLs).
    ↑TGL means   ↑   VLDL
LDL → Carry most of the body's cholesterol; a high cholesterol can mean a high LDL or HDL or both.
HDL

Total cholesterol count [108, pp. 80–81]
↑LDL is associated with atherosclerosis
↑HDL is associated with fewer heart attacks
Conclusion: Keep high-density lipoproteins high; keep low-density lipoproteins low.

	Subject A	Subject B (at greater risk for CAD)
VLDL	25 mg.	25 mg.
LDL	120 mg.	170 mg.
HDL	75 mg.	25 mg.
Total Cholesterol	220 mg.	220 mg.

Caloric Expenditure and Lean Body Mass

The percentage of fat to total weight, as shown in the following table, makes an interesting comparison in trained and untrained subjects:

	Percent of Fat in Males	Percent of Fat in Females
Athletic	5–10	15–20
Nonathletic	15	22–35

Dr. Peter Wood and his associates at Stanford University showed that sedentary men were 20 percent heavier than physically active men; and sedentary women were 30 percent heavier than physically active women. The active men ate approximately 600 calories more a day, and the active women ate about 570 calories more a day than did their sedentary counterparts. Figure 6-8 demonstrates specific blood chemistry differences between nonrunners, good runners, and elite runners.

Apparently, aerobic exercise not only burns a maximum amount of calories, but it also increases the amount of muscle per total body weight. The total body weight minus fat equals the Lean Body Mass. The Lean Body Mass (LBM), the bone and muscle, are what utilize calories. In the aging process, more of the Lean Body Mass becomes fat, even though the actual weight may not change. As the metabolizing (LBM) portion of the body becomes less, fewer calories are needed. Unfortunately, caloric intake usually does not decrease even though caloric demands are less; thus, the body gains weight on fewer calories.

If clients decide to diet without exercising, they will keep losing lean body mass even though they appear to be losing pounds. If clients exercise, even without decreasing caloric intake, the lean body mass will increase, as will caloric demand, but the percentage of fat to total weight will probably decrease.

This may not be good news to calorie and pound counters, but the resulting situation is a firm, muscular body, capable of handling even small amounts of excess poundage. The amount and tone of muscle increases, the metabolism of calories goes up, and the body becomes more efficient at utilizing food for energy.

Women, because of their lack of androgens, can gain more lean body mass and muscle without experiencing overdeveloped musculature as men do. Toning and definition of certain exercise-specific muscle groups will become apparent, however. These effects of aerobic conditioning are more subtle and longitudinal in nature than resting heart rates or venous oxygen consumption rates.

How do exercise physiologists and nutritionists arrive at a reliable lean body mass figure, short of performing an autopsy? Bone structure, height, and weight tables are relatively useless. Measuring skin folds and girth thicknesses are very indirect and nonspecific methods.

The most reliable lean body mass measurement to date is an underwater float tank scale. This method is based on the observation that fat floats. Underwater weight is very different; people with high fat percentages weigh less than well-trained clients with high lean body masses. Underwater weight is compared with conventional weight via a complex formula which derives the body density and percent of body fat which is then converted into pounds. Many more exercise laboratories are obtaining the equipment to perform such measurements. Contraindications exist for clients who fear water and those who are unable to exhale residual air from the lungs before submerging for the test.

As more scientific data is gathered on lean body weight versus total body weight, the entire concept of overweight may change. But to the present point, if weight loss is the client's goal in aerobic conditioning, the following caloric per hour expenditure table [91] may help:

Jogging	720 per hour
Bicycling	400 per hour
Swimming	500 per hour

Variable	Elite Runners (n = 20)	Good Runners (n = 8)	Non-Runners (n = 95)	Normal Range*
Total Cholesterol (ml/100ml)	175 + 26.3[+]	185 + 35.5	189 + 36.4	140 – 220
HDL Cholesterol (ml/100ml)	56 + 12.1[+]	52 + 10.9	49 + 10.5	30 – 70
LDL Cholesterol (ml/100ml)	108 + 24.5[+]	121 + 29.5	124 + 35.6	90 – 160
VLDL Cholesterol (ml/100ml)	11 + 5.2[+]	12 + 11.8	15 + 7.5	10 – 30
Total Triglycerides (ml/100ml)	74 + 25.2[+]	73 + 39.7	92 + 37.3	50 – 180
Hemoglobin (gms)	15.5 + 0.9	15.6 + 0.7	15.8 + 1.11	14 – 18
Hematocrit (%)	43.8 + 2.5[+]	43.6 + 1.7[+]	47.2 + 3.27	42 – 52
SGOT (m/ml)	35.8 + 8.2[+]	27.9 + 3.3	24.3 + 16.1	7 – 40
LDH (m/ml)	230 + 33.3[+]	204 + 19.2	169 + 29.2	100 – 225
Total Bilirubin (mg %)	1.075 + 0.43[+]	1.175 + 0.36[+]	0.744 + 0.341	0.15 – 1.00
Uric Acid (mg %)	5.80 + 0.59[+]	6.45 + 0.49[+]	6.55 + 1.14	2.5 – 8.0

* Normal ranges for young men for laboratories where analyses were performed

+ Significantly different from non-runners (p—.05)

FIGURE 6-8 Selected blood chemistries of runners and nonrunners

Reprinted with permission from Michael L. Pollock, "Cream of the Crop," *Marathoner* (Summer 1978), 32. Published by *Runner's World* Magazine Co., 1400 Stierlin Rd., Mountain View, Calif. 94043.

Ice/Roller Skating	640 per hour
Handball	1000 per hour
Squash	1000 per hour
Cross-Country Skiing	1000 per hour
Downhill Skiing	540 per hour
Basketball	1000 per hour
Tennis	500 per hour
Calisthenics	400 per hour
Walking	250 per hour
Golf	300 per hour
Softball	100 per hour
Bowling	150 per hour

In addition, the following information is required to calculate weight loss:

1 lb. body fat = 454 gm.

1 gm. body fat = 7.7 calories

454 gm. x 7.7 cal/gm. = 3,496 (or 3,500 calories per pound body fat)

Decrease in diet by 500 cal. x 7 days = 3,500 calories = 1 lb. body fat

And/or Jogging 1/2 hr. = 360 cal. x 10 days = 3,600 calories = 1 lb. body fat.

One of the most common misconceptions about exercise is the assumption that hard work is equivalent to aerobic exercise. People who report elevated pulses following heavy workouts or weight-lifting routines use the heart rate as an indicator of something it does not validly measure. The pulse records volume loads on the heart, *not* pressure (weight, resistance, intrathoracic Valsalva maneuver) loads. The more accurate measure of a training effect would be to obtain a baseline resting pulse, then proceed with 1 to 2 months of weight lifting, for example; after which time, the reduction in resting pulse if any, would be evaluated. The same procedure could then be used to evaluate an aerobic training program.

Fitness Tests

Just what does an aerobic training program consist of, how does one start and progress, and what are the contraindications?

Three tests, two of which are inexpensive in terms of both time and money, can fairly accurately determine a client's baseline level of performance, the resting heart rate, the maximum heart rate, and the comfortable training range.

The Harvard Step Test

The Harvard Step Test, routinely performed in many physiology lab classes, is described in Figure 6–9. It takes only a few minutes to perform, requires only a watch with a second hand and the ability to take a radial pulse.

The radial pulse is the one of choice, as opposed to the carotid pulse, which can actually give a falsely lower reading because of its proximity to the vagus nerve which can dampen or lower the pulse rate following exercise.

The Harvard Step Test is one of the simplest ways to evaluate cardiovascular fitness. It requires you to step up and down on a bench for a few minutes, then see how quickly your heart recovers from the effort. The version of the test described here was devised by the American Medical Association's Committee on Exercise and Physical Fitness.

1. Get a sturdy bench 12 inches high if you're under 5 feet tall, 14 inches high if you're from 5 feet to 5 feet 3 inches, 16 inches high if you're from 5 feet 3 to 5 feet 9, 18 inches high if you're from 5 feet 9 to 6 feet, and 20 inches high if you're over 6 feet tall. Step from the floor onto the bench and down again thirty times a minute for four minutes, using a metronome or having someone time you with the second hand of a watch. (If you get too tired to go on, you can stop earlier, but it will lower your score.)

2. As soon as you finish, sit quietly and take your pulse, or have someone else take it, for 30 seconds one minute after you finish, another 30 seconds two minutes after you finish, and another 30 seconds three minutes after you finish.

3. Compute your Recovery Index (RI) by using this formula:

$$RI = \frac{\text{Duration of exercise in seconds x 100}}{\text{Sum of pulse counts x 2}}$$

If your RI is 60 or less, your rating is poor; between 61 and 70, fair; between 71 and 80, good; between 81 and 90, very good; 91 or more, excellent. The test itself is quite strenuous if you're badly out of shape, so use caution and stop if you have any adverse symptoms such as chest pain or extreme difficulty in breathing.

FIGURE 6-9 The Harvard Step Test

Reprinted with permission from James F. Fixx, *The Complete Book of Running* (New York: Random House, 1977), pp. 288–89.

12–Minute or One-and-a-Half-Mile Test

The other easily self-administered fitness test is Dr. Ken Cooper's 12-minute or one-and-a-half-mile test. The original test asked the individual to run or walk for twelve minutes at a "comfortable" pace, which is taken to mean a pace at which one can comfortably carry on a conversation with a partner or with oneself. In accuracy, this test is fairly comparable to a treadmill test.

The first part of Figure 6–10 equates the test to a fitness rating scale for men and women. The second part of the figure demonstrates a way of modifying the 12-minute test by premeasuring a 1.5-mile run and then comparing the time to the age-adjusted chart. A man in the "very poor" category, for example, can increase his aerobic capacity by as much as 30 percent, following a conditioning program.

Treadmill Test

The third method of assessing venous oxygen consumption is the treadmill test. This test is expensive and time-consuming, but it is the best measure of fitness and maximum intensity. Following this test, the recommendation will usually be to exercise between 65 percent and 80 percent of maximum for sufficient conditioning. This percentage is advocated by the other two methods as well. The optimal pulse range to train at will be between 60 percent to 80 percent of maximum.

Contraindications

Contraindications to any treadmill, fitness evaluation, or training include:

Angina (uncontrolled)
Hypertension (uncontrolled)
Myocardial infarction within the last four weeks
Bradycardia
Myocarditis
Serious Arrhythmias

Once any of the tests are in progress, they should be stopped if any of the following occur:

1. Chest pain, dyspnea
2. Faintness, dizziness
3. Disorientation, ataxia
4. Patient's desire to stop
5. Decrease in systolic BP over 30 mm. of mercury
6. Negative S-T depression—2 mm.
7. PVCs: more than 2 in succession (preventricular contractions)
         more than 5 in 1 minute

It should be added that treadmill tests and aerobic conditioning programs have been developed for paraplegics confined to wheelchairs, for cardiac clients, and for the aged. Activity, fitness, and conditioning are fast becoming the right and responsibility of everyone.

Community Fitness and Conditioning Programs

Any fitness program should include the following objectives:

improvement of cardiovascular function
development of muscular strength
development of endurance
development of flexibility of joints
provision for relaxation and tension release

FIGURE 6-10 Age and sex adjusted aerobic fitness tests

From *The Aerobics Way* by Kenneth H. Cooper, M.D., M.P.H., Copyright © 1977 by Kenneth H. Cooper. Reprinted by permission of the publisher, M. Evans and Company, Inc., New York 10017.

12-Minute Walking/Running Test
Distance (Miles) Covered in 12 Minutes

Fitness Category		Age (Years)					
		13 – 19	20 – 29	30 – 39	40 – 49	50 – 59	60 +
I. Very Poor	(men)	< 1.30*	< 1.22	< 1.18	< 1.14	< 1.03	< .87
	(women)	< 1.0	< .96	< .94	< .88	< .84	< .78
II. Poor	(men)	1.30 – 1.37	1.22 – 1.31	1.18 – 1.30	1.14 – 1.24	1.03 – 1.16	.87 – 1.02
	(women)	1.00 – 1.18	.96 – 1.11	.95 – 1.05	.88 – .98	.84 – .93	.78 – .86
III. Fair	(men)	1.38 – 1.56	1.32 – 1.49	1.31 – 1.45	1.25 – 1.39	1.17 – 1.30	1.03 – 1.20
	(women)	1.19 – 1.29	1.12 – 1.22	1.06 – 1.18	.99 – 1.11	.94 – 1.05	.87 – .98
IV. Good	(men)	1.57 – 1.72	1.50 – 1.64	1.46 – 1.56	1.40 – 1.53	1.31 – 1.44	1.21 – 1.32
	(women)	1.30 – 1.43	1.23 – 1.34	1.19 – 1.29	1.12 – 1.24	1.06 – 1.18	.99 – 1.09
V. Excellent	(men)	1.73 – 1.86	1.65 – 1.76	1.57 – 1.69	1.54 – 1.65	1.45 – 1.58	1.33 – 1.55
	(women)	1.44 – 1.51	1.35 – 1.45	1.30 – 1.39	1.25 – 1.34	1.19 – 1.30	1.10 – 1.18
VI. Superior	(men)	> 1.87	> 1.77	> 1.70	> 1.66	> 1.59	> 1.56
	(women)	> 1.52	> 1.46	> 1.40	> 1.35	> 1.31	> 1.19

*< Means "less than"; > means "more than."

1.5-Mile Run Test
Time (Minutes)

Fitness Category		13 – 19	20 – 29	30 – 39	Age (Years) 40 – 49	50 – 59	60 +
I. Very Poor	(men)	> 15:31*	> 16:01	> 16:31	> 17:31	> 19:01	> 20:01
	(women)	> 18:31	> 19:01	> 19:31	> 20:01	> 20:31	> 21:01
II. Poor	(men)	12:11 – 15:30	14:01 – 16:00	14:44 – 16:30	15:36 – 17:30	17:01 – 19:00	19:01 – 20:00
	(women)	18:30 – 16:55	19:00 – 18:31	19:30 – 19:01	20:00 – 19:31	20:30 – 20:01	21:00 – 21:31
III. Fair	(men)	10:49 – 12:10	12:01 – 14:00	12:31 – 14:45	13:01 – 15:35	14:31 – 17:00	16:16 – 19:00
	(women)	16:54 – 14:31	18:30 – 15:55	19:00 – 16:31	19:30 – 17:31	20:00 – 19:01	20:30 – 19:31
IV. Good	(men)	9:41 – 10:48	10:46 – 12:00	11:01 – 12:30	11:31 – 13:00	12:31 – 14:30	14:00 – 16:15
	(women)	14:30 – 12:30	15:54 – 13:31	16:30 – 14:31	17:30 – 15:56	19:00 – 16:31	19:30 – 17:31
V. Excellent	(men)	8:37 – 9:40	9:45 – 10:45	10:00 – 11:00	10:30 – 11:30	11:00 – 12:30	11:15 – 13:50
	(women)	12:29 – 11:50	13:30 – 12:30	14:30 – 13:00	15:55 – 13:45	16:30 – 14:30	17:30 – 16:30
VI. Superior	(men)	< 8:37	< 9:45	< 10:00	< 10:30	< 11:00	< 11:15
	(women)	< 11:50	< 12:30	< 13:00	< 13:45	< 14:30	< 16:30

* < Means "less than"; > means "more than."

development of coordination and balance

development of an understanding of the role of exercise and physical activity in the maintenance of good health

provision of opportunities for social growth and development

A fitness program should consist of a twenty minute warm-up, a peak work period of from twenty to thirty minutes, and a cool down period of from five to ten minutes.

In order to motivate people to participate in such fitness activities three or more times per week, there are several important ingredients:

periodic evaluation of each person, demonstrating *concrete* results (for example, reduction in heart rates, weight loss, etc.);

interesting, new, and varied activities—such as exercising to music;

laying of a rational groundwork and philosophy of exercise that will encourage lifelong habits of activity;

relating exercise to total lifestyle changes;

recognition of achievements;

opportunities for leadership and helping others.

It would be wise for clients who are over 40 years old, who smoke, or who have any of the problems mentioned on page 215 to have a physical examination before undertaking any fitness program.

Beginners

To begin a jogging program, one should wear a watch while running from ten to fifteen minutes or for a distance of 1 mile, four to five times per week. The client should maintain comfortable breathing, and he or she should stop when the jogging becomes uncomfortable. The client may then start again when he or she feels better. For most people this difficult, sometimes painful, stage takes from two to three weeks.

Beginners should run at least three times a week with no more than two days between runs. After eight weeks, most novices should be able to run continuously for ten to twenty minutes. This varies according to individual ability, age, and condition.

After eight weeks of running, time and/or distance may be increased by about 10 percent per week. After six months, running for three to four miles, three to five days per week, should offer maximal aerobic conditioning. Warm up and cool down flexibility exercises are essential to prevent overuse injuries. For a look at some of the aerobic sports and activities that achieve the training effect, see Figure 6-11.

In summarizing recent research, a pattern exists to support the contention that certain positive preventive health measures can increase longevity. One convincing coronary artery disease risk factor reducer is aerobic conditioning. Aerobic condi-

	RUN-NING	BICY-CLING	SWIM-MING	HAND-BALL/ SQUASH	TENNIS	WALK-ING	GOLF	BOWL-ING
Physical Fitness								
Cardio-respiratory endurance	21	19	21	19	16	13	8	5
Muscular endurance	20	18	20	18	16	14	8	5
Muscular strength	17	16	14	15	14	11	9	5
Flexibility	9	9	15	16	14	7	8	7
Balance	17	18	12	17	16	8	8	6
General Well-Being								
Weight control	21	20	15	19	16	13	6	5
Muscle definition	14	15	14	11	13	11	6	5
Digestion	13	12	13	13	12	11	7	7
Sleep	16	15	16	12	11	14	6	6
Total	148	142	140	140	128	102	66	51

FIGURE 6-11 Eight sports: how much they help what

Reprinted with permission from James F. Fixx, *The Complete Book of Running* (New York: Random House, 1977), p. 39.

tioning involves consistent planned adaptation to overload (stress/exercise). The adaptive response is increased performance and strength. Stressors are increased gradually at slightly higher levels until the desired training goal is attained.

Senior Citizens

The Senate Subcommittee on Aging led Congress to amend Titles III and VII of the Older Americans Act to provide money to educate, inform, motivate, and enlist support and participation of older Americans in physical activities in order to enhance their health. [14, pp. 11–13]

Despite their paltry budgets, the President's Council of Physical Fitness and Sports and The Administration on Aging have designed a physical fitness program for older Americans. The program's goal is not only to prevent the negative effects that come with disuse, but also to promote "dynamic fitness," which involves efficiency of heart and lungs, muscular strength and endurance, balance, flexibility, coordination, and agility." [72]

Individuals are encouraged to assess themselves according to a walk-jog fitness test, not unlike those already mentioned, except in duration and intensity. The principle of gradually increasing overload is explained, and people are shown various exercises and checklists for their appropriate level. Periodic evaluations are suggested and clients are exhorted to keep moving up in levels.

This program, and others like it, is based on studies such as Herbert A. DeVries' 1970 study to improve aerobic capacity, muscular fitness, and flexibility in sixty-six male subjects with a mean age of 70. Significant findings included increased oxygen transport capacity by 29.4 percent and 35.2 percent (in two experiments), increased vital capacity by 19.6 percent, and improvements after six weeks of conditioning in percentages of (decreased) body fat, physical work capacity, and systolic and diastolic blood pressure. [35, DeVries, as quoted therein]

From this study and subsequent ones like it, it seems that the older person is definitely capable of training and that the percentage of improvement is similar to a young person's. Besides the aforementioned physiological effects, DeVries found that a fifteen-minute walk was sufficient to raise the heart rate to 100 beats per minute, and that it had a significantly greater effect than a tranquilizer (in this case, Equanil or Mebrobamate). [21] Exercise at moderate levels, then, can produce a relaxation effect in older persons.

Other Aspects of Exercise

Much criticism names jogging as one of the most efficient aerobic conditioning practices. However, some negative allegations, including the possibility of sudden death while running, arthritis, stress fractures, and the "addiction" which results in an abandonment of social roles and responsibilities, have been leveled against it. Certainly, every sport has its peculiar hazards; but joggers are plagued more by biting dogs, insensitive motorists, and muggers than by cardiac arrests!

Overuse: Athletic Syndrome

What runners and other "weekend athletes" do experience is a phenomenon called "overuse syndrome." Dyveke Spino, cofounder of Esalen Sports Center, estimates that of the twenty-six million runners in this country, 30 percent are experiencing injury at any given time. [38]

Athletes who push themselves beyond their capabilities or current levels of performance are subject to predictable injuries. These "injuries of excellence" include weekend knees, stress fractures, tennis elbows, shin splints, fallen arches, and Achilles tendonites.

Most of these distressing overuse injuries can be prevented by a well-planned, graduated exercise program, good supportive sports equipment, and sensitivity to the body's messages regarding overstretched muscles, ligaments, and incipient injuries.

One of the best preventive practices for overuse problems is stretching. Stretching must be differentiated from straining, which usually involves stretching an already stretched spindle fiber until it becomes contracted or spasms. A good rule to remember is to avoid "bouncing" warm-up exercises. Recommendations on warm-up time vary with age, condition, weather, type of exercise, etc., but average estimates range from ten to thirty minutes in length.

Physiologically, the warm-up stimulates the circulation, raises the body temperature, and enhances the efficiency of muscle contraction. It has also been proven that the heart muscle needs a warm-up. This helps ensure against myocardial ischemia, especially in cardiac clients.

Jogging requires a fairly specific set of warm-ups to increase the flexibility and range of motion of the legs, especially the hamstrings and calves, since those muscles repeat the same motion over and over.

Figure 6–12 offers a helpful set of stretching exercises, taken from Bob Anderson's book, *Stretching*. He suggests a minimum test of flexibility which involves: sitting with legs straight, fingers touching toes; sitting with legs spread, forehead on top of fists which are placed on the floor; and holding each stretch comfortably for about 50 to 60 seconds. As the body grows older, it becomes even more inflexible; therefore, the time for holding a stretch may need to be reduced to ten seconds for many aging clients.

Bonnie Friedman and Katherine Knight, nurse-runners, have organized a helpful group of preventive measures for specific running injuries. They also include some simple care instructions once an injury does occur. (See Figure 6–13 for details.)

Disuse; Immobility; Aging

If overuse poses a problem to optimal health, disuse portends slow disintegration or active negation of any physiologic gain made by the conditioning process. Disuse implies an almost intentional act. In some cases, disuse is prescribed for overuse injuries and problems. More often than not, however, disuse is a surreptitious loss of function by default.

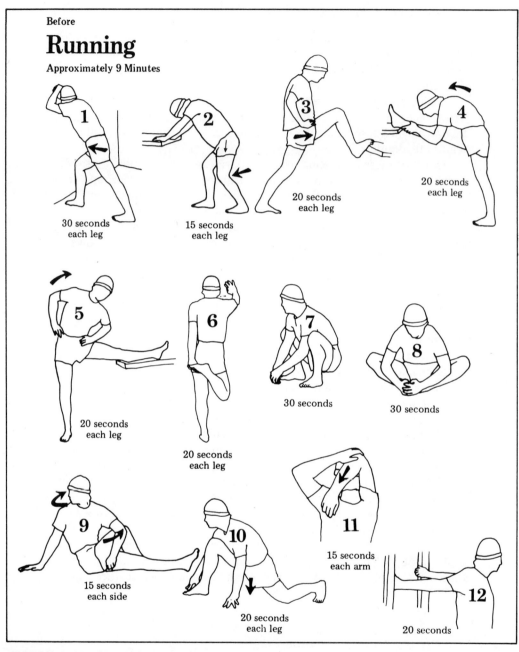

FIGURE 6-12 Stretching exercises

Excerpted from *Stretching,* copyright © 1980 by Bob Anderson; $7.95; Shelter Publications/Random House. Available in bookstores or mail from Stretching, Inc., P.O. Box 767, Palmer Lake, Colo. 80133.

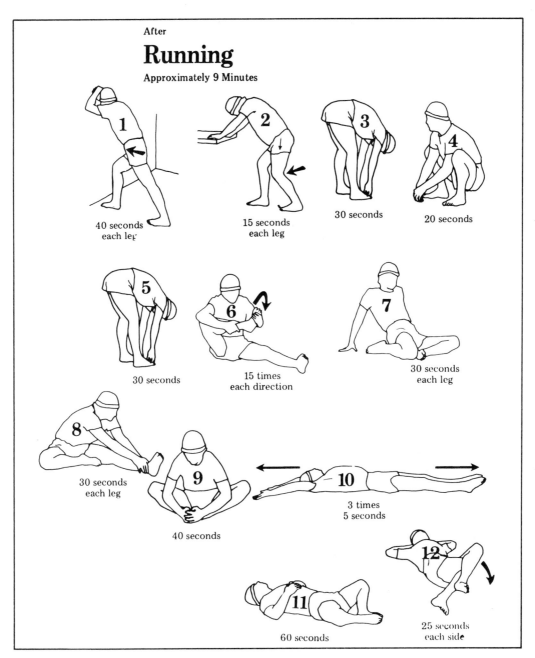

FIGURE 6-12 (continued)

FIGURE 6-13 Preventing and caring for common running injuries

Site	Prevention	Symptoms	Treatment
Knee Site of 25 percent of running injuries[1]	Stabilize the foot with well-fitting running shoes. Use heel and/or arch supports to improve fit. Cinder or any soft surface decreases the long-term wear and tear that causes most running injuries. Perform quadriceps strengthening exercises: Sit on table with legs dangling. Hang a 3–5 pound weight over ankle, extend knee and hold in locked position for 6–10 seconds. Flex knee and repeat 8–10 times. Repeat with other knee. Stretch once or twice during the run.[2]	parapatellar pain or tenderness	Don't try to run with severe pain. If you find you cannot run without great pain and a limp, rest is indicated. Look for an obvious cause—shoes, running surface. If you think you have a structural problem, seek the advice of a "running doctor," either an orthopedist or a podiatrist. Immediate treatment for most running injuries: Place ice on area 8–10 minutes following run. Use heat 3–4 times per day. For severe inflammatory response, aspirin q 3–4 h, if not contraindicated, may help.[3] If pain persists, seek medical care.
Achilles' tendon Site of 18 percent of running injuries	Wear a well-fitting running shoe with the heels in good condition. Stretch calf muscles before and after run: Facing a wall, stand 2–3 feet away with heels on ground, knees and back straight. Then lean into wall until tension is felt in calf and hamstring area. Hold for 8–10 seconds; repeat 6–8 times.	pain and tenderness with dorsiflexion and weight bearing; stiffness and pain in back of heel and ankle after a night's sleep	Rest is usually indicated. If the pain stops as you run and does not cause you to put undue stress on other muscles or change your running form, continue to run. Do strengthening and stretching exercise before and after. Be sure your shoes are in good repair. Begin your run at a slow shuffle, stop, and stretch periodically. Increase pace after warm-up.

Site	Treatment	Symptoms	Prevention
Shin Site of 15 percent of running injuries	Use running shoes with flexible foreshoe. Use a higher heeled shoe or insert a heel lift. Do wall push-up exercise (above) and shin strengthener—place weight over toes, flex foot at ankle, hold 8–10 seconds. Repeat 8–10 times.	tenderness in lower third of leg inside shin area pain on toe extension, flexion, and on weight bearing	See treatment for knee injuries.
Hip/Low Back Site of 7–14 percent of running injuries	Strengthen the abdominal muscles to improve posture and decrease irritation of sciatic nerve. Do bent-leg sit-ups (see treatment). Do hamstring stretching: place heel of one leg on chair or table with hip flexed and knee extended. Keep other leg straight with knee locked. Bring your head toward your knee until you feel pain; hold 8–10 seconds. Repeat 8–10 times with each leg.	pain radiating down buttock and posterior leg hamstring tightness	Bent-leg sit-ups prevent strain on back muscles: lie on floor with heels drawn up to buttocks. Come to a sitting position. Lie back, repeat 20 times or until unable to do more. Leg overs are helpful: lie on floor, bring straight legs over your head and try to touch floor with toes. Hold for 10 seconds. Repeat 6–10 times.[4]

[1] Henderson, Joe. First aid for the injured. Runner's World July 1977, pp. 32–36.
[2] Technical tips: thoughts on first aid. Runner's World Nov. 1977, pp. 57–61.
[3] Ullyot, Joan. Women's Running. Mountain View, Calif., World Publications, 1976, pp. 99–100.
[4] Sheehan, George. Medical advice. Runner's World. Dec. 1977, pp. 22–23.

Passive acceptance of the gradual decrease in functions as a natural outcome of aging is a prime example of disuse. The aches and pains of the early forties become the irreversible stooped shoulders and halting gaits of the middle sixties. The President's Council on Physical Fitness and Sports and The Administration of Aging describe disuse as "the mortal enemy of the human body. We know today that how a person lives, not how long he lives, is responsible for many of the physical problems normally associated with advanced age." [72]

The developmental, anatomic, and physiologic changes that occur in the aged are well-documented, as Figure 6–14 demonstrates. These effects closely parallel those imposed by immobility, which has been described by Murray and Zentner as the "unavoidable or prescribed restriction of movement in any sphere of a person's life." [64] This definition would seem to waive any degree of self-responsibility in a situation that is seemingly out of the client's control. This blind acceptance of the social parameters and timetables of aging and its subsequent increasing disuse, which bring on feelings of uselessness, is now being highly questioned. If young and middle-aged clients can forestall, and in some cases reverse, some of the effects of aging, why can't the aged do the same? One physiologic fact in their favor is that athletic ability declines slowly up to the age of sixty.

A woman's capacity to exercise declines much more slowly with age than a man's. Cardiologists testing healthy women on treadmills at the University of Alabama have discovered that the female's capacity to exercise drops only about 2 percent for every ten years of age; for their male counterparts, it is a 10 percent drop. A sixty-year-old woman should be able to do 90 percent of the physical exercise she did at age 20 before her heart reaches its maximum rate of beating. A normal male at the same age has only 60 percent of his exercise capacity left. [102]

Injuries which seem to plague younger joggers, for example, seem to be compensated for by the wisdom of careful and gradual training in the aged. Muscles and joints accustomed to years of disuse will not adapt overnight, however.

Stress fractures are a particular problem for postmenopausal women, who may be calcium-depleted. Bone meal or dolomite supplements may be needed in addition to a substitute exercise which will be less punishing on the joints and bones than jogging is. Swimming, walking, or cycling might be recommended—or even something which the Longevity Center in Santa Barbara terms "roving." Roving is a combination of walking and running at conditioning levels in which the client sets the distance goals. Time, striving, or competing is unimportant; enjoyment, variety, and individual needs are valued. [52]

Several years ago, attention was focused on foreign countries whose aged populations achieved amazing longevity. Research began on what factors contributed to the virility exhibited by the people of Soviet Georgia, Ecuador, and Hunza in West Pakistan. The Hunzahuts, in addition to benefiting from certain hereditary factors, subsist on 1,923 calories daily, of which only one percent is comprised of meat and dairy products, and engage in vigorous agrarian work conducted on steep slopes.

The Vilcabauba people also live on a low caloric, low animal-fat diet, and their level of activity in the high mountain country is staggering. The people in Soviet Georgia eat large amounts of dairy products, but primarily those that are relatively low in fat. Again, high levels of activity prevail. All the cultures mentioned claim a relatively positive outlook on the state of the world and each member of the society has a role and useful function to perform within their respective societies. [51]

The Chinese have always endorsed exercise for all ages, but especially for the aging. The Tai-Chi Ch'uan is practiced very early in the morning by the Chinese community in parks and squares from Peking to San Francisco. More will be said about this mind–body exercise, meditation, and martial art form in the next section of this chapter.

If aging is defined as a decreasing ability to survive stress, then any of the lifestyling factors contributing to increased adaptation to stress would be commended. The measurements of inability to return to normal following physiologic demands are the same as those described earlier in this section.

It is felt by some physiology of aging experts that the progressive decline in Lean Body Mass observed in the aged is due to the decrease in protoplasmic mass (potassium in muscle) and its replacement with fat and connective tissue. Can this and other so-called irreversible aging changes be modified by exercise? Hope lies in the increasing research efforts in this area.

In the last section of this chapter, an innovative human lifestyling program called Senior Actualization and Growth Experience (SAGE) will be described. Eugenia Gerard, one of the founders, describes the situation of many of the elderly who come to the program as one in which "immobility becomes a habit." [33]

In following an aerobic exercise program and the advice of Dr. Ernst Wynder, nurses and clients alike are striving "to help people die young—as late in life as possible." [109]

Misuse: Storing Tension in Target Muscles

A final aspect of activity and adaptation to stress is captured in the term "misuse." This means using the body for a purpose for which it was not designed, requiring it to perform a function for which it has not been adequately trained or conditioned.

Examples of this situation are seen in the weekend athletes who roam the parks wrenching their backs, necks, ankles, and knees. It differs from disuse in that it is *active* abuse of the body—its warning signals (pain, swelling, etc.) are ignored.

One intriguing theory, based on the work of Wilhelm Reich, of misusing the body to store tension has been proposed by psychiatrist Alexander Lowen. The basic principle is that chronic muscular tensions or "muscular armoring" result from continuing stress on the body. [56] Selyé's theory is cited by Lowen as one basis for the following observations:

1. Phase 3, or exhaustion, in Selyé's model is translated by Lowen to mean fatigue or chronic tiredness. This is interpreted as a result of continuous stresses to which people are subjected by their chronic muscular tensions. Energy otherwise available to meet ordinary stresses of living is limited because it is tied up with muscle tension.
2. The body must be tension-free in order to provide the person with sufficient energy to cope with stress. [56]

FIGURE 6-14 Anatomic changes to consider in care of aged

Copyright © 1978, American Journal of Nursing Company. Reprinted with permission from the *American Journal of Nursing, 78*, no. 8 (August 1978), 1349.

	Functional Change	Outcome
HEART	decreased stroke volume	drop in cardiac output
	slower heart rate	
	estimated left ventricular work declines at rest	
	blood flow through the coronary arteries decreases	
	myocardial ability to use oxygen decreases[1]	heart less well equipped to handle stress; with coexisting heart disease, cardiac failure and death may result
BLOOD VESSELS	smooth muscle replaced by fibrous and hyaline tissue causing decreased vascular elasticity	increased pulse pressure and systolic blood pressure
KIDNEY	renal blood flow drops at a steady rate, starting at age 40[2]	proportional reduction in glomerular filtration rate (usually measured as creatinine clearance)
	decreased fluid intake leads to decreased ability to concentrate urine	normal GFR at age 40 of 120 ml./min. falls to 60 or 70 ml./min. at age 85[3]
	ability to dilute urine decreases	BUN rises from a normal value of 9.5 mg./100 ml. at age 20 to 15–20 mg./100 ml. at age 70–80[3]

LUNGS	reduction in vital capacity and increase of residual volume; reduction of pulmonary diffusion; loss of lung recoil; and maldistribution of pulmonary ventilation/perfusion ratios—all due to change in type or quantity of fibrous proteins, collagen, and elastin in lung matrix[4]	decrease in arterial oxygen tension, less respiratory reserve in major illnesses, surgery, or trauma
	progressive weakening of respiratory muscles	reduced negative and positive intra-thoracic pressure on forced inspiration and expiration; this plus reduced expiratory flow rates account for decrease in maximum breathing capacity
GI TRACT	decreased motility of stomach and intestines reduction in intestinal blood flow[5]	constipation possible delay or slight reduction in drug absorption
	increase in gastric pH number of absorbing cells may be decreased and active transport systems may be modified	affects solubility of some drugs no data to support major change in drug absorption[6]

[1] Harris, R. Special features of heart disease in the elderly patients. In *Working With Older People—A Guide to Practice, Vol. 4. Clinical Aspects of Aging*, ed. by A. B. Chinn. (Public Health Service Publ. No. 1459) Washington, D.C., U.S. Government Printing Office, 1971, pp. 81–102.

[2] Papper, Solomon. The effects of age in reducing renal function. *Geriatrics* 28:83–87, May 1973.

[3] Cole, W. H. Medical differences between the young and the aged. *J. Am. Geriatr. Soc.* 18:589–614. Aug. 1970.

[4] Williams, M. H. Special problems in respiratory diseases. *Geriatrics* 29:67–71, June 1974.

[5] Bender, A. D. Effect of age on intestinal absorption: implications for drug absorption in the elderly. *J. Am. Geriatr. Soc.* 16:1331–1339, Dec. 1968.

[6] Crooks, J., and others. Pharmacokinetics in the elderly. *Clin. Pharmacokinet.* 1(4):280–296, 1976.

(continued)

	Functional Change	Outcome
MUSCULOSKELE-TAL SYSTEM	decrease in number and bulk of muscle fibers; muscle fibers are replaced by nonmuscular fibrous tissue	decrease in muscular strength, endurance, and agility
	density of bone decreases; in women after middle age may be related estrogen deficiency, insufficient dietary intake, and perhaps abnormalities in calcium, protein, and amino acid metabolism[7,8]	osteoporosis, osteoarthritis
HEMATOLOGICAL SYSTEM	iron deficiency anemia, probably caused by malnutrition and malabsorption[9]	iron and folate deficiency and a change in oxygen-carrying capacity
	anemia due to chronic diseases such as infection, arthritis, malignant disease	mild, normocytic and normochromic anemia
ENDOCRINE SYSTEM	insulin response or peripheral sensitivity to insulin release may be reduced	return to fasting level in glucose tolerance test is slower[3]

[7] Trotter, M., and others. Densities of bones of white and Negro skeletons. *J. Bone Joint Surg.* (Am.) 42–A:50–58, Jan. 1960.
[8] Yoshikaw, M., and others. Osteoporosis in Japan, a clinical and experimental study. In *Proceedings of the Eighth International Congress on Gerontology.* Washington, D.C., Federation of American Societies for Experimental Biology, Vol. 1, 1969, p. 225.
[9] Evans, D. M. Hematological aspects of iron-deficiency in the elderly. *Gerontol. Clin.* (Basel) 13:12–30, 1971.

Lowen's own description of people under stress emphasizes the strength of the body's language as it attempts to cope:

> They are laboring under great stress; yet they feel that if they fail to carry on, this would admit to weakness, to defeat, to their failure as human beings. In this desperate strait, they set their jaws more firmly, stiffen their legs, lock their knees and struggle on with what at times appears unbelievable will . . . in many respects, this will to carry on is an admirable quality, but it can and does have some disastrous affects on the body.[56, p. 232]

To reduce an individual's vulnerability to stress, the physical and psychic defenses against "letting down" must be worked through and released. Two sets of exercises are prescribed in Lowen's Bioenergetic Therapy to help a person get in touch with and decrease the muscular tension (see Figure 6–15). Bioenergetics is defined as "a therapeutic technique to help a person get back together with his body and to help him enjoy, to the fullest degree possible, the life of the body." [56] It serves as a bridge between activity, fitness and conditioning, and stress reduction, which is the next human lifestyling element to be discussed because it addresses *both* areas.

Perhaps one of the most important disruptive elements in Western society is the inadequate adjustment to stress, evidenced by the "misuse" phenomenon. The Alexander technique is a form of purposeful movement aimed at reducing years of misused musculature through guidance and physical manipulation. [95] It is not a meditative method, although it does involve mental control of the way in which the body reacts to stress.

F. M. Alexander, an actor born in Tasmania in 1869, regained his lost voice by learning to reteach his misused vocal musculature how to speak. Once Alexander became aware of how he had misused his own body, he began to observe how others misused theirs. He found that in modern societies the majority of people stand, sit, and move in an equally defective manner. The technique which he developed involves a nonintrusive assessment and subsequent corrective manipulation and retraining of the entire muscular system. It starts with the head and neck and moves on to the shoulders, chest, pelvis, legs, and feet.

One of the major questions scientists ask about the technique is how it works. A neurologic concept, termed "reafference," seems to help explain some of its beneficial effects. [95] The brain continuously monitors and checks the simple to complex movements of the muscles. The "feedback" evaluation is compared with the feedback expectation, and when they match, signals for correction are terminated. Apparently, lifelong misuse causes "all is correct" messages to be sent to the brain when, in fact, all is *not* correct; or, the brain may misinterpret "all is not correct" inappropriately. It is felt that this situation is environmentally—not genetically—induced.

As Nikolaas Tinbergen aptly stated upon receiving the Nobel Prize for Physiology and Medicine, "misuse, with all its psychosomatic or rather somatopsychic consequences must, therefore, be considered a result of modern living conditions of a culturally determined stress. I might add here that I am not merely thinking of too much sitting, but just as much of the cowed posture that one assumes when one feels that one is not quite up to one's work, when one feels insecure." [95, p. 25]

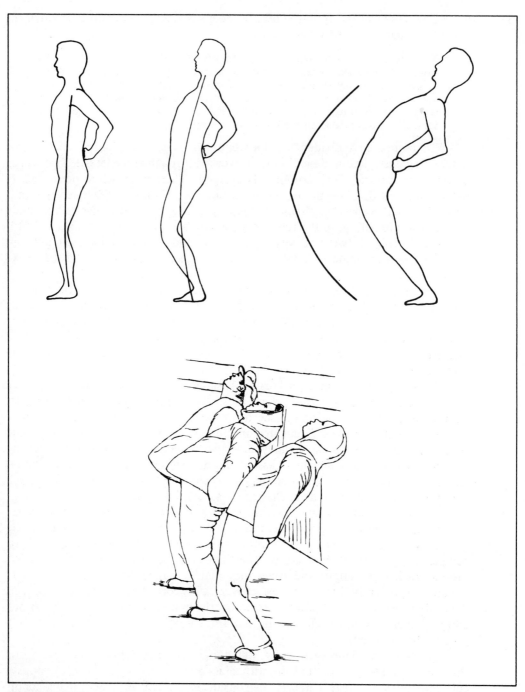

FIGURE 6-15 A comparison of Lowen's bioenergetic exercises with a Tai Chi Ch'uan exercise termed the "Taoist Arch." (Note the similarities.)

Adapted from Alexander Lowen, *Bioenergetics* (New York: Penguin Books, 1975), pp. 73–77.

STRESS REDUCTION AND MANAGEMENT

Strictly speaking, the term *stress reduction* includes any mental or physical state or practice which triggers the "relaxation response," as first described in 1971 by Dr. Herbert Benson, a Harvard researcher. The relaxation response is an innate, integrated set of physiologic changes in opposition to those of the "fight or flight" response; it can be elicited by psychologic means. Until recently, the relaxation response had been elicited primarily by meditation techniques. Research done in 1964 on Transcendental Meditators showed a decrease in their body metabolism, heart rate, and rate of breathing. These changes were distinctly different from the physiologic changes noted during quiet sitting or sleep. According to Benson, the huge variety of relaxation techniques, Eastern and Western, movement and non-movement, have four things in common—a comfortable position; a quiet environment; repetition of a prayer, word, sound, or phrase; and an adoption of a passive attitude when other thoughts come into consciousness. [104]

Application of accurate, sensitive, biofeedback instruments is yielding much more concrete information regarding this adaptive relaxation response. Just as in aerobic conditioning, certain techniques have been proven to elicit a predictable effect—in this case, a relaxation response. Attention to a daily method of relaxation has been correlated with decreased absenteeism, improved general health, lowering of blood pressure and pulse rates, and increased subjective feelings of well-being, to mention a few. [6]

Surveys exist to show that 15 percent of the American public is using tranquilizers at some point during any given year. And a recent federal study showed that both new and refill prescriptions for antianxiety drugs have more than doubled between 1964 and 1973. [8] Proponents of stress management and reduction hypothesize that routine relaxation breaks could help change the course of such polydrug abuse.

An eight-week experiment conducted by Benson and his associates investigated the effects of daily relaxation breaks on 126 manufacturing employees on five self-reported measures—symptoms, illness, performance, sociability-satisfaction, and happiness/unhappiness indices. [70, 71] The larger group was broken into three smaller groups—A, B, and C. Group A was taught a technique for producing the relaxation response; group B was instructed to sit quietly; and group C received no instructions. Groups A and B took two 15-minute relaxation breaks daily. After eight weeks, the greatest improvements on every index occurred in group A; the least improvement in group C. Although fewer than three practice periods per week produced little change, fewer than two daily sessions appeared to be *more* practice than was necessary for many of the subjects to achieve positive changes. [70, 71]

Blood pressure measurements were also taken on the workers. Even though most subjects were regularly normotensive, blood pressures were significantly lowered in group A members, with those whose readings were the highest often experiencing the greatest degree of decrease. [70, 71]

The implication drawn from these studies was that more studies on hypertensive populations might yield even greater benefits. It was concluded that the relaxation response was a particularly attractive preventive measure because it cost only the time involved to practice, had no known side effects, and was reported to be a pleasant and rewarding experience for those who practiced it regularly.

An arbitrary line will be drawn between movement and nonmovement relaxation exercise in order to facilitate organization and discussion. Several representative methods from each group will be examined in detail. The principles underlying major methods will be explained. Since so many of the stress-reduction techniques require visualization, demonstrative practice, and return demonstration, it is suggested that actual proficiency in a technique be achieved in a laboratory setting, with some initial supervision.

Nonmovement

Biofeedback

Biofeedback is a learned process in which the client uses biologic information to exert voluntary control over automatic reflex-regulated physiologic activities. (The term developed because biologic information generated by clients was fed back to them.) A physiologic function is selected and monitored. Information—such as heart rate, finger temperature, blood pressure, muscle tension, or brain waves—is translated into a visual or auditory signal which the client senses. As the client relaxes, for example, the initial high-pitched tone on the biofeedback instrument becomes lower and easier to listen to.

Apparently, when the client learns what it feels like to relax a particular function or muscle, he lets go of conscious willing and permits a state of passive volition to occur. This passive concentration culminates in a takeover by the right (feminine) hemisphere of the brain (see Figure 6-16).

Biofeedback is used to treat over fifty different psychosomatic disorders. It is particularly useful in conjunction with a wide variety of relaxation techniques. For many clients, biofeedback may help them to feel—often for the first time—discrimination between tension and relaxation. Complex mental processes, many of them not understood, are called upon to change stress responses to relaxation responses. The client learns to control "involuntary" functions, as well as to experience changing states of awareness and mental outlooks.

Most people respond to pressure by "bracing" or increasing muscular tension. Unfortunately, this muscle tension is not recognized as such, either during a stress situation, or sometimes even after its occurrence. Indeed, an enormous amount of muscle tightening has usually occurred before the client acknowledges it. Muscle relaxation is a slow process. Often, clients will attempt to "sleep it off"; this is usually ineffective since the subconscious often replays the situation and keeps the muscles tense.

Frequently, muscle tension becomes sustained at higher and higher levels, which causes the person to become hyperreactive and startle easily. Muscles may remain in a tense state until either the tension-provoking situation is removed or until it is recognized and reevaluated.

Electromyographic (EMG) biofeedback indicates that the muscles are great expressors of mind-body activities. Significant reductions in muscle tension have

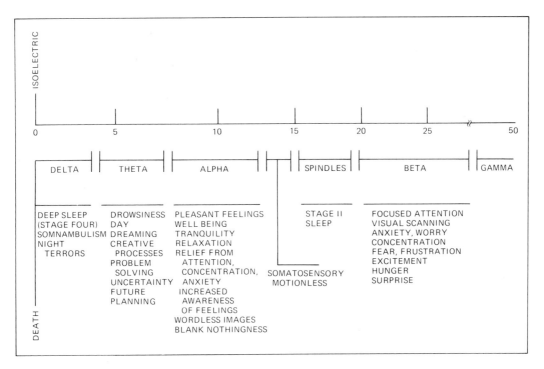

FIGURE 6-16 Emotions and behavioral states associated with various bands within the spectrum of EEG activity stabilized as steady states using EEG biofeedback

Reprinted with permission from Gary Schwartz and David Shapiro (eds.), *Consciousness and Self-Regulation,* vol. II (New York: Plenum Press, 1978), p. 407 Figure 2.

been obtained via relaxation or meditation techniques. No highly controlled interventions that force muscles to relax or change, such as drugs, deep massage, or electrical shocks, are used. Instead, relaxation and meditation techniques intuitively and cognitively, passively and subconsciously, affect the cerebral mechanism that makes the muscles respond. [9, p. 31]

An internal feedback mechanism sustains the stress reaction by relaying information on the stress-reactive systems to the central nervous system, where it is available for cerebral interpretation into the emotional and cognitive reactions to stress. Let's discuss two methods which can be applied to alter this destructive self-perpetuating course of events.

The first method—counseling, in the form of self-counseling, crisis intervention, and coping skills training—has been in use for years. (These methods will be discussed further in the Interpersonal Coping section of this chapter.) Basically, useful information is introduced to the client which offers a different interpretation of the stress situation or which adds some stress-reduction mechanisms to the client's coping repertoire.

The second method uses biofeedback to supply purely physiologic information to the client about the degree of muscular or visceral tension present. What makes this method highly intrapersonal is that the client learns to control and normalize his or her own physiologic activities. Only the client can understand and "control" the involuntary functions of his or her body.

An interesting side effect of learning to become aware of muscle tension—eventually, *without* biofeedback—is that clients also become acutely aware of what caused and what continues to cause that response to occur. In many cases, clients begin to understand the mental processes and stress responses involved.

Autogenic Training

One of the most effective and well-researched relaxation methods is Autogenic Training. The name implies what the technique accomplishes—self-regulation of autonomic functions.

Autogenic Training Phrases

My right arm is heavy.
My right arm is heavy.

My left arm is heavy.
My left arm is heavy.

My right leg is heavy.
My right leg is heavy.

My left leg is heavy.
My left leg is heavy.

My arms and legs are heavy and warm.
My arms and legs are heavy and warm.

Heartbeat calm and regular.
Heartbeat calm and regular.

Breathing calm and regular.
Breathing calm and regular.

My center is warm.
My center is warm.

My forehead is cool.
My forehead is cool.

My neck and shoulders are heavy.
My neck and shoulders are heavy.

Autogenic Training, as developed over fifty years ago in Germany by Dr. Johannes Schultz, involves the linking of a few verbal formulas with corresponding mental images to trigger the body's automatic self-regulatory tendencies to maintain peace, harmony, and homeostasis. All four of Benson's conditions for relaxation (see page 233) are employed by the training, which also utilizes a pattern of specific body positions, as illustrated in Figure 6–17. [104]

After assuming the positions, one mentally recites a series of eight "phrases," each of which has its own image or visualization (see below). A light hypnotic state is induced. One "set," as pictured in the figure, takes approximately fifty seconds to complete. The usual requirement is for three sets (or a triplet) to be completed four times a day (12 to 15 minutes per day). The client is asked to keep a log (Figure 6–18) which is used by the trainer or nurse to discuss progress, modifications, and feelings about the training and its effects on the client's life.

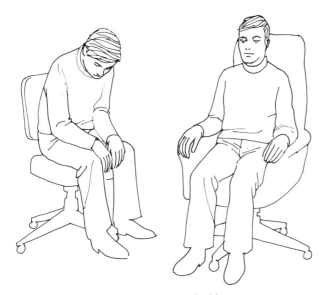

The Standard Sitting Position

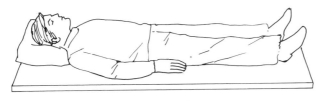

The Lying Position

FIGURE 6-17 Autogenic training positions

Once the basics of the technique are mastered, additional phrases may be added to the original ones. These usually take the form of a positive effect desired—an affirmation. Autogenic training can be used for creative thinking and problem solving, self-contemplation, free association, and dream work.

Jacobson's Progressive Relaxation

A popular relaxation method, called Progressive Relaxation, was developed by Edmund Jacobson in the late 1920s. The client tenses a muscle and then relaxes it

Name:			Date:
TRIPLET #	TIME OF DAY	DURATION OF TRIPLET	COMMENTS ON EVENTS DURING THE A.T. EXERCISES
1			
2			
3			
4			
additional observations			

(Use space below for further comments and remarks on any noticeable specific or general changes in yourself.)

_____

_____

_____

_____

_____

FIGURE 6-18 Autogenic training log

momentarily, thereby consciously observing the two different bodily sensations. They begin to sense the difference between the two feelings as they respond—either to a trainer or to a tape recording. A typical excerpted response follows:

> Sit quietly in a comfortable position.
> Take a deep, slow breath.
> Hold the breath for several seconds.
> Slowly exhale.
> Take another deep, slow breath.
> Hold the breath and pull your toes toward your head, tightening your leg and calf muscles.
> Feel the tension.
>
> Breathe out and let go completely.
>
> Take another deep, slow breath.
> Hold the breath and make a fist with both hands.
> Feel the tension.
>
> Breathe out and let go completely.
>
> Take another deep, slow breath.
> Hold the breath and bite down as hard as you can, tightening your jaw muscles.
> Feel the tension.
>
> Breathe out and let go completely.

Each set of muscles is tensed and relaxed until the entire body has been covered. (Figure 6–19 shows a shortened version of Progressive Relaxation.) The original exercise is usually done in a reclining position and requires up to one hour to complete, which presents a problem for many busy people who simply can't spare such a lengthy block of time.

Progressive Relaxation and Autogenic Training are usually advocated and practiced by a very determined, persevering group of followers; thus, in a sense, both techniques are self-selective and those who can adhere to the regimen involved claim excellent results. But what about the average, unmotivated person who feels the occasional need to relieve tension? For such people, several relaxation techniques have been adapted from other more orthodox methods, as, for example, yoga. Let us examine some of these techniques.

The Feeling Pause

The first of these techniques was designed by Samuels and Bennett in *The Well Body Book*. The University of California at Berkeley adapted it to their student population's needs and included it in their student Health Service Manual. A description of this "Feeling Pause" technique follows:

Purpose: To release muscular tension, and to facilitate an overall relaxation response.

Concept: Muscles are tightened and then released which promotes deep relaxation because of the "pendulum effect".

Caution: Tighten down less heavily on areas with recent strain or sprain.

Procedure:

1) *Preparation*

2) *4 part breath-* inhale through abdomen; hold for 5 seconds; release all at once; sink as you breathe easily.

3) *right arm-* inhale; hold breath and tighten entire arm by making fist; tighten fist, wrist, forearm, bicep as you lift entire arm six inches into the air; release breath all at once as arm flops down; allow arm to sink; roll arm slightly and compare to left arm. Repeat.

4) *left arm-* repeat procedure with left arm twice. Compare how arms feel vs. the legs.

5) *right leg-* inhale; hold breath and tighten entire leg by pointing toe; tighten toes, foot, calf, thigh and right buttock as you lift entire leg into the air; release leg all at once as leg flops down; allow leg to sink; roll leg gently and compare to left leg and arms. Repeat.

6) *left leg-* repeat procedure with left leg twice.

7) *abdomen-* inhale (less fully); hold breath and tighten by making a "hard stomach"; release breath all at once; compare to arms and legs. Repeat.

8) *chest-* inhale up into chest; hold breath and tighten the muscles below the armpits (pectorals); release breath all at once; compare to abdomen. Repeat.

9) *shoulders and back-* inhale; hold breath and tighten shoulders by raising them up as if to cover the ears in shrugging gesture; release breath all at once as shoulders return to original state of rest; allow shoulders to widen and lower by reaching hands gently for feet; sink; compare to torso. Repeat.

10) *neck-* inhale; hold breath and tighten by raising head up six inches and *gently* tensing back neck muscles until mild trembling is felt; release breath all at once as head flops gently to original position; sink; compare to shoulders and back. Repeat.

11) *face-* inhale; hold breath and tighten by bringing entire face to a point at the tip of the nose as the eyes squint and lips pucker in a kissing gesture; release breath all at once; allow face to expand and relax; sink; compare to neck. Repeat.

12) *conclusion-* gently allow hands to move and give yourself a face massage-take care of yourself as you give attention to your hairline, forehead, eyebrows, eyes, temples, ears, nose, cheeks, mouth, chin; work your way back up the face checking each of these areas; run your fingers through your hair from the roots all the way out as you pull any remaining tension from your entire body out through your scalp and into your hands; "throw" tension far away by shaking hands vigorously; Sink, float, drift . . .

FIGURE 6-19 Progressive relaxation: a shortened variation

The feeling pause is a natural response which all of us use, to some degree, nearly every day of our lives. It is that moment when we pause briefly to close off messages from the world around us, or outside us, so that we can get in touch with feelings that come from ourselves. Classically, it is similar to the moment of scratching your head as you ponder. That same response can be expanded within your consciousness, and once expanded, provides you with a mental tool for making choices for ease in your life.

Find a comfortable place and position. Close your eyes. Take a slow, deep breath, inhaling through your nose. Allow your chest and your abdomen to expand as you breathe. Feel the fullness of your lungs and abdomen, as they fill with air. Now hold your breath for a moment. Then exhale slowly and enjoy the feelings of the air moving out through your nostrils. Feel your chest and your abdomen relax. Take another slow, deep breath, inhaling through your nose. Enjoy the luxury of this breath as though you were inhaling the delicious scent of spring blossoms. Feel your chest and abdomen become full. Then exhale slowly, feeling your chest and abdomen relax. Do this 3 or 4 times.

Now let yourself breathe normally.

Feel your feet and legs. Imagine them becoming very heavy. Imagine your buttocks, back, shoulders, arms, hands, and head becoming very heavy. Imagine them being too heavy to lift. Enjoy this feeling of heaviness for a moment.

Now imagine what it would be like to move into outer space. Imagine yourself drifting weightlessly. Imagine the deep pure blue color of space all around you. Imagine how the earth looks far in the distance.

Imagine stars and planets moving past you in the distance. Imagine yourself into space of diffuse white light, as bright and ethereal as a distant star. As you approach this light, it increases in size until you feel yourself surrounded by its glow. Being in this light you feel that you are bathed in the feeling of tranquility and clarity.

If disturbing thoughts or feelings enter your mind as you are in this feeling pause state, allow them to pass by you just as you imagine planets and stars passing you by on this voyage. Let these thoughts and feelings fade into the distance, leaving them behind you in the same way that you imagine a comet disappearing over the horizon.

Stay in this mental space for as long as you wish. Enjoy it as a tranquil resting space to which you can go any time you wish. When you want to return to your everyday state of mind, simply open your eyes.

After this exercise, you may become acutely aware of physical and psychological pain, aches, and tension. You may also be very receptive to creative thoughts and suggestions. [101] *

Palming

Another exercise with yogic origins is "palming," used for relieving eye strain and for improving vision. The client sits on the floor or at a table or desk, draws up the knees, and keeps the feet flat on the floor and slightly apart. The palms are rubbed together as if to generate heat and are then placed over the closed eyes. The

* Reprinted with permission from The University of California Berkeley Student Health Service Manual (1977), by Hal Z. Bennett.

fingers of the right hand should be crossed over the fingers of the left hand, which is placed on the forehead. The color black is visualized if desired. The elbows should rest on straight knees and the head should not be bent. Deep breathing should be maintained throughout.

Visualization

A great number of the relaxation exercises assume the ability to visualize. A brief look at the development of visualization and imagery reveals some interesting points. The use of visualization in healing has been recorded as early as in the cuneiform of the Babylonian Empire. And yet, throughout history, the definition of visualization has eluded the deductive processes. It is a conscious experience involving perceptual and emotional participation and the ability to maintain focus on one object of concentration, as in right-hemisphere-dominated thinking.

Visualization maintains concentration on one object and gives to one who practices it, the following qualities—alertness, clarity of thought, identification with the object and a feeling of participation in the visualization and a feeling of wholeness. [80, p. 65] The usual visual descriptive categories do not apply to visualization. The person has no vested interest in the image; no biases or attitudes are imposed on it. There is no difference between the visualization and the person. During the experience, a visualization supersedes time, space, description, or analysis.

The information received during a visualization seems to come from a source other than the person himself. This purity of vision brings with it enormous energy, which can be sensed by and transmitted to other people. Descriptions are very inadequate. The nurse and client will need to begin with some concrete relaxation and visualization exercises and gradually move toward more intricate ones to understand and experience visualizing.

A technique called "guided imagery" is used by such people as Ruth Carter Stapleton in the "healing" of people with psychologically debilitating problems. Carl and Stephanie Simonton have claimed amazing results with cancer clients through guided visualization. Certain types of laying-on-of-hands therapies rely on the healer's forming an image of what he or she hopes to achieve in balancing the client's energies.

All these examples demonstrate the use of imagery and are basically parapsychological phenomena. Put more simply, all these techniques involve the creation of a positive self-image, something that has been advocated for years by such people as Norman Vincent Peale. The term PMA (Positive Mental Attitude) is used with great frequency to describe peoples' world views in which they shape the world around them in a kind of visualization.

Scientific research is desperately needed in this area since there has been and can be so much charlatanism in psychic and spiritual phenomena. In all these meditative states, the alpha brain wave pattern can be recorded on an electroencephalograph (EEG). The four cycles of brain waves and their associated activities are shown in Figure 6–16.

Movement

Yoga

Yoga is a system of physical, mental, and spiritual development based on the Sanskrit root word *yaj,* meaning to join or unify. Both the Hindu Yoga (500–1500 B.C.) and the Taoist Tai-Chi Ch'uan are movement modes learned by rote *imitation* of the master or teacher. The mind is emptied of thoughts and filled only with slow, rhythmic movements which can lead to the same feeling of peace as in meditation. The mind experiences the intuitive right-dominant hemisphere. It is perfectly alert, senses all stimuli, but chooses to focus on the movement and breathing.

Yoga is divided into several different methods of achieving the same goal, that is, unity with the Supreme Consciousness:

1. Karma Yoga (work and action)
2. Juana Yoga (knowledge and study)
3. Bhakti Yoga (devotion and selfless love)
4. Mantra Yoga (repetition of certain invocations and sounds)
5. Raja Yoga (yoga of consciousness—highest level)
6. Hatha Yoga (positions and breathing—basic level)

The yoga postures pictured in Figures 6–20 and 6–21 are intended to promote function of the entire organism—respiration, circulation, digestion, elimination, metabolism, etc., and to affect the working of all the glands and organs, of the nervous system, and of the mind. This is achieved by doing deep breathing while the body is placed in the various postures. A sense of awakening, balance, and stamina are achieved as one moves through the exercises which are modeled after the natural movement of various animals. Relaxation is viewed as an art, breathing as a science, and control of the mind over the body as a means of harmonizing body, mind, and spirit.

Tai-Chi Ch'uan

Tai-Chi Ch'uan, with its fifteen-century history, is considered to be the supreme martial art form in China. It combines the slow rhythmical movements of Yoga with the alertness and singleness of purpose of a war dance. The movement patterns are reminiscent of a dance routine. Each movement is designed to balance the flow of Chi through the meridians (also used in acupuncture) and to balance the Yin and Yang polarities.

The motion is very slow and controlled. Students of Tai-Chi say they experience peace, stimulation, "tingling" in the extremities, and heat. Continued practice of Tai-Chi is believed by the Chinese to guarantee longevity.

The manner of movement is regulated by the principle of Yin and Yang. It is the interplay and harmony of opposites—firmness and softness, strength and lightness, insubstantiality and substantiality, activity and passivity, motion and quiescence.

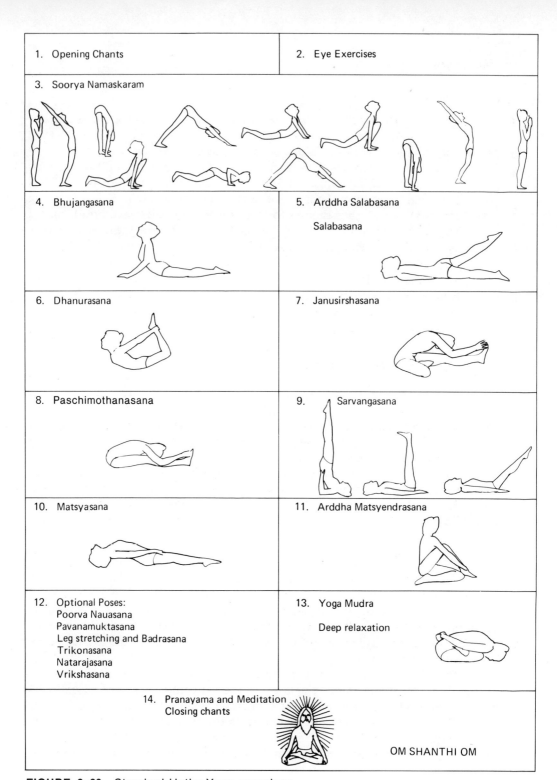

1. Opening Chants	2. Eye Exercises

3. Soorya Namaskaram

4. Bhujangasana	5. Arddha Salabasana Salabasana

6. Dhanurasana	7. Janusirshasana

8. Paschimothanasana	9. Sarvangasana

10. Matsyasana	11. Arddha Matsyendrasana

12. Optional Poses:
   Poorva Nauasana
   Pavanamuktasana
   Leg stretching and Badrasana
   Trikonasana
   Natarajasana
   Vrikshasana
	13. Yoga Mudra
	
	   Deep relaxation

14. Pranayama and Meditation
   Closing chants

OM SHANTHI OM

FIGURE 6-20   Standard Hatha Yoga exercises

STANDARD HATHA YOGA EXERCISES

1. Opening Chants.
2. Eye exercises (vertical, horizontal, diagonals, half circles, full circle both ways), 8–10 times each.
3. Soorya Namaskaram - Sun Worship, 3-4 times each.
4. Bhujangasana - Cobra Pose, 2 times; concentration between shoulder blades.
5. Arddha Salabasana - Half Locust Pose, 2 times each leg; concentration lower back. Salabasana - Locust Pose, once; concentration lower back.
6. Dhanurasana - Bow Pose, once; concentration entire spine.
7. Janusirshasana - Head to Knee Pose, once each side; concentration lower back and legs.
8. Paschimothanasana - Forward Bending Pose, once; concentration lower back and legs.
9. Sarvangasana - Shoulder Stand, once for at least 3–5 minutes; concentration thyroid gland.
10. Matsyasana - Fish Pose, once; concentration thyroid gland.
11. Arddha Matsyendrasana - Half Spinal Twist, once each way.
12. Optional poses.
13. Yoga Mudra - Yogic Seal, once for at least 30 seconds, deep relaxation (tighten and relax all muscles, watch breath, watch mind).
14. PRANAYAMA (deep breathing; kapalabhati—diaphragmatic breathing—3 rounds; Nadi Suddhi—nerve purification—alternate nostril breathing) and OM SHANTHI OM (closing chant).

The self-defense aspects of Tai-Chi are based on nonaggression and nonopposition. The key is strategy without the exertion of awkward force or strength. This attitude is consistent with some of the nonmovement meditative practices.

Each movement involves the alternate shifting of the body weight from one leg to another and is synchronized with breathing. Performance is slow, light, calm, and effortless for the fifteen to thirty minutes that an entire "set" takes to complete. Disadvantages of the technique are that the movements are difficult to remember and it cannot be self-taught.

An abbreviated version of Tai-Chi Ch'uan has been developed, which is called Tai-Chi Chih. Only six movements are involved and they take only five to fifteen minutes to perform. This simplified method supposedly brings about all the healthful benefits of Tai-Chi Ch'uan, but can be quickly self-taught from a book. [93]

Head Rotations. 1) Sit comfortably in a chair, keeping the spine erect and your hands resting on your knees. 2) Now, simply lower your chin toward your chest. 3) Then lower your right ear toward your right shoulder. 4) Next, drop your head backward gently. 5) Then, lower your left ear toward your left shoulder . . . Remember, do not strain. This exercise is designed to limber the neck and relieve tension.

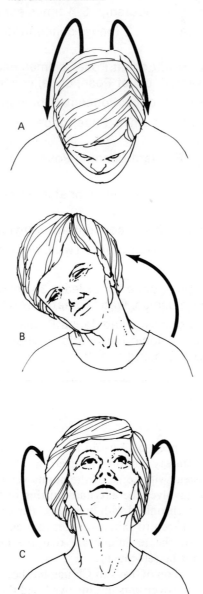

A

B

C

FIGURE 6-21   Yoga head rotations

Figure 6–22 illustrates a fifteen-minute series of Tai-Chi warm-up exercises called the "Eight Precious Set." These exercises prepare a student for the more complex Tai-Chi Ch'uan movements. They, too, give the student the feelings of warmth, energy, and tingling, and they are a good preparation for any athletic activity. Each exercise is aimed at toning and stimulating a particular group of organs.

Massage

Massage is a generic term encompassing hundreds of manipulative techniques for helping the body to relax, release tensions, balance energy flow, and soothe the being with gentle caring. Tappan describes massage as the systematic and scientific manipulation of the soft tissues of the body through gliding, percussing, compressing, or vibrating. [94, p. 3]

Massage has been practiced in the Orient for thousands of years. In China and Japan, it is combined with the knowledge of acupuncture points and called Shiatsu.

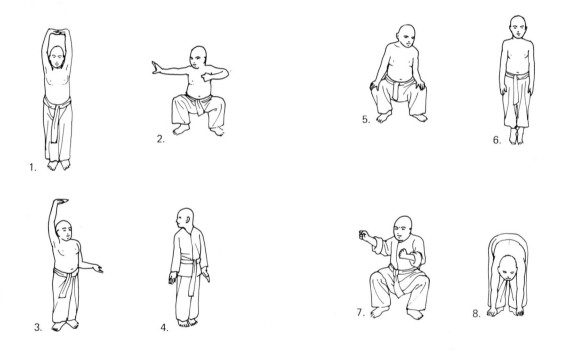

1. OVERALL STRETCH (8X)
2. PULL BOW AND ARROW (16X—LF & RT)
3. STOMACH STRETCH (16X—LF & RT)
4. NECK ROTATION (16X—LF & RT)

X = times; LF = left; RT = right.

5. UPPER TORSO ROTATION (16X—LF & RT)
6. CLASP HANDS AND STRETCH (8X)
7. PUNCH (16X—LF & RT)
8. SERIAL STRETCH (8X)

FIGURE 6-22 Tai-Chi Ch'uan: The Eight Precious Set

Nurses have traditionally been taught the French massage strokes of *effleurage* (gliding), *petrissage* (light pinching and kneading), *tapotement* (striking and gentle pounding), *friction* (compression), and *vibration* (shaking). [94, p. 3]

Massage induces relaxation and relieves pain and muscle tension. It has been suggested that massage may have the ability to stimulate the production of the peptide, endorphin. Within this class of endorphins exists the enkephalins which may be neurotransmitters for pain impulses.

Rogers feels that the increase in the levels of enkephalins accounts for how acupuncture and acupressure work. [94] The systems are based on the energy pathways or meridians which provide vitality and nourishment for all the vital organs. A successful attempt to relate the Western systems of anatomy and physiology to the meridians has been proposed. Perhaps further research on the function of enkephalins will help to explain this relationship more fully.

Zone Therapy, Reflexology, and Foot Massage

Although acupuncture is thousands of years old, it rarely used the feet as treatment sites, although points were identifiable on them. In 1913, Dr. William H. Fitzgerald brought "Zone Therapy" to the United States while directing the Nose and Throat Department of St. Francis Hospital in Hartford, Connecticut. His discovery was that applied pressure and massaging of certain zones had a definite effect in bringing about normal physiologic functioning in all parts of the zone treated, no matter how remote this area might have been from the part on which the treatment was performed.

Zone therapy is a method of massaging and applying pressure with the thumbs, fingers, and heel of the hand, or with a special vibrating device, which produces a reflex action on other organs or tissues of the body through the nerve endings in the soles of the feet (see Figure 6–23). Problem areas are found by locating small nodules of crystal-like formation under the tissues of the skin on the sole of the foot.

There are many ways to stimulate reflex action to the nerve endings and to the flow of blood throughout the body. Some of these methods are general massage, zone therapy, various forms of hydrotherapy, and vibration.

A normal treatment takes approximately twenty minutes, unless pain is experienced by the client or some contraindication—such as an ulcerated area or blood clot—is discovered in history or examination.

The massage should be given in a low rotary-like motion, not using the flat ball of the thumb as much as the lateral aspect. The pressure should be firm but gentle at first, and gradually increased with as much pressure as the client is able to tolerate comfortably. The thumbnails should be filed quite low.

It is important to enlist client participation and feedback as the nurse progresses so that problem areas can be properly assessed and appropriate history-taking can ensue. If a client complains of tenderness in the arch of the foot, for example, questions regarding past or current history or symptoms of urinary tract infections or problems would be indicated. The client might also experience a sensation in his or her bladder rather than in the foot itself. This, too, should be followed up.

Reflexology is based on the idea that there are nerve or (electro-magnetic) energy connections between all parts and organs of the body which connect with the feet. By pressing firmly on the spot on your foot which corresponds to your problem organ you can have a positive influence on the ailment, possibly by improving the circulation to that organ by stimulating the energy and nerve connections.

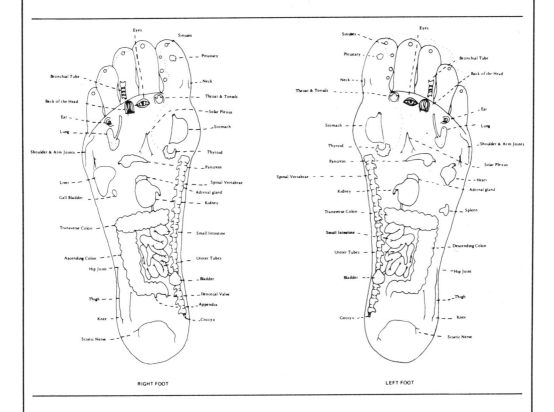

Press in all over the soles, tops and sides of your feet with your thumbs. Press firmly and hard. Some points will feel good or neutral, and some may be quite sore. Check the foot chart for the connected organ or body part to see if there are any problems in the connected area. Because you can stimulate all parts of the body simply by working on the feet, a reflexology foot massage is very refreshing, for yourself or for someone else.

FIGURE 6-23   Foot reflexology chart

Reprinted with permission from Anne Kent Rush, *Getting Clear* (New York: Random House, 1973), p. 140.

As with many of the Chinese medical techniques, the research substantiating the technique is largely found in the testimonies of practitioners and their clients rather than in validated studies. Since the method does not lend itself to assessment of nerve pathways via dissection, it is difficult to explain why it works according to Western anatomical standards.

What most practitioners will agree to is the beneficial effects of the foot massage—relaxation of nervous tension, increase of blood and lymphatic circulation, and resultant feelings of stimulation and well-being.

One of the simplest, most clearly written books about the techniques and purposes of massage is *The Massage Book* by George Downing. [24] In it, he lays out some easy-to-follow hints about massage in general:

1. Apply pressure when you do massage.
2. Relax your hands. A brief relaxation exercise before the massage might help.
3. Mold the hands to fit the contours over which they are passing.
4. Maintain an evenness of speed and pressure as long as steadiness and confidence are not sacrificed.
5. Explore and define the underlying structure of the body of the person being massaged.
6. Use weight rather than muscles to apply pressure.
7. Once contact has been made with the client's body, try not to break it until the massage or exercise is completely finished.
8. Do massage with the entire body, not just the hands.
9. Pay attention to the body mechanics of standing, sitting, or kneeling to prevent muscle straining.
10. Always remember that the person being massaged is a person, not an intricate muscle and bone machine. [24, pp. 27–31]

Above all, practitioners should feel free to experiment with new techniques and styles, and to encourage feedback from the client regarding what works best for him or her. Involve the client in the process. Foot massage, particularly, lends itself to self-massage techniques that can be easily adopted if the person can assume the crossed-legged position. Family members can easily be taught how to perform massage on each other. More will be said about touch as one of the most primitive and effective forms of communication, caring, and healing in later chapters of this book.

Hand massage follows the same principles of zone therapy as foot massage. Hand massage is often less threatening to a client in the early phases of a therapeutic relationship. The hand is easily accessible and carries fewer social taboos than the foot. The diagram in Figure 6–24 depicts the reflexology of the hand quite accurately.

Acupuncture and Acupressure

Acupuncture and Acupressure make use of hands-on healing to tone and sedate different organs and parts of the body by stimulating certain points along energy pathways called *meridians*. For nearly five thousand years, the Chinese have used acupuncture as therapy for all kinds of ailments. Sometimes needles are used

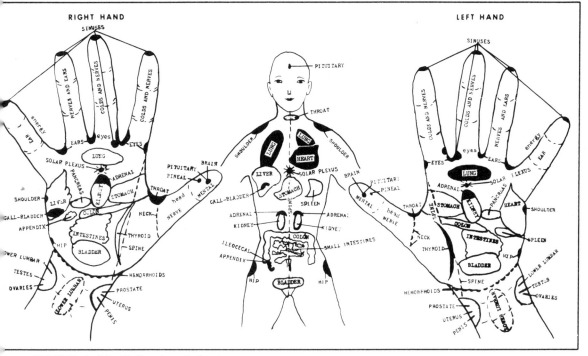

FIGURE 6-24 Reflex hand chart

Reprinted with permission from Mildred Carter, *Hand Reflexology: Key to Perfect Health* (West Nyack, N.Y.: Parker Publishing Co., Inc., 1975), pp. 27–28.

with electrical stimulation; sometimes only simple pressure or massage is necessary. The acupuncture meridians are numerous and each has varying numbers of points along it. Twelve major meridians exist and are briefly outlined in Figures 6–25 and 6–26. The meridians are of differing lengths and govern different organs.

Meridians coursing the front of the body are yin; those traversing the back are yang. Meridians which have their origin in the earth (lower) are yin; those originating in the heavens are yang (see the arrows in the two figures). There are over 600 points along the meridians, and it takes years of study and practice to learn to use them for healing purposes.

Touch for Health

A method of healing and health promotion based on acupuncture meridians, kinesiology, and chiropractic is called Touch for Health. A beginning knowledge of this technique can be mastered in one weekend.

Touch for Health is a method of attaining and maintaining natural health using acupuncture, touch, and massage to improve postural balance and reduce physical and mental pain and tension.

Mankind is seen as a structural, chemical, and spiritual or psychological being. There must be a balance between the three. The methods presented touch on all three aspects, but the emphasis is more on the structural, since this seems to be the most neglected area. Touch for Health involves touching and massaging the

LIFESTYLING   **251**

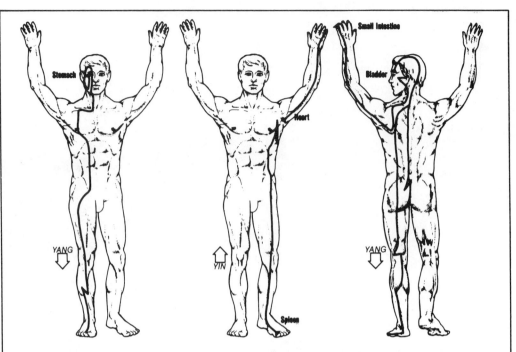

MERIDIAN MASSAGE

MERIDIAN MASSAGE brings up body energy and gives the spirits a lift, too. You can do it fully clothed, of course. And while this model begins with the Stomach Meridian - actually, you can begin with any meridian. Face your subject and use both hands to run the right and left sides simultaneously.

STOMACH MERIDIAN: Start under pupil of eye - go straight down to jaw; circle up, around face to frontal eminences - drop straight down over eye to clavicle - go out to sides to directly above nipples; then down over chest - jog in at stomach and cut at hips - down legs, outside kneecaps and go 'out' at second toe.

SPLEEN: Start top outside tip of big toe - go up inside of leg and straight up, veering outside chest to arm crease - then halfway back down rib cage and 'out'.

HEART: Start in armpit - go down inside arm, over palm and 'out' the inside little finger.

BLADDER: Part One/Start inner corner of eyes - up over head and down back either side of spine to below waist - jog up and in toward spine to mid-back - down between buttocks and 'out' to either side. Part Two/Start top of shoulder on path already run - out to mid-shoulder blade - down back and back of leg behind ankle bone and 'out' on little toe.

KIDNEY: Start on ball of foot - up sole to back of ankle bone - circle back down over the heel - continue straight up inside leg to breast bone - 'out' on clavicle.

CIRCULATION/SEX: Start outside nipples and go up and around arm crease - down inside arm and 'out' middle finger.

TRIPLE WARMER: Start at third (ring) finger - up outside arm over elbow to behind the ear lobe - circle up back of ear and around to top forward ear connection - go forward to the

FIGURE 6–25 Meridian massage

Reprinted with permission from *In Touch for Health*, 4, no. 8 (August 1979), Newsletter published by Touch for Health Foundation, 1174 N. Lake, Pasadena, Ca. 91104

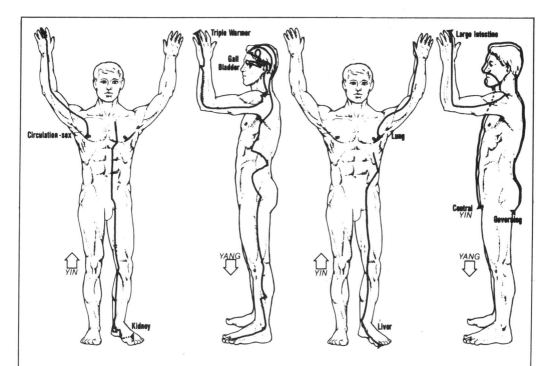

GALL BLADDER: Start outer corner of eyes - back to orifice of ears - up toward the crown of head - circle forward and down over temples and back to base of skull. Now - forward over top of head to frontal eminences - back same path to base of neck. Across back of shoulders, forward under arms to side of rib cage - half circle back, down and come forward on the hips - down outside legs in front of ankle bone and 'out' the fourth toe.

LIVER: Start inside big toe - up inside leg to hip bone - backward on hip; up around the waist and forward to rib cage - 'out' under nipples.

LUNG: Start upper chest in line with arm crease - down inside arm in line with thumb and out over thumbnail.

LARGE INTESTINE: Start tip of first finger - go up outside of arm - over shoulder and in to base of throat - up face and in to midline under base of nose - back and 'out' at flare of nostrils.

CENTRAL: Start at pubic bone - up body midline - 'out' at lower lip.

GOVERNING: Start base of spine - up and over head - down over nose - 'out' at upper lip.

And that's MERIDIAN MASSAGE - a great way to give a person needed energy and 'lift'!

FIGURE 6-26 Meridian massage

Reprinted by permission from *In Touch for Health,* 4, no. 8 (August 1979), 7. Newsletter published by Touch for Health Foundation, 1174 N. Lake, Pasadena, Ca. 91104

body and the muscles, using their functions, their relative strength and weakness, and how they work in the body, to get the body into better balance.

Pain is the final alarm before some life-threatening malfunction takes place. Just prior to the pain and malfunction, there are signs and symptoms which can be recognized. One of these is a weakening of the muscles and a change in the posture. Individuals must learn to listen and to feel what is going on in their bodies and be able to correct the minor problems before they develop into serious illnesses. Using Touch for Health methods helps prevent malfunctions and pains from developing, as well as correct the reason for the pain and allow the life force to flow uninterrupted throughout the body.

Using applied kinesiology, the muscle-balancing massage, therapists test clients for specific muscle weaknesses and treat them. They are not just treating muscles, they are treating the whole body. The body is all one unit with many different systems and functions. Some of the muscles are more related to some specific organ, they may share a lymph vessel or an acupuncture meridian, for example. When the muscle is improved by restoring the energy flow of these systems, this also gives relief to the organ which is sharing that system.

There are many ways to look at the body and just as many different kinds of judgments to be made about it. A doctor uses a number of diagnostic methods. Some of them are simple enough that with practice, lay people can learn what they can do for themselves to help maintain their own health care. Testing the functions of the muscles themselves is one of the most effective ways of evaluating the structural balance to be achieved.

Reading the body language is one way to become aware of what is happening with the body. Balance is evaluated. Both halves of the body should be symmetrical. There shouldn't be any unusual protrusions. How do the clothes fit on the body? Are they twisted to adhere to a twisted waist, a misplaced hip or vertebra?

How to test muscles. It is important to test only the first couple of inches of the range of the muscle action, applying the pressure gradually and releasing it gradually. With a great or sudden force, even a strong muscle could be overcome. *Retesting* is also necessary once the muscle has been reevaluated.

In order for the muscles to perform efficiently, all the energies from all systems in the body which affect that muscle must be able to flow freely. If, for any reason, this energy is cut off or turned off, then the muscle weakens. With the application of kinesiology, the energy flow is restored with the reflexes of the different systems. These reflexes act like electrical switches in turning on or off the energies to the muscles.

Neuro-lymphatic massage points. The energy to the lymphatic system is regulated by what is called neuro-lymphatic reflexes, located mainly on the chest and back. These reflex points act like circuit breakers or switches that get turned off when the system is overloaded. The location of the reflex points does not seem to correspond to the position of the lymph glands, but they are related. The points vary in size. Some are palpable, can be felt, and others are not. They are usually tender spots, and the tenderness is usually greater in the front of the body than in the back. The reflexes or areas which are found to be the most sore seem to be the ones in greatest need of massage.

To work on the neuro-lymphatic reflexes for a muscle that has been found to be weak, points on the body that are shown for that muscle are found. [See Figure 6–27] Treatment requires moving around the point with the fingers using a deep massage, and keeping this pressure for 20–30 seconds. The amount of tenderness can be an indication of the extent of the problem. It is important that if the person being treated becomes too uncomfortable and wishes to stop, his judgment be respected. The tenderness will decrease as treatment progresses over several days. When the reflexes have been turned on in this way, the blockage in the energy of the lymph flow to the organ and muscle is relieved and the weak muscle will have improved in strength when retested.

Neuro-vascular holding points. Neuro-vascular holding points are located mainly on the head. These points, for strengthening a muscle, require simple contact with the pads of the fingers, merely touching and slightly stretching the skin. A few seconds after contact is made, a slight pulse can be felt at a steady rate of 70–74 beats per minute. This pulse is not related to the heartbeat, but is believed to be the primitive pulsation of the microscopic capillary bed in the skin. After a pulse has been felt on both sides and it has become synchronized, then the neuro-vascular points may be held for about 20 seconds or up to 10 minutes, depending on the severity of the problem. This appears to improve the blood circulation to both the muscle and the related organ, and the weak muscle will have increased strength when retested.

Meridians. Acupressure vessels, or meridians, are located throughout the body. They contain a free-flowing, colorless, non-cellular liquid which may be partly actuated by the heart. These meridians have been mapped and measured by modern technological methods, electronically, thermatically, and radioactively. With practice, they can also be felt. There are specific acupuncture points along the meridians. These points are electromagnetic in character and consist of small, oval cells called Bonham corpuscles, which surround the capillaries throughout the body. There are some 500 points which are being used most frequently in a definite sequence, depending on the action desired. Using the flat of the hand will give better coverage, but it is only necessary to come within 2 inches of the meridian, either off to the side or even above the skin over clothing, for it to be effective. Tracing can be done quickly, but it is sometimes more beneficial when done with more care. Retest the muscle, and if it is not stronger, try tracing in the opposite direction, except for the heart meridian.

New muscles are chosen, perhaps those related to some current health problem, and familiarity with the tests is developed. Whenever a weakness is encountered, that muscle is looked up and one or two of the treatment techniques are used. The muscle is always retested and a chart is kept of which muscles are being worked on. It is important to become aware of what is happening with the body and how using these techniques can fit into everyday life, and the importance of the involvement of the whole family in maintaining each other's health and well-being. [96]

Rolfing

Another body therapy gaining popularity is rolfing, a technique of manipulating deep fascia tissue to liberate pain, anger, etc., and to allow the body to resume its normal healthful stance. The technique, which might be likened to deep painful massage, originated with Ida Rolf, a physician, whose theory combines components of the Alexander Technique with some osteopathic techniques.

Stress-Reduction Programs

In addition to the number, intensity, and duration of stressors a person must face, past experiences with comparable stressors strongly shape the type of response experienced. Negative arousal symptoms have been enumerated as one response, and

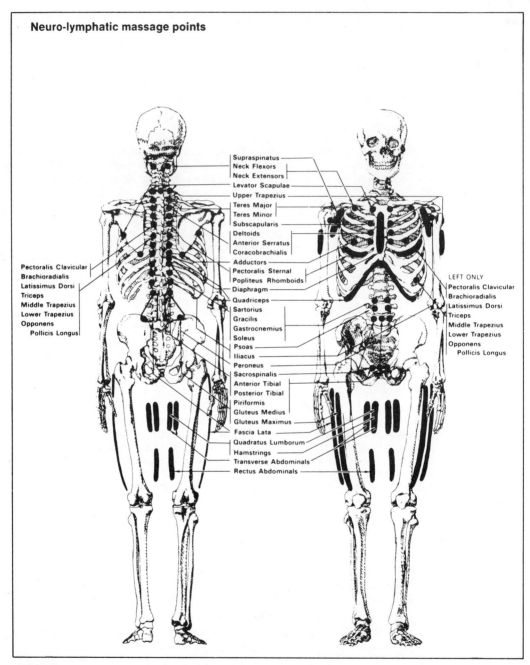

Neuro-lymphatic massage points

Supraspinatus
Neck Flexors
Neck Extensors
Levator Scapulae
Upper Trapezius
Teres Major
Teres Minor
Subscapularis
Deltoids
Anterior Serratus
Coracobrachialis
Adductors
Pectoralis Sternal
Popliteus Rhomboids
Diaphragm
Quadriceps
Sartorius
Gracilis
Gastrocnemius
Soleus
Psoas
Iliacus
Peroneus
Sacrospinalis
Anterior Tibial
Posterior Tibial
Piriformis
Gluteus Medius
Gluteus Maximus
Fascia Lata
Quadratus Lumborum
Hamstrings
Transverse Abdominals
Rectus Abdominals

Pectoralis Clavicular
Brachioradialis
Latissimus Dorsi
Triceps
Middle Trapezius
Lower Trapezius
Opponens
Pollicis Longus

LEFT ONLY
Pectoralis Clavicular
Brachioradialis
Latissimus Dorsi
Triceps
Middle Trapezius
Lower Trapezius
Opponens
Pollicis Longus

FIGURE 6-27   Neuro-lymphatic massage points

Reprinted by permission from *In Touch for Health,* 4, no. 8 (August 1979), 5. Newsletter published by Touch for Health Foundation, 1174 N. Lake, Pasadena, Ca. 91104

certain ego defenses (for example, denial, repression, etc.) unconsciously come into play to alleviate anxiety temporarily. When the stressful situation becomes a conscious event, an individual may ignore the problem, seek temporary diversion, or actively attempt to resolve it. A few fear-specific stress-reduction programs that can assist the person in actively coping with stress are described in the following section.

Coping Skills Training

Current interest in coping centers around coping skills training which is based on Goldried, Swinn, and Richardson's work in deep muscle relaxation and systematic desensitization (such as the type used in the clinical example on page 263). Meichenbaum and Cameron have taken these techniques and developed a "stress inoculation" program. [23] The principle is that if people learn how to respond inappropriately to a stressful situation, they can teach themselves (or be taught) to change a stress response to a relaxation response.

The first step is to learn some form of relaxation similar to the techniques thus far enumerated in this section of the chapter. Slipping into a relaxed state should become second nature in order that it may be called upon at a moment's notice. A form of breathing relaxation is a good backup form, for example.

Next, a Subjective Unit of Distress hierarchy is formulated in which typical personal stress situations are listed and ranked. In a relaxed state, the least stressful scene is visualized (sights, smells, etc.). Any signs or feelings of tension act as the signal to relax. Once an image or situation can be faced comfortably, the next situation is approached. At the end of four or five days, the list should be complete, and the individual should work through it two or three times.

Stress-coping thoughts comprise the next level of coping. A stressful situation is called up, along with psychophysiologic and behavioral responses. Finally, mental self-statements, such as those suggested by the rational emotive therapy exercise presented in the self-responsibility section of this chapter, are used. Some stress-coping thoughts for use in times of stress to quiet negative arousal have been formulated by Meichenbaum and Cameron. [20, as quoted therein, p. 124]

1. *Preparation:*
   There's nothing to worry about.
   I'm going to be all right.
   I've succeeded with this before.
   What exactly do I have to do?
   I know I can do each one of these tasks.
   It's easier once you get started.
   I'll jump in and be all right.
   Tomorrow I'll be through it.
   Don't let negative thoughts creep in.

2. *Confronting the stressful situation:*
   Stay organized.
   Take it step by step; don't rush.
   I can do this; I'm doing it now.
   I can only do my best.

Any tension I feel is a signal to use my coping exercises.
I can get help if I need it.
If I don't think about fear, I won't be afraid.
If I get tense, I'll take a breather and relax.
It's OK to make mistakes.*

The final phase is to practice all the steps using real situations until relaxation becomes an automatic response in times of stress.

Coping and Crisis Intervention

Despite a person's own problem-solving skills, certain maturational and situational crises can prove too much for him to handle. It is at this point that the nurse or professional helper's assistance is sought. The nurse is asked for help in assessing the extent of the crisis state in the client.

It is important to isolate the precipitating event in a crisis. What was the final incident that went beyond the individual's ability to handle the situation? How is the person responding to the problem? Is the person realistic and oriented, able to problem solve, or is he immobilized?

Crisis anticipation, identification, and prevention were mentioned in the preceding chapter. The interpersonal process of helping someone cope with crisis is often called *crisis intervention,* which is a short-term helping process that focuses on the resolution of an immediate problem through the use of personal, social, and environmental resources. Nurses are constantly called upon to participate in crisis anticipation and resolution as part of their helping, healing role.

Aguilera and Messick have designed a crisis intervention model which is used by many different health professionals to assess and assist the person experiencing acute stress. [1] Figure 6–28 outlines this helpful paradigm.

Some basic guidelines for helping a person in crisis follow:

Show acceptance of the person and establish a positive, concerned relationship.

Help the person confront the crisis by talking about his present feelings of denial, anger, guilt, or grief.

Help the person confront the crisis by taking it in manageable doses.

Recognize denial as a normal reaction.

Explain the relationship between the crisis situation and his present behavior and feelings. Help him understand that his emotions are normal within the context of crisis.

Help the person find facts rather than speculating or guessing.

Explore past life occurrences only in relation to the existing crisis.

Avoid giving false reassurance.

Don't encourage the person to blame others for the crisis event.

Anticipate that people facing loss may behave in a grossly maladaptive way.

Explore coping mechanisms.

* Adapted from D. Meichenbaum and R. Cameron, "The Clinical Potential of Modifying What Clients Say to Themselves," in *Self-Control: Power to the Person,* eds. M. J. Mahoney and C. E. Thoreses (New York: Wadsworth, 1974).

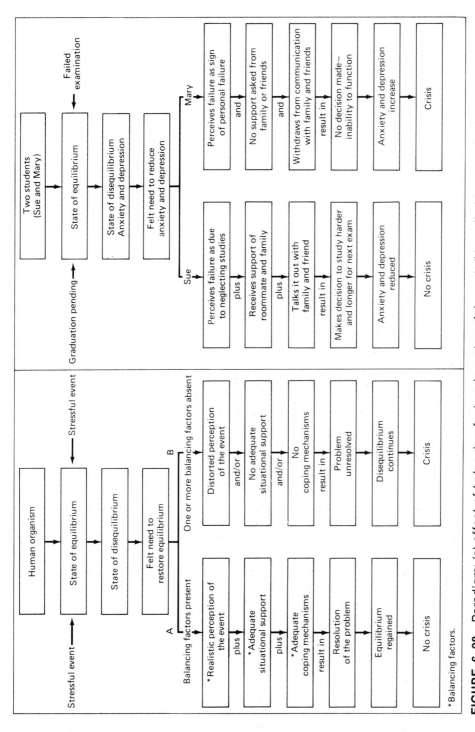

FIGURE 6-28 Paradigm: (a) effect of balancing factors in a stressful event; (b) applied to case studies

Reprinted from Donna Aguilera and J. Messick, *Crisis Intervention: Theory and Methodology*, 3rd ed. (St. Louis: C. V. Mosby, 1978), pp. 68–69.

Strengthen or reinforce previously learned behavior patterns that can be effective but are not presently being used.

Clarify and reemphasize the person's responsibility for his own behavior, decisions, and way of life.

Help the person establish necessary social relationships and change personal behavior accordingly.

Assist the person in making and accepting help.

Techniques which aid effective crisis assessment include:

A straightforward approach with simple, direct questions.

The ability to "walk in another person's shoes."

The ability to grasp the depth of another's despair and to share the feelings that this evokes.

Finally, having the courage not to run away from frightening experiences, such as suicide threats or attempts.

Now let's examine some general rules which can help clients adapt to environmental stressors, which can aggravate or precipitate a crisis. First, the predictability of a stressor affects the degree of response to it. [88] When an irritant is identified and brought into consciousness, a deliberate response can be incorporated, thus reducing the long-term stressful effects. Examples to illustrate the point abound, for example, in working situations in which loud, periodic noises or discharges of fumes or fibers occur. Second, the social context in which stress occurs is important. A boyfriend's outburst at his fiancée in the midst of a family gathering, for example, will have heavier repercussions than the same argument carried on in the privacy of their own quarters.

Finally, the feeling of control over a stressful situation (for example, driving home in the rush-hour traffic) is a key factor in coping. [88] If a client can opt to take a bus or to leave the office at a non-rush-hour time, he will feel as if he has modified the situation.

Crisis anticipation and intervention are primarily preventive nursing measures aimed at helping clients protect themselves from further complications and stress. Nurturative and generative aspects of nursing care are naturally incorporated into any plan of care as innovative coping strategies are devised with the client. At various stages of crisis work, the nurse is also called upon to utilize healing, soothing, and relaxing therapies which can be viewed as nurturative. All three interrelated aspects of nursing care are employed to promote wholeness.

Support Systems and Groups

Coping with stress invariably involves some type of support system. This support can be in the form of another person or group. Many of the consciousness-raising groups of the 1960s and 1970s embodied the group-support concept. Spinoffs of this movement encompass a huge range from psychotherapeutic groups to interest groups rallying around a specific need, issue, or cause with very specific short-term goals.

Three of the hundreds of groups specializing in holistic approaches to self-growth, awareness, and responsibility were described in Figure 2-5 on pp. 61–62. These groups are offered as courses at such centers as Esalen, located in Big Sur, California, where this type of activity has been in operation for over twenty years. The focus of all support groups is to enhance the individual, family, or group's ability to deal effectively with challenge.

Support systems may be of several types. The most spontaneous example is the family, which typifies informal care giving. An informal support system is one in which distance and objectivity are not present. [11] Authentic mutual and reciprocal advice and opinions are extended. Organized supports are composed of a community of interest-based groups which do not have professionals directing the care giving. Alcoholics Anonymous is a good example of such an organization.

Religious denominations make up a third source of group support. The power of such groups should not be underestimated. Strong bonds often exist and charitable endeavors include helping individuals and families in times of crisis.

Professionals can be involved with these formal and informal support systems in several ways:

1. by initiating or helping to organize new support systems inside community institutions where they are needed;
2. by organizing new support systems in the outside community;
3. by consulting with and educating organizers and other key members of organized support systems; and
4. by consulting with and educating members of unorganized supportive networks within the community. [11]

Clinical Applications of Stress Management and Lifestyle Modification

Earlier in this chapter, various stress-management methods were mentioned. Basically, any therapeutic stress-reduction program will involve the following:

1. The identification of the relevant responses to stress the person experiences. This should include a description of the immediate anxiety reaction. This can be done by reconstructing a particularly stressful situation and determining the responses, coping and defense mechanisms, both effective and ineffective, and support systems available and/or utilized.
2. Identification of subsequent cognitive, behavioral, and physiologic reactions which maintained the anxiety level.
3. Application of the most efficient and efficacious techniques to eliminate the immediate reactions and training the client in self-control skills that preclude the recurrence of stress-maintaining reactions. [82, p. 273]

The following list contains some common manipulations used to reduce the stress response. Items are listed in terms of which response components are their focus.

1. *Physiologic reactions:* relaxation therapies; systematic desensitization; implosive therapy; and biofeedback;

2. *Cognitions:* rational emotive therapy; semantic conditioning; self-instructions; modified self-verbalizations; thought stopping; placebo and expectancy manipulations;

3. *Overt behaviors:* reinforcement of approach behavior; response prevention; modeling; and contact desensitization. [82, pp. 278-79]

A theory of self-control of stress responses that requires an *interpersonal therapeutic relationship* has been proposed by Donald Melchenbaum. "A cognitive theory of self-control" is composed of three stages—self-observation, incompatible thoughts and behaviors, and cognitions concerning change. [82]

In stage one (*self-observation*), the clients observe their own behavior. They are shown how to monitor their own thoughts, feelings, and interpersonal behaviors. This can be done with self-recording tools, such as journals, flow sheets, and checklists. With help, clients begin to pinpoint maladaptive events and inappropriate reactions.

Clients and clinician go through a series of steps, such as interviewing, testing, and homework assignments, in which clients come to gain a different view of their behaviors and emotional disturbances. As self-awareness increases, clients gain a sense of control of their emotional states and behaviors. They begin to see their contribution to their own experiences and their responsibility in the shaping of their responses to others. Both nurse and client need to understand their thoughts, feelings, and behaviors, and being able to explain these things helps clients to feel more in control of their lives.

In stage two, (incompatible thoughts and behaviors), clients begin to visualize and initiate new behaviors. These activities are incompatible with older maladaptive patterns. This incompatibility in itself will raise anxiety levels and necessitate stage three (*cognitions concerning change*), in which stage the nurse and client reinforce new desired behaviors and clients begin to generalize through new application concepts to other areas of their lives.

During the transitions among the three stages, clients come to identify their anxiety arousal as helpful rather than destructive signaling. Any of the signs of a stress response, such as sweaty palms, increased heart and respiratory rates, or muscle tension, become cues to use the coping techniques which have been gained through practice.

The resultant change in mental attitude may in itself change the client's negative arousal automatic responses. The developer of this theory labels this change as one of "learned resourcefulness," replacing a sense of "learned helplessness." Thus, even a negative arousal state is not as important as what clients say to themselves about that state that causes either effective coping and resolution or gradual self-destruction through increasingly higher anxiety maintenance.

It appears that although Emile Coué's famous self-statement, "Everyday in every way I'm getting better and better," [16] may have some benefit in changing cognition and behaviors, the more detailed a set of mental instructions is, the better. This confirms the approach used in later stages of Autogenic Training in which clients are given very specific instructions about (1) the exact response desired; (2) under what conditions they will perform the response; and (3) the need for a positively stated phrase to describe the desired outcome.

Now let's examine an example of an application of intrapersonal lifestyle modification:

A 20-year-old, well-adjusted nursing student came to her instructor seeking self-help assistance for a persistent fear of needles. This fear was impeding her professional functioning in the delivery room of a busy, metropolitan hospital where she was beginning her clinical nursing experience.

J. was observing a delivery in which a medication was being administered intravenously, when she began to feel flushed and experienced some alarming visual sensations. The room seemed to "expand and shrink" and she began to feel herself swaying and falling. She was assisted to a chair where she lost consciousness for several seconds.

Reviewing the incident, J. stated that she had witnessed births, bleeding, and surgery before and had felt no sense of dread related to these occurrences. She was able to isolate the actual piercing of the skin by a needle as the major irritant. She recalled her first personal experience of the fear of needles during an early childhood immunization. Since that time, any sight of a needle brought on the aforementioned symptoms. She had discussed this problem with her mother, but had received no professional help until this visit.

J. had been participating in an Autogenic Training group for six weeks and had successfully used it to clear up some stress-related acne. She asked if she could incorporate a phrase for needles.

A desensitization hierarchy was designed by J. with the therapist's assistance. The lowest level irritant—a picture of a needle—to the highest level—a large needle piercing her own skin—were pictured. Pictures of other levels (including tuberculin patch test needles and intercutaneous and subcutaneous injection visualizations) were interspersed between the lowest and highest pictures on the scale.

The procedure went as follows:

1. The autogenic phrases were repeated three times.
2. At the end of the third series of AT phrases, the following was added:
   "Needles are not important to me."
   "Needles are not important to me."
3. The student first pictured herself in a safe, warm cocoon, similar to a see-through bubble. The student was asked to picture a needle—the hub, the shaft, the bevel from the safety of the bubble. In her mind, she was to pick it up, feel it, handle it. The accompanying instructions were:
   "Even though the needle is being handled, it is as if it is not your hand that is being touched by it. You are safe and warm in your cocoon (which J. had previously visualized created for herself), observing your hand picking it up and handling the needle. Although it is your hand, it doesn't affect you. It is as if you are watching your hand from your cocoon. Let any feelings you are experiencing wash over you as you remain safe and warm, observing, in your cocoon. Feel the warmth and relaxation flowing through you."
4. Now move on to the next image in your mind.
5. Each image was explored in the same manner—the nurse trainer speaking aloud as J. followed until an image began to cause discomfort. J. indicated this by raising her index finger.
6. At this point, the nurse and student returned to the most recent comfortable image and concluded.
7. J. was to repeat this proceduce four times a day independently, keep a log of her responses, and return in two days.

J. advanced to Image 4 on Day 1 and Image 8 on Day 3. She completed the rest of the images on her own. A week later she reported that she had donated blood and observed the whole procedure without experiencing any negative symptoms. She felt she had mastered this fear and looked forward to giving injections, administering IVs, and so forth, during the next semester.

This uncomplicated example demonstrates the use of some of the stress-reduction techniques that have been mentioned. Nurses need to practice these techniques with professional supervision before attempting them on clients. Actual or simulated application training is an important aspect of stress-management training. Exposing clients to stress or anxiety-producing situations and evaluating coping responses to them is one test of the training's efficacy.

A clinical situation that demonstrates intrapersonal and interpersonal aspects of lifestyle management follows:

Susan is a 19-year-old nursing student who is entering the clinical rotation portion of her education. She has always been slightly overweight and finds herself constantly nibbling during periods of stress. Susan has gained five pounds during the first two weeks of school and she is very discouraged. She has never sought professional help for her weight problem before, but she decides to investigate the student health center's weight management program.

In an holistic nursing approach, the nurse will collaborate with the staff nutritionist to assess the eating and activity patterns, the physiologic and psychosocial factors contributing to and maintaining the overweight, and the education regarding the causes and risks of overweight. Following this assessment, using various self-assessment and objective goals, a weight management program would be designed with Susan, which would focus on the following goals:

1. changing long-term eating behaviors (*Self-Responsibility and Environmental Modification*)
2. lowering caloric intake (*Nutrition*)
3. increasing caloric expenditure (*Fitness*)
4. decreasing tension surrounding school (*Stress Management)*

The table on pp. 264–65 contains a variety of different strategies for each goal. Several methods may need to be tried in each (lifestyle) area. The long-term goal for Susan is to incorporate a series of lifestyle modifications stemming from a conscious change of attitudes and behaviors which will gradually alter not only her lifestyle but also the quality of her life.

In selecting which methods will work best for her, Susan may need to evaluate less holistic approaches to weight loss, such as diet pills, protein-sparing drinks, hormones, or even acupuncture. Each approach should be evaluated from an overall long-range point of view. Criteria for evaluating might include:

1. Does it address any of the lifestyle elements?
2. Does it make claims of overnight success, but no long-term behavior change?
3. Does it satisfy the client's needs (immediate *and* future)?
4. Does it help the client take control over the weight program, or does it perpetuate dependence on a person, pill, technique, or machine?

Typical Overweight Program Alternatives

Client should choose one alternative from each lifestyle element.

Lifestyle Elements	Technique	Components	Comments on Effectiveness
Self-Responsibility and Intrapersonal Environment Action	Behavioral Modification —Self-monitoring —Environmental changes	Patient learns to observe eating behaviors through record-keeping, and to make changes in his environment and behavior that result in a smaller energy intake. Focus is on the behaviors related to food, not the food itself.	Fairly effective, especially in terms of long-term weight loss. Weakness is that some clients may uncover psychologic problems that must be dealt with. Requires much motivation and attention, especially in the beginning.
		Through techniques of covert conditioning or internal control, mental suggestions for eating behavior change are made.	These techniques are successful in reducing food intake only for as long as they are maintained. Have a tendency to become less strong with time.
Fitness & Conditioning	Exercise	Aerobic, energy-expending exercise is most effective for cardiovascular training, improvement of muscle tone, and improvement of psychologic well-being.	Effective as an addition to calorie-reduction program to cause greater weight loss. Alone can produce weight loss of ½ lb. per week if done daily. Positive aspect of a weight control program. Helps to control appetite in overweight persons.

(continued)

Typical Overweight Program Alternatives (continued)

Lifestyle Elements	Technique	Components	Comments on Effectiveness
Stress Management (AT, TM, PR)	Aversive conditioning —Hypnosis —Positive imagery	Relaxation response elicited and suggestions for restructuring response to stress made in alpha state to unconscious	Motivated clients can achieve long-term as well as immediate effects from relaxation training
Nutrition	Low carbohydrate, high protein diets, high or moderate in fat (ketogenic) —Pennington Diet, 1953 —"Calories Don't Count Diet," 1961 —The Drinking Man's Diet, 1964 —Dr. Stillman's Diet, 1967 —Dr. Atkin's Diet, 1972 —Scarsdale Diet, 1979	Diet usually 1000 cal. or less, with less than 50 Gm. CHO. Protein is usually 120 Gm. or more. Based on fact that if CHO restricted, body metabolizes ketones, which decreases hunger and causes diuresis and water loss. Usually low in calories because one cannot eat enough protein to make up for calories previously obtained from carbohydrates.	Effective for short-term weight loss. Unappetizing, so patients cannot stay with it. Do not know effects of long-term ketosis. Does result in less hunger and menstrual dysfunction, but may include aggravation of gout and osteoporosis. Short-term losses of 2 to 3 lbs. per week are seen; much is due to water loss. Long-term weight loss is from calorie deficit. Can cause increase in blood fat and cholesterol levels.
	Balanced low calorie diets —Many names and variations —Weight Watchers Diet	Protein meets the RDA, carbohydrate is moderate, and fat is low. Calories restricted, but usually not less than 1000 cal. Carbohydrate at least 80 Gm. Protein 1.0 Gm/kg. IBW.	Diet continues to meet the RDA. Carbohydrates prevent ketosis. Patient usually experiences hunger. Diet can be made to fit in with existing eating patterns; can be lifetime change. Weight loss due to calorie deficit is 1 to 2 lbs. per week.

Adapted with permission from L. Kathleen Mahan, "A Sensible Approach to the Obese Patient," *The Nursing Clinics of North America*, 14, no. 2 (June 1979), 229–45. (Philadelphia, Pa.: W. B. Saunders Co.)

COMMUNITY COPING:
ENVIRONMENTAL AND POLITICAL AWARENESS

The fifth human lifestyling element is environmental and political awareness and action. It effects and is effected by the other four elements—self-responsibility, nutrition, fitness, and stress reduction. The four basic elements can be looked upon as part of the internal and interpersonal environment of the nurse and client. Personal health patterns relative to these four areas will effect the individual's internal health status. Interpersonal lifestyle modifications, implemented on a massive scale, can change the health statistics of a group, a community, or even a nation, as exemplified by the Barefoot Doctor's Movement in the People's Republic of China. (Motivated workers from the community were successfully trained to perform primary care in their villages and thus changed the health status of that group and the nation.) There are other external environmental factors that must be addressed, not only on a personal basis, but on a nationwide and international community basis as well. Such issues as pollution and nuclear radiation come immediately to mind as examples.

The external environment includes all those events and influences which effect the individual, family, and community in relation to soil, air, water, plants, animals, and other human and nonhuman resources. Governmental agencies, such as The Occupational Safety and Health Administration (OSHA) and the Environmental Protection Agency (EPA), have been established by the United States Congress to deal with environmental health hazards.

Most large corporations and industries have occupational health programs whose goals are largely geared toward preventive health measures and early detection of job-related illnesses. Research is constantly being conducted on new substances and their effects on workers and the environment.

As societal demands for food and energy increase, the problems of safe fertilizer, pesticides, and synthetic fuel alternatives become more complex. The issue is one of expediency. What substances can most quickly fulfill a given need with the least damage and fewest side effects? Can these side effects be predicted, limited, and modified?

Examples of mismanagement of environmental untoward effects in the drug industry abound. Designing drugs that can best produce the desired effects with the fewest side effects is the goal, but in the case of diethylstilbestrol (DES), a synthetic hormone used to prevent miscarriage in the 1950s and 1960s, we have a classic example of achieving such a goal *without* knowledge of deleterious *long-term* side effects—in this case, vaginal cancer. [37] The daughters of the DES mothers of the 1950s have become the population at risk for vaginal cancer in the 1970s and 1980s. Technology and science are quickly discovering the payment for short-sighted modification of even the *cellular* environment.

Pollution and nuclear radiation do not respect local or national boundaries. It is insufficient for individuals or professionals to be concerned only about their immediate environments. Shortages of oil and food reserves can effect the welfare of huge populations across the globe. Humankind is increasingly being exposed to the benefits and costs of an era of scientific technological thinking; more humanistic and spiritual philosophies are called for. (The creation of an holistic world view will be touched upon in Chapters 8 and 10.)

A look at the physicochemical external environment can yield countless cases of transgressions against humankind and the environment. The National Institute of Occupational Safety and Health (NIOSH) lists 12,500 substances with at least some toxic properties.

On a nationwide level, the environment and ecology movement has generated governmental response in the formation of the National Environmental Protection Act, which established the Environmental Protection Agency (1969), the Clean Air Act (1970), the Water Pollution Control Act (1972), and the Toxic Substances Act (1976). Individual states, for example, California and Oregon, have developed even more stringent environmental protection legislation.

Population control is another hotly debated environmental-moral issue. Despite tremendous opposition, federal support of family planning and abortion services continued, with a resultant decline in birth rates and maternal morbidity rates. Financial support for abortions has recently been withdrawn, however.

Considered in the environmental awareness question are the socioeconomic, moral, and political conditions which effect the intra-, inter-, and community systems. Altering socioeconomic indicators of health is an amazingly complex task involving everything from changing the unemployment patterns of a neighborhood, providing decent housing for the elderly and day-care centers for working mothers, to altering the criminal justice system. Nurses have the professional obligation to become just as involved in a community housing problem, for example, as in a health screening program. (See the Wellness Inventory in the appendices to assess your own level of environmental awareness.)

Included in the moral climate of health is the public attitude toward health. National policies and programs on health *should* reflect the spirit of the people. If the public is demanding a health care system that is not only cost accountable but also caring, then public policy should mirror that goal. If people want to assume more responsibility for their own health and health care decisions, then the laws should ensure that right.

Governmental Policies and Programs

It is difficult enough for some people to go along with current concepts of health promotion and disease prevention on an individual level, incorporating the ideas outlined in this chapter. The degree of complexity and difficulty increases as the number of people involved in any group attitude or behavior change increases. The community sector of health is perhaps the most challenging aspect of coping.

The community attempts to cope in several major ways. The first and most fundamental way that communities deal with their problems is through their voluntary or private organizations. These range from neighborhood church groups to the American Heart Association. Often private or voluntary agencies will receive a grant from an official health organization if it is meeting a community need consistent with governmental goals.

The second way is through the federal government and its official agencies and departments, funded by the taxpayer's money. The major department effecting health on the federal level is the Department of Health and Human Services. The Secretary is one of the nine Secretaries who comprise the President's Cabinet. The Secretary administers countless numbers of programs which affect the health of the nation. The monies for these projects are siphoned down through federal, state, and local bureaucracies.

Of the national health budget, only 2 to 2.5 percent is spent on disease prevention and control, only 0.5 percent for health education, and only 0.5 percent for improving the organization and delivery of health services. The national budget for environmental-health research is approximately 0.25 percent of total health expenditures. [44, 45]

An area of community concern which deserves more funding for research and counseling is the biologic-genetic component of individual high-risk groups (for example, sickle cell carriers, Tay-Sachs carriers). Preventive nursing can play a large part in the screening, diagnosis, and parental decision-making process regarding the conception, birth, and care of children with genetic or congenital abnormalities.

Finally, balancing governmental support of self-help and self-care programs and projects focusing on wellness and the "worried well" may render more long-term personal and fiscal benefits for the community than the billions poured into acute-illness-oriented specialty care, which benefits so few.

One attempt at guaranteeing a continued thrust toward health promotion and a more holistic orientation toward health care has been Public Law 93–641, The National Health Planning and Development Act, enacted in 1975. One of the "national health priorities" listed in the Act states that federal, state, and area health planning and resource-development programs and national health planning goals should include:

"the promotion of activities for the prevention of disease, including studies of nutritional and environmental factors effecting health and the provision of preventive health care services." [and]

"the development of effective methods of educating the general public concerning proper personal (including preventive) health care and methods for effective use of available health services." [90]

One of the few federally funded community approaches to promoting wellness in high-risk populations is demonstrated in the following listing of supplemental food programs administered by the United States Department of Agriculture:

School lunch and breakfast program

Supplemental food service

Child-care food program

Food stamps

Commodity distribution

Special supplemental food program for women, infants, and children (WIC)

In addition, the DHHS administers the Title III Program, the National Nutrition Program for the Elderly, which is one step toward meeting some of the nutritional needs of this long-neglected group.

It behooves nurses to become more familiar with these programs and their eligibility requirements. The nurse is often the referral agent and resource to clients who are eligible for these and other federal programs. Community-based organizations and self-help groups often qualify for goods and services of which they are frequently unaware.

Private and Cooperative Programs

Senior Actualization and Growth Exploration (SAGE)

One striking example of a holistic wellness lifestyle modification program which is partially funded by governmental and foundation grants is the SAGE (Senior Actualization and Growth Exploration) Project in Berkeley, California. [33]

The program originated in 1975 with twelve senior citizens and several dedicated professionals with interests in gerontology and holistic health who felt that growing old could be a creative growth process. This project combined all the lifestyle elements previously discussed plus a focus on interpersonal group communication process, study and work.

Activities of seniors in the SAGE project include yoga, Tai-Chi, movement, breathing, massage, exercise, dance, meditation (with or without biofeedback), assertiveness training, discussion and group process work, guided imagery, and much more.

Nurses need to initiate, stimulate, and support groups such as SAGE in nursing homes and extended-care facilities, in community centers for mothers with young children, in schools for faculty and students, in adult education classes, and in retirement preparation groups. The "worried well" are not always found in public health centers and hospital outpatient departments. The nurse engaging in such preventive and generative activities will have to search out the hidden populations in need of innovative coping strategies.

Aerobic Dance

The Young Men's and Women's Christian Associations (YMCA and YWCA) sponsor aerobic dance and fitness classes. Local city parks and recreation departments often co-sponsor programs such as "Dancergetics," an aerobic fitness program choreographed to jazz, disco, classical, and western music. Such programs can be found in the San Francisco Bay area, Salt Lake City, Utah, and in other states throughout the country.

The hour-long group programs usually follow a similar pattern:

1. Warm-up stretching. (*warm-up*)
2. Warm-up dance routines. (*peak work*)
3. Aerobic dance routines. (*peak work*)

4. Floor exercises. (*cool down*)
5. Relaxing exercise. (*cool down*)

Such programs are financed by individual participants and the cooperating agencies. This is only one example of an innovative application of fitness to life situations meeting needs of people attempting to optimize their health.

The Northern California Conference on Occupational Stress

The first Northern California Conference on Occupational Stress (May, 1980) was sponsored by several local and international unions to discuss stress in the workplace and its relationship to personal life. Among other items, the conference addressed the potential California ballot initiative which requires employers to give "stress" days off, to provide stress reduction services, and to set up stress committees that would have input into reorganizing stressful work conditions to promote health and a more harmonious, relaxed environment.

The Self-Care Movement

Certainly the entire self-care movement can and will be considered in any and all of the arenas of intra-, inter-, or community systems coping with and adapting to stress.

Self-care by its very name begins with clients who place themselves somewhere on the activity-passivity grid (described in Chapter 1), with self-care as the ultimate goal. Almost every client and nurse exhibits self-care in some aspect of his or her lifestyle whether it be in their job settings, their interpersonal relationships, or their health care.

The self-care movement originated from the belief that very few clients had the opportunity or support system to pursue this goal even if they desired it. In its broadest sense, self-care could encompass any individual or group attempts at attaining total responsibility for every aspect of self-growth and development.

The lifestyle elements of self-responsibility, nutrition, fitness, stress management, and environmental awareness on the wellness end of the health continuum particularly lend themselves to lay self-care. Self-care management also encompasses both episodic and chronic illness. This discussion of self-care will revolve around healthy persons seeking information about maintaining and optimizing their current wellness status, preventing illness and chronic degenerative diseases, and safely problem solving a variety of common health-illness situations.

Self-care has been defined by Lowell Levin as a process whereby a lay person functions on his/her own behalf in health promotion and prevention and in disease detection and treatment at the level of the primary health resource in the health-care system. [54]

Self-help in social settings has included group therapy, psychotherapeutic communities, and common interest self-help groups such as Alcoholics Anonymous, Colostomy Clubs, etc. These groups have attributed much of their success to their dissemination of mutual information, experience sharing, and group support and structure. Health collectives utilizing this self-help idea began appearing in the late 1960s and many have survived to form an ever-growing alternative grass roots level health care system.

Self-care has long been associated with folk practices that are unscientific, unresearched, and sometimes hazardous to health. Regardless of what the medical establishment thinks of self-care, it exists at some level in all individuals, families, and cultures, and it is presently experiencing an upsurge in popularity because of spiraling costs and distrust in and incompetency of other conventional services. Self-care is only as good as the knowledge, motivation, and competent problem solving of the individual. [54]

Self-care is not merely an intrapersonal phenomenon. Even if a person does not require professional services, some form of self-care education must occur in order for the person to best perform the four roles of self-care, that is, prevention, self-diagnosis, self-medication/self-treatment, and participation in professional care when necessary. [54, John Fry as cited therein]

Self-care involves interest, participation, decision making, and political action in determining public policy and programs regarding health. Although lifestyle changes are largely a personal issue, most potential and real health problems involve some degrees of social/economic/political change. Nutrition labeling is one example of public and political input into the quality of the food supply. Personal health behavior effects the family, support network, and community. Communities can be assessed regarding their level of self-care and self-determination.

One community, professional, and political argument against self-care is that it is being misused by those who would limit development of innovative technological advances and improvements in health care delivery. Certainly, the focus on medical technology has been the thrust in health care in recent years. Self-care may, in fact, cause a shift in emphasis in health resource development toward educational resources, for example.

Parts of the professional community are understandably threatened by the inevitable changes that will occur in the professional-client relationship, with the client moving from passive recipient to active participant. Professional education will have to change to prepare practitioners well-versed in interpersonal negotiation and contracting for health with a motivated, questioning client who is cognizant of his rights. The myth of the professional as "pill fairy" is fast being exploded. Self-care does not imply that its advocates never get sick or never consult the health care system. Self-care proponents are really preprimary caregivers surveying their own day-to-day health within given parameters. The clients are the first to detect minor deviations from their own norms. They have the background and willingness to interpret their information in light of their own experience. Only the client can answer the question, "What meaning does this feeling, symptom, illness, have for me?"

Self-care leads to the apparent conclusion that lay people know far too little about evaluating and improving their health via lifestyle modification before they become ill. Self-care includes effective coping with illness through the appropriate use of health-care facilities.

One novel self-health idea sponsored by Blue Shield and the Mendocino County, California, Office of Education, is to offer a $500 bonus to those of its 218 employees who stay healthy. Blue Shield covers any medical expense over $500, but if an employee doesn't use up the $500 deductible the Office of Education has set aside for him, he may pocket the total or balance at the end of the year. In the meantime, the fund for the 218 employees involved is generating interest on the remainder of the unused money—in this case $50,000. Claims have been cut back by 60 percent. Big employers and legislators are becoming interested in this amazingly simple stimulus for people to stay well. Program administrators claim that for the first time employees are actively attempting to maintain health through lifestyle modification programs such as jogging and fitness clubs. [42]

Professional care is seen as supplementary to lay self-care. The trend toward self-care is part of a resurgence of populism in every area of American life. Individuals are reasserting more control over their own lives. Other aspects of this campaign include women's rights, progressive education, self-sufficiency skills (such as home and auto repair), political campaigning, reform, participatory democracy, tax reform, and appropriate technology. [19]

In summary, people want to take health into their own hands and to have enough knowledge to cope with minor health problems. The proliferation of health cooperatives and self-help and self-care groups all demonstrate this desire.

The Women's Self-Help Movement

A specific description of the what and why of women's self-help will demonstrate the use of groups to foster self-health assessment and awareness, coping with interpersonal relationships, developing a support system, and promoting political consciousness and informed political action.

The concept of self-help is a holistic one because it enables women to view their bodies as integrated entities, over which they possess self-knowledge and control.

The emphasis in women's self-help has been on speculum use, breast exam, and education about what a healthy body is and how it can be maintained. Anatomy and physiology, sexuality, vaginal and cervical conditions, pregnancy and childbirth, menopause and aging, and most important, self-knowledge as well women, are some of the other things that are discussed in women's self-help groups.

These groups give women a forum in which to share information and anxieties, as well as a specific place to learn how to use speculums, to determine what to look for in self-exam, and to experience doing bimanual exams. After women have acquired these skills, group leaders feel that they will be able to demand good health care. Self-help proponents do not advocate using the knowledge and skills gained through self-help as an exclusive alternative to treatment from medical professionals, but rather, it is felt that getting to know more about themselves makes women more powerful and effective when they do seek care or assistance from the established health care system.

The primary function of a women's self-help group is to initiate bodily self-knowledge removed from myth, misinformation, and medical mystique. Women are encouraged to become familiar with their bodies throughout their cycles. One way is through frequent speculum exams performed throughout their cycles; vaginal, cervical, and external changes are recorded, as well as what is happening in the rest of the body. This enables each woman to become aware of the changes that occur in each stage of her cycle. Findings are compared and repeated; exams are done among the group; and an appreciation of the differences in how each individual woman's body functions and of what is normal and healthy are determined.

One of the beauties of self-help is that it can be done by anyone, anywhere. The groups originated when one woman took home a plastic speculum following a visit to her gynecologist and used it to look at herself. She showed her friends and together they all began to discover more about their own bodies. The members of the self-help function group of the Berkeley's Women's Health Collective, for example, do not view themselves as paraprofessionals engaged in teaching a class; rather, in these self-help groups, they facilitate discussion and offer resources and support to a group of women who are engaged in self-taught education, reeducation, and consciousness raising. Training focuses on demonstrating techniques to facilitate this process, familiarizing themselves with the sources of information available, and assuring themselves that they have an accurate understanding of content.

Following an introduction to the concept and purpose of self-help, as well as to the philosophy, politics, and services of the collective (whether for a one-time drop-in group, presentation, or ongoing group), the topics of discussion are decided upon by the group as a whole. The ongoing groups usually consist of about eight women and two function members, and may meet for an average of five times. They have provided self-help for lesbians, pregnant women, women prostitutes, older women, disabled women, and other distinct groups in order to focus on the particular issues of concern to differing groups of women, all done within an atmosphere of maximum supportiveness.

Some other topics included in self-help group discussions are venereal disease, birth control, herbal and holistic remedies for common female complaints, nutrition, abortion services and how to evaluate them, PAP smears, healthy body work for women, menstrual extraction, lesbian health care, feminism, sterilization, hysterectomy, mastectomy, DES and estrogens, client rights, and how to deal with doctors.

Nurses can perform a valuable function as group resource persons and facilitators of the group communication process. They have the informational background, communication, caring, and problem-solving skills to contribute greatly to women and self-help groups' needs for self-knowledge, self-growth, and self-determinism, and indeed, nurses are often the chief referral resource for a client seeking such self-help.

REFERENCES FOR CHAPTER 6

[1] Donna Aguilera and J. Messick, *Crisis Intervention: Theory and Methodology,* 3rd ed. (St. Louis: C. V. Mosby Co., 1978).

[2] Terence Anderson, "New Horizons for Vitamin C," *Nutrition Today,* 12, no. 1 (January/February 1977), 6–13.

[3] Marian Arlin, "Controversies in Nutrition," *Nursing Clinics of North America,* 14, no. 2 (June 1979), 199–214.

[4] Werner Baumgartner and others, "An-

tioxidant Effects in the Development of Erlich Ascites Carcinoma," *AJCN,* 31, no. 1 (March 1978), 457–65.

[5] Nedra B. Belloc and Lester Breslow, "Relationship of Physical Health Status and Health Practices," *Preventive Medicine,* vol. 1 (192), no. 3 (August 1972), 409–21.

[6] Herbert Benson, John F. Beary, and Mark P. Carol, "The Relaxation Response," *Psychiatry,* 37, no. 1 (February 1974), 37–46.

[7] Herbert Benson, *The Mind/Body Effect* (New York: Simon and Schuster, 1979).

[8] Gail Bronson, "For Many, Tranquilizers Are a Way to Deal with Fears and Frustration," *The Wall Street Journal,* western ed., p. 1, 1979.

[9] Barbara B. Brown, *Stress and the Art of Biofeedback* (New York: Harper & Row, 1977).

[10] Gerald Caplan, *An Approach to Community Mental Health* (New York: Grune and Stratton, 1961).

[11] Gerald Caplan, *Support Systems and Community Health* (New York: Behavioral Publications, 1974).

[12] Mildred Carter, *Helping Yourself with Foot Reflexology* (West Nyack, N.Y.: Parker Publishing Co., 1969).

[13] Mildred Carter, *Hand Reflexology: Key to Perfect Health* (West Nyack, N.Y.: Parker Publishing Co., 1975).

[14] C. Carlson Conrad, "When You're Young at Heart," *Aging,* no. 258 (April 1976), 11–13.

[15] Kenneth H. Cooper, *The New Aerobics* (New York: Bantam Books, 1975), pp. 16–31.

[16] Emile Coué, *The Practice of Autosuggestion* (New York: Doubleday, 1922).

[17] Norman Cousins, "The Mysterious Placebo, How Mind Helps Medicine Work," *Saturday Review,* October 1, 1977, pp. 9–12.

[18] Edward T. Creagan and others, "Failure of High-Dose Vitamin C Ascorbic Acid—Therapy to Benefit Patients with Advanced Cancer," *NEJM,* 301, no. 13 (September 27, 1979), 687–90.

[19] Robert DaPrato, "The Trend Toward Self-Care," *San Francisco Sunday Examiner and Chronicle,* June 19, 1977, p. 12.

[20] Martha Davis, Elizabeth Eshelman, and Matthew McKay, *The Relaxation and Stress Reduction Workbook* (Richmond, Ca.: New Harbinger Publications, 1980).

[21] Herbert A. DeVries and G. M. Adams, "Electromyographic comparison of single doses of exercise and meprobamate as to effects on muscular relaxation," *American Journal of Physical Medicine,* 51 (June 1972), 130–41.

[22] Herbert A. DeVries, *Vigor Regained* (Englewood Cliffs, N.J.: Prentice-Hall, Inc., 1974).

[23] "Do Women Need Iron Supplements?," *Consumer Reports* (September 1978), 502–04.

[24] George Downing and Anne Kent Rush, *The Massage Book* (New York: Random House, 1972), pp. 27–31.

[25] Rene Dubos, *Man Adapting* (New Haven: Yale University Press, 1965), p. 261.

[26] Wayne Dyer, *Your Erroneous Zones* (New York: Avon Books, 1976), pp. 15–16.

[27] Erik P. Eckholm, *The Picture of Health* (New York: W. W. Norton & Co., 1977), pp. 43, 68, 76.

[28] Ellen Buchman Ewald, *Recipes for a Small Planet* (New York: Random House, 1975).

[29] Benjamin Feingold, *Why Your Child is Hyperactive* (New York: Random House, 1975).

[30] John Feltman, "Antioxidants, Aging, and Cancer," *Prevention,* 30, no. 7 (July 1978), 62–67.

[31] James F. Fixx, *The Complete Book of Running* (New York: Random House, 1977), pp. 23–27.

[32] Bonnie J. Friedman and Katherine Knight, "Running for Life, Health, and Pleasure," *AJN,* 78, no. 4 (April 1978), 602–07.

[33] Eugenia Gerard, Sage Foundation Videotape, 1976.

[34] Coleen P. Greecher and Barbara Shannon, *American Dietetic Association Journal,* 70, no. 4 (April 1977), 368–72.

[35] Raymond Harris and Lawrence J. Frankel, *Guide to Fitness After Fifty* (New York: Plenum Press, 1977).

[36] "The Herbs and the Heart," *Nutrition Review,* 34, no. 2 (February 1976), 43.

[37] Arthur L. Herbst and Robert E. Scully, "Adenocarcinoma of the Vagina in Adolescence," *Cancer,* 25, no. 4 (April 1970), 745–57.

[38] Holistic Health: The Renaissance Nurse Symposium, April 19 and 20, 1980.

[39] Wen-Shan Huang, *Fundamentals of Tai Chi Ch'uan,* 2nd ed. (Hong Kong: South Sky Book Co., 1974).

[40] Richard Hyatt, *Chinese Herbal Medicine, Ancient Art and Modern Science* (New York: Schocker Books, 1978).

[41] Frederick Fletcher Hyde, "The Origin and Practice of Herbal Medicine," *Mims Magazine* (February 1978), pp. 127–36.

[42] John Jacobs, "Stay Healthy, Earn a Reward," *San Francisco Sunday Examiner and Chronicle,* no. 27, July 6, 1980, p. 1.

[43] Donald W. Kemper, "Medical Self-Care: A Stop on the Road to High Level Wellness," *Health Values: Achieving High Level Wellness,* 4, no. 2 (March/April 1980), 63–68.

[44] M. Kirsten and others, "Health Economics and Preventive Care," *Science,* 195 (February 4, 1977), 457–62.

[45] John H. Knowles, ed., *Doing Better and Feeling Worse* (New York: W. W. Norton & Co., 1977).

[46] Hans Kraus and Wilhelm Raab, *Hypokinetic Disease—Diseases Produced by Lack of Exercise* (Springfield, Ill.: Charles C Thomas, 1961).

[47] Frances Moore Lappé, *Diet for a Small Planet* (New York: Ballantine Books, 1972).

[48] Michael C. Latham and Francisco Cobos, "The Effects of Malnutrition on Intellectual Development and Learning," *AJPH,* 61, no. 7 (1971), 1307–24.

[49] Denis Lawson-Wood and Joyce Lawson-Wood, *Acupuncture Vitality and Revival Points* (Devon, England: Speight Press, 1975).

[50] Richard S. Lazarus, "Psychological Stress and Coping in Adaptation and Illness," *International Journal of Psychiatric Medicine,* 5, no. 4 (Fall 1974), 321–33.

[51] Alexander Leaf, "Getting Old," *Scientific American,* 229 (September 1973), 43–52.

[52] Jon N. Leonard and others, *Live Longer Now* (New York: Charter Books, 1974), p. 181.

[53] Lowell Levin and Eugene Bender, *The Strength in Us* (New York: New Viewpoints—A Division of Franklin Watts, 1976).

[54] Lowell Levin, Alfred Katz, and Erik Holst, *Self-Care—Lay Initiatives in Health* (New York: Prodist, 1979).

[55] D. M. Lithgow and W. M. Politzer, "Vitamin A in the Treatment of Menorrhagia," *South African Medical Journal,* 51, no. 7 (February 12, 1977), 191–93.

[56] Alexander Lowen, *Bioenergetics* (New York: Penguin Books, 1975).

[57] Henry C. Lu, trans., *The Yellow Emperor's Book of Acupuncture* (Vancouver, B.C.: The Academy of Oriental Heritage, 1973).

[58] L. Kathleen Mahan, "A Sensible Approach to the Obese Patient," *Nursing Clinics of North America,* 14, no. 2 (June 1979), 229–45.

[59] William A. McGarey, *Acupuncture and Body Energies* (Phoenix, Ariz.: Gabriel Press, 1974).

[60] David Mechanic, "Stress, Illness, and Illness Behavior," *Journal of Human Stress,* 2, no. 2 (June 1976), 2–6.

[61] Benjamin F. Miller and Claire B. Keene, *Encyclopedia and Dictionary of Medicine, Nursing and Allied Health* (Philadelphia: W. B. Sanders Co., 1978).

[62] Carolyn L. Morris, "Relaxation Therapy in a Clinic," *AJN,* 79, no. 11 (November 1979), 1958–59.

[63] Lester M. Morrison, "Serum Cholesterol Reduction with Lecithin," *Geriatrics,* 13, no. 1 (January 1958), 12–19.

[64] Ruth Murray and Judith Zentner, *Nursing Concepts for Health Promotion* (Englewood Cliffs, N.J.: Prentice-Hall, Inc., 1979).

[65] National League for Nursing, *Stress: Making It Work For You* (New York: National League for Nursing, 1977).

[66] "Nutrition Research," *American Dietetic Association Journal,* 70, no. 4 (April 1977), 368–72.

[67] Anita L. Owen, Gemma Lanna, and George M. Owen, "Counseling Patients about Diet and Nutrition Supplements," *Nursing Clinics of North America,* 14, no. 2 (June 1979), 247–68.

[68] Linus Pauling, *Vitamin C, The Common Cold, and the Flu* (San Francisco: W. H. Freeman & Co., 1978), p. 208.

[69] Kenneth R. Pelletier, *Toward a Science of Consciousness* (New York: Dell Publishing Co., 1978), p. 143.

[70] Ruanne K. Peters and others, "Daily Relaxation Breaks in a Working Population: Effects on Self-Reported Measures of Health, Performance, and Well-Being," *AJPH,* 67, no. 10 (October 1977), 946-53.

[71] Ruanne K. Peters and others, "Effects on Blood Pressure," *AJPH,* 67, no. 10 (October 1977), 954-59.

[72] The President's Council on Physical Fitness and Sports and the Administration on Aging, "The Fitness Challenge . . . in the Later Years," (Washington, D.C.: Administration on Aging, 1975).

[73] Ira Progoff, *At a Journal Workshop* (New York: Dialogue House Library, 1975).

[74] Richard H. Rahe and Ransom J. Arthur, "Life Change and Illness Studies: Past History and Future Directions," *Journal of Human Stress,* 4, no. 1 (March 1978), 3-15.

[75] Judith M. Richter and Rebecca Sloan, "A Relaxation Technique," *AJN,* 79, no. 11 (November 1979), 1960-64.

[76] Karl Robert Rosa, *You and AT* (New York: Saturday Review Press/E.P. Dutton & Co., 1973).

[77] Walton T. Roth, "Some Motivational Aspects of Exercise," *Journal of Sports Medicine,* 14, no. 1 (March 1974), 40-47.

[78] Bengt Saltin, "Physiological Effects of Physical Conditioning," *Medicine and Science in Sports,* 1, no. 1 (March 1969), 50-56.

[79] Mike Samuels and Hal Bennett, *The Well Body Book* (New York: Random House, 1973), p. 1.

[80] Mike Samuels and Nancy Samuels, *Seeing With the Mind's Eye* (New York: Random House, 1975).

[81] Gary E. Schwartz, "Biofeedback, Self-Regulation, and the Patterning of Physiological Processes," *American Scientist,* 63 (May-June 1975), 314-24.

[82] Gary E. Schwartz and David Shapiro, *Consciousness and Self-Regulation,* vol. I (New York: Plenum Press, 1976).

[83] Gary E. Schwartz and David Shapiro, *Consciousness and Self-Regulation,* vol. II (New York: Plenum Press, 1976), p. 401.

[84] Bob Sevene, "How to Begin Running," *Runner's World* (June 1979), 48-51.

[85] George Sheehan, *Dr. Sheehan on Running* (Mountain View, Ca.: World Publications, 1975), p. 103.

[86] David Shottenfeld, "Alcohol and Tobacco," *Nutrition Today,* 13, no. 5 (September/October 1978), 8-9.

[87] T. A. Simons and others, "Treatment of Hypercholesteremia with Oral Lecithin," *Australian and New Zealand Journal of Medicine,* 7 (June 1977), 262-66.

[88] Jerome E. Singer and David C. Glass, "Making Your World More Livable," *Blueprint for Health,* XXV, no. 1 (Chicago: Blue Cross Association, 1974), 59-65.

[89] Mary J. T. Smith and Hans Selyé, "Reducing the Negative Effects of Stress," *AJN,* 79, no. 11 (November 1979), 1953-55.

[90] Anne R. Somers and Herman M. Somers, "A New Framework for Health and Health Care Policies," papers on the National Health Guidelines: Conditions for Change in the Health-Care System (Washington, D.C.: USGPO, September 1977), 15-19.

[91] "Sports Report," *Well-Being Magazine,* no. 16 (1976), 12-14.

[92] Irwin Stone, *The Healing Factor: Vitamin C Against Disease* (New York: Grosset & Dunlap, 1972).

[93] Justin F. Stone, *Tai Chi Chih* (Albuquerque, N. M.: Sun Publishing Co., 1974).

[94] Frances M. Tappan, *Healing Massage Techniques* (Reston, Va.: Reston Publishing Co., 1978).

[95] Nikolas Tinbergen, "Ethology and Stress Diseases," *Science,* 185, no. 4145 (July 5, 1974), 20-27.

[96] John Thie, *Touch for Health* (Marina del Rey, Ca.: De Vorss and Co., 1973).

[97] David Van Thiel and others, "Ethanol Inhibition of Vitamin A Metabolism in the Testes: Possible Mechanism for Sterility in Alcoholics," *Science,* 186, no. 4167 (December 6, 1974), 941-42.

[98] Gregory S. Thomas, "Physical Activity and Health: Epidemiologic and Clinical Evidence and Policy Implications," *Preventive Medicine,* 8, no. 1 (January 1979), 89-103.

[99] Joan Ullyot, *Women's Running* (Mountain View, Ca.: World Publications, 1976), p. 150.

[100] United States Senate Select Committee

on Nutrition and Human Needs, "Nutrition and Health," (U.S. Government Printing Office, December 1975).

[101] University of California, Berkeley, *Student Health Service Manual* (Berkeley, Ca.: The Regents of the University of California, 1977).

[102] *The Wall Street Journal,* western ed., vol. C, no. 47, March 8, 1979, p. 1.

[103] John White and James Fadiman, eds., *Relax* (New York: Dell Publishing Co., 1976).

[104] Kerr L. White, "Prevention as a National Health Goal," *Preventive Medicine,* 4, no. 3 (September 1975), 247–51.

[105] Roger J. Williams, *Nutrition Against Disease: Environmental Prevention* (New York: Bantam Books, 1973).

[106] Sue Rodwell Williams, *Essentials of Nutrition and Diet Therapy,* 2nd ed. (St. Louis: C. V. Mosby Co., 1978), p. 58.

[107] John D. Williamson and Kate Danaher, *Self-Care in Health* (London: Croom-Helm, 1978).

[108] Peter Wood, "Running Away from Heart Disease," *Runner's World* (June 1979), 78–81.

[109] Dr. E. L. Wynder, quoted by Don Ardell, "From Omnibus Tinkering to High-Level Wellness," *AJHP,* 2, no. 2 (October 1976), 19.

[110] John Yudkin, "Dietary Fat and Dietary Sugar," *Lancet,* II, no. 7357 (August 29, 1964), 478–79.

Chapter 7
communication

CHAPTER OUTLINE

CHAPTER OBJECTIVES

1. Define communication and list the four essential biopsychosocial processes necessary for any communication to occur.
2. Describe the five elements present in any communication model.
3. Explain three major areas of study in nonverbal communication.
4. Evaluate intrapersonal communication style using the chapter checklist.
5. Describe four listening skills used in nursing and list one example of each.
6. Correctly use and label six therapeutic communication techniques in a self-composed nurse-client interaction.
7. List six barriers to communication.
8. Define the nursing interview, describe its purposes, and list the conditions necessary to facilitate a productive interview.
9. Compose a real or simulated process recording, identifying verbal and nonverbal communication, an analysis of the interaction, the techniques demonstrated, and the effectiveness of the interaction.
10. List four task-oriented and four group-maintenance functions which aid in establishing an effective group.

COMMUNICATION

Definitions

Communication has been defined as all the processes, verbal and nonverbal, conscious or unconscious, by which one mind may affect another. The very derivation of the word implies that two persons are coming together, sharing information and feelings, and *transacting* dynamically in the communication process. In communicating with others we use all the capacities we have to sense, perceive, interpret, understand, feel, and express. [19] Communication is the dynamic process which synthesizes all these capacities, abilities, motives, and goals.

Discussion of the communication process in nursing must of necessity be limited to its purposes and application in the context of the nurse-client relationship. Examination of the nurse's own communication patterns will precede study of the interpersonal and group communication process. Review of the therapeutic relationship will focus on holistic Rogerian and Transactional Analysis theory as described in earlier chapters. Certain specific directive and nondirective communication techniques will be explored.

The nursing interview will be viewed in some depth as a prime example of use of communication skills in nursing. Initiating, maintaining, and terminating the nurse interview, consciously avoiding certain hindrances and blocks to communication will be demonstrated. Learning from each nurse-client transaction will be emphasized. A method for recording, analyzing, and improving communication skills is suggested.

Application of communication theory and processes to groups and to the community will be briefly discussed. References to public or mass communication will be made, and professional communication channels will be looked at. Suggestions for the use of communication to teach and to change will be reserved for Chapters 9 and 10.

The process of communication fits into a holistic nursing framework from several points of view. Smuts' notion that all parts relate dynamically to each other and to the whole is characteristic of the fluid transactional quality of communication. This ever-changing aspect of communication has stimulated researchers to use the words "black box" to describe the unknown variables that enter into every transaction between a sender (encoder) and a receiver (decoder). [24] The complexity of one person, with all his or her unknowable needs and motives, trying to interact with another with a different set of needs and wants in fluctuating environments, times, and spaces can, at times, resemble an Eastern puzzle.

Zen monks don't even attempt to untangle the riddles of communicating. They cope by creating other riddles or *koans* to express the unfathomable nature of words and language. A holistic view of communication should incorporate some Zen ideas, namely the inadequacy of relying on mere words to convey meaning and the need for *nowness,* as the following poems illustrate:

Pure and fresh are the flowers with dew,
Clear and bright is the singing of the birds;
Clouds are calm, waters are blue.
Who has written the True Word of no letters?

Lofty are the mountains, green are the trees,
Deep are the valleys, lucid are the streams;
The wind is soft, the moon is serene.
Calmly I read the True Word of no letters.
[32, p. 264]

Living in the here and now is behaviour derived from the Zen experience. Guilt and anxiety are children of the past and future. To the extent that a person dwells upon the should-have-been or might-be of life at the expense of living life in the reality of the present, he suffers. [6, Thomas Keefe as quoted therein]

Besides being able to "see" beyond the immediate communication into the depths of meaning, the holistic nurse acknowledges information outside the realm of usual communication, that is, clairvoyance, psychic-reading, healing, psychometry, telepathy, clairaudience, and automatic writing. Although research on these forms of communication is forthcoming, this spiritual aspect of communication is being viewed with less skepticism than previously.

Finally, the holistic nurse recognizes the communication process as the most potent tool for change that he or she possesses. Appropriate use of communication can persuade and stimulate attitude and behavior changes in self, clients, and communities.

Study of communication theory and technique warrants as much attention in nursing as do the behavioral, social, and biological sciences. Communication theory crosses disciplinary boundaries and draws from psychology, sociology, neurophysiology, anthropology, linguistics, and ecology. [24] Part of the difficulty in interpreting communication research is that it comes from each of the aforementioned disciplines, each of which has its own terminology and point of view.

The vocabulary problem is small indeed compared to transcultural communication which supersedes much more than jargon and language differences. In transcultural communication, variables such as time, personal space, use of touch, nonverbal communication, and the relationship of what is said to what is meant, may determine the nature and outcome of the entire relationship. [35]

The Process of Communicating

A first look at communication must begin with the biopsychosocial processes needed for every communication to occur—sensation, perception, symbolization, and transmission. The sense organs pick up external and internal stimuli and processes select, organize, interpret, and perceive them through the nervous system to the brain, the center of all perception. [24, pp. 28–32] *Perception* specifically involves attending to a specific sensation, ordering it, transforming it into a symbol, and comparing the symbol to others stored in the memory. [24, p. 33]

Two principles have importance for behavior modifiers and communicators in health. First, if a sensed stimulus is perceived as a threat, it may be ignored (for example, attempting to describe someone who has robbed you); and second, persons can only take in one sensation at a time and attend to it (for example, two different pains are impossible to give equal concentration to). [24, p. 33]

Symbolization is part of the perceptive process by which persons compare the sensation to their systems of values, beliefs, and past experiences or frames of reference. This makes each person's interpretation of the data unique. It also makes changes in the system a complex matter. The most coherent information on this internal frame of reference is that of cognitive dissonance, which describes the responses of individuals confronted by information that is unfamiliar or unlike their own. If persons are forced to consider dissonant or threatening information, they are placed in a state of tension because they cannot hold two inconsistent pieces of information. [24, p. 37] This then motivates individuals to close out all potentially dissonant information or to modify their belief systems. Nurses need to recognize that this process occurs continuously as they introduce new concepts to clients, especially those that require belief and behavior changes.

Finally, *transmission* refers to the expression, verbally and/or nonverbally, of the message to be communicated. This does not guarantee that communication will occur, however.

Zen masters feel that one of the mistakes human beings make is to confuse an experiential fact with its expression in letters which are only "conceptual shows of the fact." [32, p. 23] Master Eisi's comment typifies a Zen explanation of the language problem: "Affirmatively speaking, all the sutras are Zen expressions. Negatively speaking, there is not a word that can be a Zen expression." [32, p. 28]

A Communication Model

All communication must have the following five elements, as depicted in Figure 7–1:

1. A sender or encoder.
2. The message itself.
3. A receiver or decoder.
4. Feedback: the receiver's message to the sender.
5. Context: the setting or environment surrounding the communication.

If communication were as simple as this model suggests, it would be relatively easy to carry on a transaction. Unfortunately, no model is really unidimensional and many of the aforementioned variables need to be taken into account. In addition to time, space, culture, etc., people only communicate approximately 10 per-

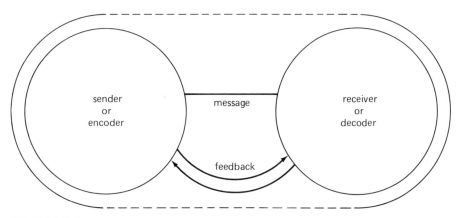

FIGURE 7-1

cent of their true meaning verbally. The rest is transmitted nonverbally through voice, posture, actions, gestures, touch, and body language.

COMPONENTS OF COMMUNICATION

Nonverbal Communication

The point has been made that clients and helpers need to become more in tune with their bodies and with the right-hemisphere-dominated feminine aspects of their personalities. Tuning in to nonverbal communication and becoming an astute observer of the body's messages will help nurses see beneath the mask of fear in clients and help them to trust their own intuitive faculties.

Body Language—Kinesics

Alexander Lowen's theory of bioenergetics has been alluded to in Chapters 4 and 6. What Lowen, Alexander, and other body therapists believe is that "the body does not lie" even if verbal communication belies it. Nonverbal communication has been studied for a relatively short period of time, but three major categories have been established. The first area is that of *body language,* the study of which is termed *kinesics.* As an individual grows and develops, the correspondence or congruence between verbal and nonverbal messages becomes less and less. It has been estimated that incongruency between verbal and nonverbal behavior may occur up to two-thirds of the time.

"Reading" nonverbal behavior involves sensitizing ourselves to facial expression, eye contact, body position, posture, body movement, and gestures, and interpreting those messages. In our western culture, certain gestures signify close-mindedness or fear (crossed legs or arms), authority (standing above the level of the receiver), evasiveness or lying (avoiding eye contact). Clients under stress can exhibit characteristic behaviors, such as hyperactivity, inability to maintain eye contact, twitching, and rapid speech patterns. Clients in pain or those experiencing fear, grief, or anger all exhibit behavior the nurse must become aware of.

Touch

The second category of nonverbal behavior is *touch,* which has been explored in Chapters 3 and 4 of this text. It is worth repeating that touch is an essential part of human development from conception through old age. Jourard has observed that "wellness" ensues from having one's individuality respected and acknowledged, and that being heard and touched by a person who cares seems to reinforce identity, mobilize spirit, and promote self-healing. Deprivation of touch has been correlated with difficulty in directed thinking, anxiety, and distorted perception [17, p. 39]

Frederick Leboyer views frequent infant massage as essential as food to healthy development. He has captured the technique that women in India use and is teaching it to American and European women:

> Here you are, looking at each other.
>
> At every moment, your massaging must be sensitive and responsive to the slightest flutter of this new being. You will be holding an unbroken dialogue. Not in words, of course! True communication, true communion, is silent, as you know. Speak with your eyes. Speak through your hands.
>
> Let it all flow from you heart.
>
> Be *here*, live *now*, completely!
>
> For if your mind is on other things, the baby will know it immediately. The whole thing would become merely mechanical, a mere exercise, easy, boring, and empty. [31]

The laying-on-of-hands is, of course, touch with the intent to heal—a therapeutic modality of which we have yet to grasp the extent.

Proxemics

Proxemics is the study of space in human transactions, and it constitutes a third area of nonverbal communication. The concept of territoriality is considered within this rubric. Much of the research is applied from animal behavior studies. Territory fulfills needs for identity, security, and stimulation [21, Robert Ardrey as cited therein, p. 49]. It is now becoming apparent that the quality of personal space is a facet of healing. Color, structural and geometric design, textures, sound, light, scents, temperature, the presence of living things, art, air quality, and the influence of what the Chinese called the Five Elements—earth, metal, water, fire, and wood—all contribute to an individual's sense of health and comfort in space.

Personal space is the area or "energy field" immediately surrounding and protecting a person. Hall has indentified four basic distances for certain transactions:

1. Intimate distance (6″–18″ space between people; parents and children, lovers).
2. Personal distance (1 1/2 ft.–4 ft.; close friends).
3. Social distance (4 ft.–12 ft.; behind desks, counters, or tables, during business and social transactions).
4. Public distance (12 ft.–25 ft.; speaker and audience). [24, p. 63]

Written Communication

Another form of nonverbal communication is written communication. This hardly fits the definition of communication because one of the essential components—feedback—is missing. The receiver is not obligated to give feedback, and nonverbal feedback cannot be observed. The receiver gets an opportunity to restructure thoughts cognitively without having to contend with feelings that might belie true response.

Much of nursing traditionally involves very limited written communication, as typified by charting. (This area will be addressed in the section on problem solving through written records and care plans presented in Chapter 8.) Suffice it to say that in nursing the only communication that occurs on a frequent basis between caregivers in the institutional setting is often written. The continuity of client care hinges on the clarity of this written communication. Therefore, a method for insuring follow-up of client needs via the written word is of utmost importance.

Other forms of written communication include poetry and artwork which, in the case of communication disorders—for example, certain types of schizophrenia, aphasia, autism, and chronic brain syndromes as seen in some of the aged—is often the only method of communication. Interpretation of this type of symbolic communication requires additional preparation and practice.

Verbal Communication

Verbal communication encompasses all the symbols people speak when they communicate, which range from grunts to seven-syllable words arranged in complex sentence patterns. When one considers jargon, slang, double meanings, jokes, wit, sarcasm, hyperbole, and other linguistic techniques, the interpretation of meaning can become a true challenge. The inadequacy of language to communicate thoughts and feelings is well-expressed by D. T. Suzuki:

> The contradiction so puzzling to the ordinary way of thinking comes from the fact that we have to use language to communicate our inner experience which in its very nature transcends linguistics. [8, Suzuki as quoted therein, p. 45]

Time

Time is another important concept bound up with communication. It is in this dimension that the Zen of communication strongly parallels recent communication research. Hinduism chose myth as the form in which to express the paradoxes of reality. Buddhists and Taoists exposed mystical experiences through contradictory *koans* and *haikus*. And the more one thinks about the statements these poems make, the less sense they make, and that is precisely their purpose—to stop the left-dominated linear thought process and to prepare the learner to enter the nonverbal, nonlogical world of inner reality.

Zen's purpose is not to accumulate abstract knowledge, nor to carry on a philosophical discussion, but rather to live the concrete life of the moment, termed *oneness*.

Attempting to analyze the patterns of causal relationships can lead to missing the spontaneous joy of valuing each moment for itself. Constantly comparing one's own ideal with reality leads to unnecessary suffering. Living in the now avoids the disappointment stemming from contrasting events to the might-have-beens. This concept relates to some of the ideas contained in self-responsibility. It is also characteristic of a Type B personality, which is not preoccupied with future events.

Purposes of Communication In Nursing

Some of the main purposes of understanding and utilizing the communication process in nursing follow:

1. to initiate, maintain, and terminate the nurse-client relationship;
2. to gain information via the nursing interview related to clients' health and lifestyles and to help clients learn more about themselves during the course of the interview;
3. to help clients learn more about health and high-level wellness behaviors;
4. to counsel clients seeking it and to help nurse and client handle emotionally charged issues and feelings;
5. to stimulate change in both nurse and client toward health and wholeness;
6. to communicate with co-workers and interdisciplinary helpers to ensure quality caring of clients and to facilitate change in the health care system and society.

INTRAPERSONAL COMMUNICATION

Although communication is by definition an *interpersonal* process, there are certain aspects of good communication which need to be evaluated intrapersonally. The nurse must have a sound knowledge of communication theory and application skills. This can only be achieved by assessing one's own communication style, practicing new interpersonal techniques, evaluating them in light of current research, reviewing and modifying them according to valid criteria, and reapplying them to continuously improve the quality of the nurse-client relationship.

Exploring Feelings

The first part of assessing communication patterns is to look at feelings toward self, because this will effect and shape feelings toward others. We can look at our own communication process by questioning and reflecting on our interactions, by a written replay and analysis of our interactions (process recording), by videotaping ourselves in action, and by soliciting the honest feedback of people we trust. In Chapter 4 we explored our feelings of self-esteem and self-worth. Take a few minutes now to reexperience attitudes toward yourself, your family, and your life. It is important that nurses, in particular, feel "okay" about themselves before they initiate communication with someone who is not feeling well and/or who is trying to seek help to change.

Exploring one's feelings is not a very easy task. Human beings are born with emotions that are closely connected to the state of the body and mind. As societal conditioning toward rational control of feelings—especially negative ones—predominated development, we learned to suppress and divorce ourselves from the way we felt. It is a commonly held misconception that a person can think *or* feel, but cannot do *both*. Emotions and "vibrations," as psychics term them, are often the truest and earliest indicators of what is going on in a situation. Often the rational mind muddies the waters by intellectualizing a very basic bit of intuitive information. An exercise, suggested by Daniels and Horowitz, helps nurses and clients to sensitize themselves:

Difficult Feelings

Students and nurses often cite the following "difficult" feelings:

1. *Feelings of being no good.* This attitude stems from the way we grew up and developed our self-esteem. Sometimes we ourselves can change our negative self-feelings to positive ones; sometimes we (and our clients) need to ask for help.

2. *Feelings of not being able to do things or of putting ourselves down because we can't grasp something as quickly as we'd like.* Communication skills in nursing are a prime example of an area in which students feel frustrated and incompetent. Honest expression of these feelings to someone who can give support, positive suggestions, and lots of trial-and-error learning opportunities is one good way to start building confidence.

3. *Feelings about not being able to* do *something about a situation.* This frequently happens when a student tackles a big nursing problem for the first time and finds no easy solution. An Eastern approach might be to admit that not all problems have solutions, or not the ones we think they should have. Sometimes, expressing the exasperation to the appropriate person moves the responsibility for solution closer to the *real* responsible person.

4. *Feelings of not being able to accept affection from others,* which may also stem from a childhood that lacked sufficient touching and "stroking." Reworking these feelings and understanding their bases is often the first step toward change.

5. *Hostile and guilty feelings* that appear for no apparent reason require a lot of work. There are written resources on the subject and groups which help individuals "get in touch" and "deal" with their anger.

6. *Feelings of helplessness and passivity* often plague students and nurses, especially when they find themselves working and learning in authoritarian environments. Assertiveness training has been one method of helping people cope with these feelings.

Expressing Emotions

Gerard Egan offers the following guidelines for expressing emotions appropriately in order that we may more fully enrich our lives:

1. Emotions are a legitimate part of being a person. We should not apologize for having feelings, including negative ones.

2. The emotions one person experiences in response to a situation are not necessarily the

same as another person's. One person's feelings are not better than another's. Because one client is angry at a spouse's death and another is relieved, does not make one better than the other.

3. Only expressing the positive emotions of joy, peace, and satisfaction is not preferable. Experiencing the whole range of feeling positive and negative is felt to be appropriate.

4. Emotions should not be used to manipulate people's or groups' feelings of grief. For example, pain in a person can engender pity and relief of responsibilities by others.

5. Deal with emotions as they occur. Don't let feelings pile up and get suppressed for another time or they may explode when you least expect it. If a feeling is too difficult to express, at least admit that it's bothering you and you can't find a way to articulate it right now.

6. Assert your right to an emotional response. Don't apologize for the way you feel and don't punish another person who challenges you. Express yourself without making others feel guilty. [11, pp. 74–75]

Evaluating Your Own Communication Style

Nurses should take the time to take stock of communication style by answering questions such as the following:

1. Do I like spending a lot of time with people, or do I prefer being by myself, or somewhere in between?
2. What do I like in other people? What do I dislike?
3. Do I let others know what I want from them? Do I tell them directly, or do they find out in indirect ways?
4. If I care about others, how do I show it? Do others know I care about them?
5. Am I good at understanding others and at letting them know I understand?
6. Do I respect others? How well do I communicate that respect?
7. Am I real with others, or do I play games and act phony at times?
8. Am I open with others? willing to talk about myself?
9. Can I confront others without overpowering or punishing them?
10. Do I ever discuss the strengths and weaknesses of a relationship with another?
11. Do I make attempts to meet new people? How does it feel?
12. Am I an active listener—listening carefully, then responding?
13. Do people come to me for help or to discuss problems? How does it make me feel?
14. Does closeness frighten me? If so, what about it frightens me?
15. Which emotions do I express easily to others, and which ones do I swallow or hide?
16. Can others tell what I'm feeling?
17. Do I use my emotions to control others?
18. Do I think it's "ok" to be emotional with others?
19. Which emotions do I enjoy in others? Which ones do I fear?
20. What do I do when others keep their emotions locked up inside themselves?
21. Does feeling left out and lonely play much of a part in my life?
22. If I feel rejected, how do I try to handle my feelings?
23. Do I feel responsible for what happens in my relationships with others, or do things just "take their course"?

24. Do I want to grow in my interpersonal relationships?
25. Am I willing to work, risk, change, in order to get involved with others?
26. Can I let others be themselves?
27. Is it important for me to be myself when with others?
28. Am I too cautious or too careful in relating to others? What do I fear?
29. How do I get along with people who have opinions and views that differ from mine?
30. Do I have any prejudices toward others? Do I acknowledge them?
31. Do I share my values with others? [11, pp. 15–19] *

Empathic Feelings and Nursing

When nurses are transacting with depressed, distressed clients, kindred feelings are often triggered off within themselves as they try to relate empathically with clients. Nurses can choose either to turn off those feelings and dissociate themselves completely from the client or to stay involved. Nurses need to recognize that the negative feelings which they are picking up may be projected onto them from the client. If we are already experiencing some insecurity and anxiety, these additional negative assaults may cause inappropriate anger for the situation. If old feelings haven't been resolved, they may compound and spill over into a totally unrelated situation.

Nurses often feel the weight of the client concerns which they bear daily. Sometimes the nurse assumes that the client wants much more from him or her than is actually being communicated. Since nursing contends with so many problems that are not immediately resolved, an overwhelming feeling of helplessness may result. Oftentimes nurses overreact to what the clients' simple needs may be. Basically, clients recognize that the nurse is not a replacement or responsible for their own self-healing abilities. Often clients are simply asking to be treated as persons, to be understood, listened to, and involved in mutual decision making.

Working Through Strong Feelings

Some methods for protecting ourselves as we are working through a strong feeling in a nursing situation have been devised by a nurse-transactional analyst:

1. Let your spontaneous feeling happen inside yourself. Be aware of it. Observe with your Adult ego state how you feel. This takes the edge off.
2. Tell yourself with your Nurturing Parent that it is okay to feel that way and you don't have to act on it right now.
3. As soon as possible tell someone you trust how you feel. Ask them to validate you.
4. Think about it. Are you ready to drop it now? Or do you want to ventilate it later?
5. Do you want to act on it? How can you do that without getting into trouble? [12, pp. 114–15]

* From Gerard Egan, *You and Me: The Skills of Communicating and Relating to Others.* Copyright © 1977 by Wadsworth, Inc. Reprinted by permission of the publisher, Brooks/Cole Publishing Company, Monterey, California.

In Chapter 4, Transactional Analysis was discussed as a method of facilitating development and human relationships. Transactional Analysis asks nurses what expectations they have of themselves in the nurse role. Do nurses feel that they are supposed to feel warm, loving, and friendly and not express anger, fear, or sadness? Do certain things about nursing frighten or disgust them, for example, surgery, needles, pain, death? Having these feelings is not wrong. If abortion repulses a nurse she is entitled to her feeling and to the appropriate expression of it. Nurses have the right to request an assignment change or to seek another position if they disagree with policy. Nurses do not have the right to vent their feelings on the client who is requesting objective information. There is an enormous difference between the nurse who allows herself feelings of doubt and grief and the one who protects herself from all emotions by covering them with a cold, unfeeling demeanor.

Communication Patterns in Response to Threat

In assessing one's own communication style and the communication patterns of others, it may be helpful to recall Virginia Satir's classifications of typical communication patterns that occur when a nurse or client is reacting to stress and/or threat to self-esteem. Any classification runs the risk of inflexibility and stereotyping, but may be useful if used as a general guide. Look at the following four patterns. Do you see yourself in any of them? Can you understand the annoying behavior of another by examining the underlying fear and feelings of inadequacy?

1. The *placating pattern* is characterized by verbal agreement with any message received. Disagreement or anger is prevented at all costs. The message conveyed both verbally and nonverbally is, "My purpose here is just to make you happy." The verbal messages often include lots of apologies. A client who is a placater is often sending out the message, "I'm helpless; take care of me." This type of response is inconsistent with the idea of taking responsibility. To teach assertiveness and take-charge skills to a placater is a true challenge.

2. The *blaming pattern* is typified by verbal tirades and by finding fault with everyone else. The blamer never takes responsibility and is invulnerable to question or criticism. Internally, the blamer is frightened of being wrong and incompetent and seeks to prevent mutiny by being a tyrant. The blamer's body language is the picture of a person under stress. In a client this behavior may take the form of phrases such as, "If only that nurse hadn't . . ." or "That doctor really makes me mad; one day he tells me to do one thing and the next day he changes it completely . . .no wonder I'm so messed up."

3. The *computing pattern* is frequently used by healing professionals to protect themselves legally and emotionally. Computing usually contains a lot of six-syllable jargon, "um, er, a's," and transitional words such as "in reference to that point," or "weighing all the factors in such a complex situation," or "it appears that . . ." Computing is the epitome of the left-dominated rational hemisphere in action. The receiver of the communication is usually left standing with mouth open,

wondering how to interrupt such a barrage of information with a simple question. Computers very rarely own up to feelings by using the word "I." They are eternal observers of life, too frightened to get involved.

4. The *distracting pattern* is a decoy tactic in which an attempt is made to divert attention from the self in the hopes that the threat will go away. Distracters usually try to sidetrack a group with comments or questions that are completely irrelevant and which take everyone off on a tangent. The hidden message is often, "I want someone to notice me, but I don't know how to do it," or "If I keep your attention long enough, maybe I'll be able to get from you what I need, which is someone to care." [29]

All these patterns have one thing in common—feelings of low self-worth. When a person uses any one of these responses, it is usually part of a habitual pattern of communication learned in early childhood. In Transactional Analysis, placating and distracting might be considered part of the Child ego state; computing and blaming part of the Parent ego state. In any case, occasional use of these responses is part of normal transacting, but continuous reliance on these patterns only serves to reinforce feelings of low self-esteem. If communicating in nursing did nothing more than help both the nurse and client to recognize these patterns as ego-defensive strategies which do not facilitate constructive change, a major goal would have been achieved.

If the four response patterns indicate low self-worth, then what pattern signifies a safe, secure, competent sense of self-esteem? Satir calls it a *leveling response;* Tranactional Analysis calls it the Adult ego state. Leveling does what it says—it flows, it is congruent (verbal, nonverbal, feeling), honest, and free. It is a meaningful, open transaction in which appropriate experiences are shared and understood. Weaknesses and strengths are acknowledged and helpful supportive resources are sought out. The communication is clear and simple. The next section of this chapter will elaborate on the leveling response, broadening it to include certain attitudes and specific ways of communicating with colleagues and clients to develop effective relationships.

INTERPERSONAL COMMUNICATION

All communication by definition is interpersonal or dyadic. The basic process of communication has been described. Perception is felt to be an essential component and becomes crucial in interpersonal transactions. Interpersonal perception involves beliefs and thoughts about people and feelings and behavior towards them. When we encounter a client for the first time, we begin to make judgments about him or her which may effect the relationship until its termination. How we look at our value judgments is an *intrapersonal* task. [1]

Judgments about the other person have been classified as static and dynamic. Static judgments are stable, ongoing aspects of the person—such as ethnic background, religious or political persuasion, sexual orientation, appearance, etc.

Dynamic judgments are those made about transitory aspects of that person, which can change readily and rapidly—for example, verbal content, facial expression, vocal qualities, and body position. Such judgments may easily be false if the person consciously, unconsciously, or while under duress, conceals the person he or she really is. This is called *masking*, and it is not always deliberate. One frequently seen example of masking is the person who is suffering physical or psychic pain, and yet, attempts to cover it up with a smile or a flippant remark.

The nurse needs to recognize that all judgments made about the other person temper or control the behavior of the other to a certain extent. If a client senses the nurse's nonacceptance of his value system, for example, that client may cover certain aspects of himself which he knows the nurse might frown upon or reject. What ensues is a very complicated game of "keep away," which yields false information and perceptions on the part of both the nurse and the client. Some static judgments which hinder open communication are stereotyping, thinking that first impressions are lasting impressions, concerning oneself excessively with certain traits such as cleanliness or style of dress, and automatically attributing positive qualities to people whom the nurse likes or vice versa.

Refraining from value-laden judgments involves another side of self-responsibility and caring. It means the nurse does *not* take responsibility for the action of a client, and it also means not making automatic assumptions about another. Adequate information must be gathered from a variety of sources over a period of time before conclusions about the client may be drawn. The nurse is responsible only for her own behavior; the client is not a reflection on the adequacy of her care, and the client's behavior is *not* a statement about the quality of the nurse-client relationship.

Interpersonal communication is the basis for initiating, maintaining, and terminating the nurse-client relationship. This involves countless transactions with the client, family, friends, other health personnel, and various community agencies. It is essential that the nurse's communication to all immediate and extended members of the health care team be clear, concrete, effective, efficient, and relevant. Most health care problems could be alleviated, if not solved, through effective communication techniques, some methods of which will be presented later in this section. The goal of any therapeutic communication is to convey empathy, congruency, and positive regard (as described by Carl Rogers in Chapter 3).

Therapeutic Communication

Rogers has contributed a valuable communication technique, classified as the nondirective Rogerian approach. This nondirective technique has revolutionized therapeutic communication and is consistent with such holistic concepts as self-responsibility, humanistic caring, development of human potential, creative coping with stress, and maintenance of a nonjudgmental attitude toward the communication process. Nurses who have placed themselves in the roles of mother-surrogate, advisor, moralizer, or lecturer have had particular difficulty in cultivating Mayeroff's kind of patience which is required for this kind of communication. Therapeutic communication is not standard social communication. There have been efforts to incorporate this therapeutic communication style into everyday relationships. Nurses and students often claim the style is false to their own way of communicating and forces them to be "phony" in their interactions. Like any new technique, therapeutic communication must be practiced and tailored to suit the personality of the practitioner using it and the client. It does not work for everyone, but at least it gives the client a chance to ventilate feelings in a safe environment. In addition, a few other positive outcomes may occur:

1. Both nurse and client learn that even "bad" feelings are "okay" and are not directed at any particular person.
2. Being heard and understood helps the client to feel cared for and worthwhile.
3. Clients begin to listen when they feel they have been listened to.
4. Clients begin to find their own solutions when they realize they aren't going to be handed any ready-made advice. They begin to assume responsibility for their lives.
5. Nurses become more acceptant of clients' feelings and attitudes. They realize that certain problems are really the clients' concerns and that trying to solve a person's problems for them places an unnecessary burden on all involved. For many nurses this is a very difficult concept to accept. The counselor role of the nurse is difficult to learn, but provides relief in the long run.
6. Clients are unique. They have their own ways of solving problems and expressing themselves. Therapeutic communication allows this to happen. [14]

Developing Listening Skills

The first step in effective therapeutic communication is simple listening—taking in or attending, as Dolores Krieger calls it. All the things that you know about body position, kinesics, proxemics, body language, tone of voice, gestures, eye contact, and so forth, come together as you quietly take all these things in, regarding the other person. The nurse's body language must communicate openness and relaxation. When setting oneself up to communicate, one should face the person squarely, adopt an open posture, lean toward the client, maintain eye contact, and appear relaxed without seeming indifferent. [11]

Silence

It is important to observe both nonverbal and verbal messages. Having all this to do, beginning nurses find it all they can do to maintain a conversation. Actually, one of the keys to listening is silence. Instead of the uncomfortable strained silence which the nurse anticipates, just a simple "letting be," without cluttering the environment with a distracting response, can convey the nurse's interest, acceptance, trust, and acknowledgment of the client's right to share whatever he or she may wish.

Listening to a client contains an enormous quality of nowness (in the Zen sense). The nurse has no prior judgments about the client, nor does he or she attempt to fit the client into his or her own belief system. [6] Passive listening can be a form of meditation, in which the client becomes the object of concentration rather than of breathing or a phrase. David Brandon eloquently describes this nowness in listening:

> Nowness closes no doors. It involves an openness which throws away fears and expectations. It opens itself to risks, to new learning, experiences and interpretations. It declares "I am ready to see you in a social way. I wish to put no boundaries on what you might say or do." [6]
>
> . . .by being receptive, noninterfering, nondemanding and letting be. By hushing our own voice, the client may begin to hear his own inner voices. [6, Abraham Maslow as quoted therein, p. 68]

Obviously, silence is not the only kind of listening or communication would not occur.

Passive Listening

Another level of listening, which takes the form of acknowledgment of the receipt of the message and encourages the client to continue, is what Gordon terms "empathic grunting" or "uh-huh," "I see," or "Go on." Nonverbal congruent communication involves leaning forward, frowning, and smiling appropriately.

Active Listening; Listening for Feelings

The type of listening which requires the most skill is active listening, which mirrors the client's previous message. Active listening first requires an accurate decoding of the client's message into a feeling, and the subsequent feeding back of that feeling to the client to examine it in a different way. Perhaps this "feeding back" is done in the form of a question; the client then confirms the accuracy of the nurse's interpretation by saying something like, "Yes, that's really how I feel," or "Yes, I *am* angry," or "You're right."

How do nurses attune themselves to decoding messages into feelings? They can practice by doing exercises such as the one found in Figure 7–2, or in real-life situations with friends, family, and eventually, clients.

In order to use active listening techniques with children, colleagues, or clients, some basic attitudes must be adopted which may appear at first to be self-evident, but if the listener has not incorporated them, active listening will not take place. These attitudes include the following:

1. The nurse must truly want to hear the client. If the nurse is rushed or busy with another priority, it should be stated at the beginning of the interaction, for even a child can detect preoccupation on the part of the listener. It is more honest to state: "I'm really pressured right now, Jonathan, and I know this is something that deserves some undivided time and attention. Can I come back and discuss this with you at a more convenient time?"

2. If a client's concern is expressed at an inopportune time due to circumstance, mood, or so on, choose a time when you really want to talk about it and are ready to give your energy to it. The statement in item (1) may be used in this situation as well.

3. When Rogers stated acceptance as a part of the caring relationship, he meant just that—genuine acceptance of *any* feeling that the client happens to express. If the nurse is really repulsed by a certain feeling or statement expressed by a client, she should first decode the message to accurately read its underlying feeling. If the nurse is still disgusted about the client's attitude, she should not attempt to be therapeutic in that situation. Her disapproval, disgust, etc., will effect her verbal and nonverbal communication and invalidate the entire transaction. Nurses need to be sensitive to their own value systems and blind spots. A judgmental nurse should not be counseling clients who conflict with her value system if she cannot operate without letting her feelings "block" the communication.

4. The nurse must honestly trust in the client's own ability to express feelings, work through them, and arrive at some solution or resolution.

5. Feelings, especially passionate ones of anger, hatred, and love are transitory and subject to change. A client's hurtful hostility can turn, within minutes, to

FIGURE 7-2 Listening for feelings (a communication exercise)

Reprinted with permission from Thomas Gordon, *Parent Effectiveness Training* (New York: David McKay, Co., Inc., 1970), pp. 307–09.

DIRECTIONS: *Children communicate to parents much more than words or ideas. Behind the words often lie feelings. Following are some typical "messages" children send. Read each separately, trying to listen carefully for feelings. Then in the right-hand column, write the feeling or feelings you heard. Discard the "content" and write in only the feeling—usually one or several words. Some of the statements may contain several different feelings—write in all the main feelings you hear, numbering each different feeling. When you have finished, compare your list with those in the Key, scoring each item according to the scoring directions.*

Child Says	Child is Feeling
EXAMPLE: I don't know what is wrong. can't figure it out. Maybe should just quit trying.	(a) Stumped. (b) Discouraged. (c) Tempted to give up.
1. Oh boy, only ten more days until school's out. 2. Look, Daddy, I made an airplane with my new tools! 3. Will you hold my hand when we go into the nursery school? 4. Gee, I'm not having any fun. I can't think of anything to do.	

5. I'll never be good like Jim. I practice and practice and he's still better than me.
6. My new teacher gives us too much homework. I can never get it all done. What'll I do?
7. All the other kids went to the beach. I don't have anyone to play with.
8. Jim's parents let him ride his bike to school, but I'm a better rider than Jim.
9. I shouldn't have been so mean to little Jimmy. I guess I was bad.
10. I want to wear my hair long—it's my hair, isn't it?
11. Do you think I'm doing this report right? Will it be good enough?
12. Why did the old bag make me stay after school, anyway? I wasn't the only one who was talking. I'd like to punch her in the nose.
13. I can do it myself. You don't need to help me. I'm old enough to do it myself.
14. Arithmetic is too hard. I'm too dumb to understand it.
15. Go away; leave me alone. I don't want to talk to you or anybody else. You don't care what happens to me anyway.
16. For awhile I was doing good, but now I'm worse than before. I try hard, but it doesn't seem to help. What's the use?
17. I would sure like to go, but I just can't call her up. What if she would laugh at me for asking her?
18. I never want to play with Pam anymore. She's a dope and a creep.
19. I'm sure glad that I happened to be born the baby of you and Daddy rather than some other parents.
20. I think I know what to do, but maybe it's not right. I always seem to do the wrong thing. What do you think I should do, Dad, work or go to college?

FIGURE 7-2 (continued)

SCORING KEY:
Listening for Feelings

DIRECTIONS:

Give yourself a 4 on those items where you feel your choices closely match those on the Scoring Key.

Score yourself a 2 on items where your choices only partially match or where you missed a particular feeling.

Give yourself a 0 if you missed altogether.

1. (a) Glad.
   (b) Relieved.
2. (a) Proud.
   (b) Pleased.
3. (a) Afraid, fearful.
4. (a) Bored.
   (b) Stumped.
5. (a) Feels inadequate.
   (b) Discouraged.
6. (a) Feels job is too hard.
   (b) Feels defeated.
7. (a) Left behind.
   (b) Lonely.
8. (a) Feels parents are being unfair.
   (b) Feels competent.
9. (a) Feels guilty.
   (b) Regrets his action.
10. (a) Resents interference of parents.

11. (a) Feels some doubt.
    (b) Not sure.
12. (a) Angry, hateful.
    (b) Feels it was unfair.
13. (a) Feels competent.
    (b) Doesn't want help.
14. (a) Frustrated.
    (b) Feels inadequate.
15. (a) Feels hurt.
    (b) Feels angry.
    (c) Feels unloved.
16. (a) Discouraged.
    (b) Wanting to give up.
17. (a) Wants to go.
    (b) Afraid.
18. (a) Angry.
19. (a) Grateful, glad.
    (b) Appreciates parents.
20. (a) Uncertain, unsure.

YOUR TOTAL SCORE _____

HOW YOU RATE IN RECOGNIZING FEELINGS:

61–80   Superior recognition of feelings.
41–60   Above average recognition of feelings.
21–40   Below average recognition of feelings.
0–20   Poor recognition of feelings.

acceptance or relief if he or she is given the proper outlet and response. Active listening helps sender and receiver to recognize the real focus of an emotion and removes it from a person-to-person battle of wills.

6. The client must be seen as a separate and unique person—not as an extension of the nurse's will or goals. This relates to humility in caring and requires the nurse to step back and not do or learn *for* the client unless absolutely necessary. [13, pp. 59–60]

Active listening also requires flexibility, true concern for the other person's way of living, and a willingness to change. The nurse must be secure in herself to allow herself to be drawn into the client's world and to see it as he does.

The Understanding Response

Active listening is one of a variety of therapeutic communication techniques that are incorporated into what Berstein has described as the "understanding response." In the understanding response the health professional attempts to comprehend the client's point of view and communicate that comprehension to the client. Several communication skills will be discussed, but the chief methods for completing the understanding approach are through the use of reflection of feeling, restatement, clarifying feelings, eliciting feelings through broad opening statements, and focusing and summarizing techniques.

Therapeutic Communication Techniques

Some examples of therapeutic techniques follow:

Accepting	"I understand."
Recognition of Person	"Sue, you've changed your hair."
Stroking	"I really like it with those red highlights."
Offering Self	"Mind it I have a cup of tea with you?"
Broad Opening Statement	"Is there anything on your mind?"
Making Observations	"You appeared tense in exercise class this A.M."
	Client: "I was as tight as a drum until I broke a sweat after the first 20 minutes."
Restatement	*Nurse:* "Tight as a drum?"
	Client: "Yeah, you know, all my muscles were stiff like I slept wrong or did some heavy exercise. The only muscle I remember straining was my TMJ (temporal mardibular joint) arguing with my mother last night!"

Reflection	*Nurse:* "You're angry with your mother?"
	Client: "All I did was ask for the car for the weekend so my friends and I could go skiing."
Seeking Clarification	*Nurse:* "Could you go back a few steps and explain some of the preceding events which might add to some understanding of what happened?"
	Client: "Everytime I try to do something like this on my own my mother treats me like a 5-year-old!"
Translating or Decoding Feeding Back Feelings	*Nurse:* "You sound as if you're hurt and that your mother doesn't trust you."
	Client: "Yeah, and I've never given her one reason not to trust me either."
	Nurse: "Could there be other reasons why your mother is so firm about this?"
	Client: "Well, my other sister was killed in an automobile accident 3 years ago when she was my age . . .maybe that has something to do with it."
Summarizing and Seeking Validation of Perceptions	*Nurse:* "OK, let's see if I've got this right. You've stated that your mom is almost irrational when it comes to your borrowing the car for social reasons, but she lets you run errands in it. You see her refusal as an attempt to keep you as a little girl and you feel you can handle responsibility at your age.
Encouraging a Plan of Action	"Can you think of some ways to resolve this problem that you and your mother are having?"

Communicating Understanding to Clients

How can nurses communicate understanding to their clients? Some possibilities are as follows:

1. by using plain and understandable language;
2. by making sure that the tone of voice and manner of speaking are congruent;
3. by allowing the person's message time to sink in before responding;
4. by responding to each new idea rather than waiting until the end of the discussion and focusing on only one thought; and

5. by responding to both feelings and content. Not every therapeutic conversation needs to revolve around reflection of feelings alone. There are many content areas with which the nurse can also help the client. [11]

Barriers to Communication

Most barriers to communication are not physical, but a few—such as sensory, perceptual, and expressive disorders that include hearing and sight impairments, stroke, brain dysfunction, or absence of the organs involved in speech—can contribute to a dysfunctional communication process. Special care must be taken to enhance the person's ability to communicate, whether that entails locating a translator, making sure that a communication aid is within reach (for example, a chalkboard for a postlaryngectomy client), that a hearing aid has batteries, or that a pair of dentures fit for proper speech. Other physical barriers to communication include noise or distractions.

Berstein lumps all blocks to communication into four categories—the evaluative, reassuring, hostile, and probing responses. [4] In actuality, all the responses require that a value judgment be made by the receiver which would serve to discredit the feeling the sender is expressing, for example:

Client: "I really wish my doctor would give me some more information on whether I can walk on this sprained ankle or not."

Nurse: "Don't worry, he'll be here in good time and everything will work out just fine." (*evaluative and reassuring*)

Some specific nontherapeutic techniques follow:

Nontherapeutic Communication Techniques	Nurse's Statements
Advising	"Good morning, Jean. You really shouldn't be looking like a sad sack, you have so much to be thankful for."
Overly approving	"That's right, put a smile on your face."
"Why"-ing	"Why are you frowning, anyway?"
Agreeing, disagreeing, or disapproving	"I think everyone has a right to pout, but not on the day they're taking their new baby home."
Evaluative	"It's not a very good start to motherhood, you know."
Defending	"I think your husband looks like he'll be a big help to you—don't say things against him."
Making Stereotyped Comments	"This is just postpartum depression. You mothers all come out of it sooner or later."
Changing the Subject	"Now what would you like me to do with these gorgeous flowers?"

One direct technique usually used in interviewing can be used non-therapeutically—probing. Probing actually involves trying to focus in on a particular problem or group of complaints or signs. It is asking for more information about a topic, for example, "Tell me a little more about your pain," or "Describe this pain for me in detail in your own words." It becomes nontherapeutic when its use is inappropriate, for example, "Exactly how did your father die?", or when the timing is poor, for example, "You mentioned that your father is in the coronary-care unit. Have you seen the latest film on cardiopulmonary resuscitation?"

Missing or not picking up on themes, key words, ideas, or feelings can block communication. Intellectualizing, moralizing, and advice-giving are other tactics which set up barriers to communication. Hays and Myers have stated that "the nurse's role, in her communication with a patient, is to guide the patient . . .while learning herself. To do this she must provide a relationship in which the patient is given the opportunity to learn about his difficulties in living, to discover the sources of his difficulties and his present discomfort, and to identify other patterns of behavior which will both alleviate these difficulties and meet his needs." [25]

There are many more ways to block communication than just tuning out, misinterpreting, or focusing on the wrong feeling. Satir mentions that effective "being with" in communication takes a kind of clairvoyance to sense what it is the person is trying to say. If the rules of communication are followed and if we begin by checking or validating our perceptions, our batting average can improve considerably. There are always those special people close to the person who often know exactly what the person means even when a client is comatose, and such people should be utilized. Clairvoyant powers can be developed to assist in communication interpretation. Other esoteric assessment measurements, such as graphology (handwriting analysis), are gaining credibility in this country after having been widely accepted elsewhere as guides to interpreting communication.

For the time being, nurses need to be scrupulous in their assessment of a client's communication processes because they are the keys to any problem solving, teaching, or change that will occur in the nurse-client relationship.

The Nursing Interview

An *interview* is a serious, purposeful communication between two people, in which one participant gives information and the other seeks it. A *nursing interview* denotes any interaction, either verbal or nonverbal, between a nurse and a client which focuses on the health needs of the client or family. The interview is the major vehicle for conducting a positive nurse-client relationship as well as for serving as the basis for most assessment, diagnosis, and treatment.

A good interview elicits the following:

1. the necessary history;
2. the extent of psychological difficulties;
3. the reaction of the client to a particular health or illness event which has caused him to come for help; and

4. an opportunity for the client to learn something about himself so that health needs may be identified and ways of meeting them determined.

Conditions for a Productive Interview

Certain basic conditions are necessary to facilitate a productive interview. They are:

1. active listening;
2. a rapport between client and interviewer;
3. freedom from interruption;
4. psychologic privacy; and
5. emotional objectivity.

All of the therapeutic communication techniques mentioned in this text are suggested with the addition, in some cases, of probing and direct questions.

The purpose of the interview dictates the formality of approach and types of questions to be asked. In a health history, very direct questions, or even a self-responding questionnaire, are used. Direct questions usually require a *yes*, or *no*, or monosyllabic response. This usually elicits no information other than the necessary history. The nurse-client relationship is not furthered, but astute observation of the client's behavior may reveal some information about the client's true self.

Principles of Interviewing

In contrast to the direct approach is the open interview which begins with a broad subject and then gradually moves toward the specific. After a sense of trust has been established, questions usually progress from less to more personal. *Yes*-or-*no*-response questions are avoided, and questions are phrased to avoid bias (*not*, for example, "But you've quit smoking now, haven't you?").

Nurses should remember that interviewing in nursing takes place constantly, not just in the waiting or examining room of a clinic, but anytime the nurse requests information from a client or follows up on a client's leading statements. Murray points out that what the nurse learns about the client is not nearly as important as what she can help him to learn about himself. Reflective responses give both nurse and client an opportunity to replay a comment and to become aware of its underlying meaning. All human behavior has purpose and meaning and may have a particular significance for a client which only he can determine.

The nurse who is self-aware and self-acceptant does not need to impose her unmet needs and goals on the client, thus guiding him toward her own goal achievement. Carl Rogers asks:

> Do we respect [the client's] capacity and his right to self-direction, or do we basically believe that his life would be best guided by us? Are we willing for the individual to select and choose his own values, or are our actions guided by the conviction (usually unspoken) that he would be happiest if he permitted us to select for him his values and standards and goals? [23]

Process Recording

One exercise that nurses, counselors, and sociologists have all tried and tested for years in order to help analyze and improve their therapeutic communication skills is the process recording exercise. A process recording is a written recording of a significant portion of what goes on between the nurse and the client. These interactions are the actual experiences with the patient and any other persons involved in the situation. The record includes *anything* that occurs—whatever is said or done and any other relevant aspects of the environment, as well as the apparent effects of these things.

The process recording is intended to help the nurse to:

1. communicate effectively with clients;
2. identify feelings and needs so that they may be constructively directed;
3. identify the client's feelings, needs, and problems; and
4. assist the client in identifying these needs and problems and in working with them.

Guidelines for writing a process recording include the following:

1. Identify the purpose of the interaction. This may emerge as the interaction progresses or it may be identified by the nurse in advance. (Or the initial purpose may have to be modified in light of what takes place.)
2. Write a short introduction telling a little about the client and the situation being recorded.
3. Write the interaction as soon as possible after it takes place. Include both the verbal and nonverbal behavior. Use four columns: one for the patient's responses, one for the nurse's responses, and one for an analysis of the interaction. The fourth column is used to identify the principles of communication that applied, techniques that were used, and if the criteria of accuracy, relevancy, efficiency, and effectiveness were met.

Nurses should periodically analyze their own interaction patterns via some tool, for example, videotape, peer evaluation, role play, and so on. Communication skills need constant practice and improvement; they represent the helper's most important resource.

Rules for Effective Nurse-Client Communication

The nurse, when communicating with a client, must:

1. make clear verbal and nonverbal statements to others;
2. be in touch with self, attitudes, beliefs, and feelings;
3. observe others as different from self and any other person;
4. behave toward others as people separate from self and unique;
5. view differences as an opportunity to learn rather than as a threat to one's own value system.

6. deal with interpersonal situations as they exist, not as how the nurse would like them to be;
7. take responsibility for all feelings, thoughts, and perceptions rather than attributing them to someone else; and
8. be practiced in communication skills which can clarify, receive, and check the meaning of communication between the nurse and client. [30]

A Checklist for Therapeutic Nurse-Client Interactions

In a therapeutic interaction the nurse:

1. creates an environment in which clients can safely look clearly and objectively at themselves and their behavior;
2. is not afraid to ask questions, and models a clear, straightforward communication style for the client;
3. makes observations on the client's verbal and nonverbal presentation of self;
4. asks for and gives information in a nonjudgmental, congruent manner;
5. builds client self-esteem through valuing statements and stating client strengths; for example, "You handled that difficult situation well.";
6. establishes collegial relationships—that is, *both* are learners;
7. welcomes questions and checking on meaning of statements;
8. emphasizes good motivation in client, but states use of communication techniques as inappropriate, irrelevant, inefficient, or unclear when observed;
9. elicits suggestions for positive strokes toward others. ("How could you show Jim that you cared for him?");
10. sets ground rules of interaction, for example, no interrupting, three-minute time limit, etc.;
11. does not set up a defensive response. ("You really came across as hostile toward Jim, didn't you?");
12. makes negative emotions "okay" to express;
13. handles sensitive material carefully;
14. interprets unclear communications and suggests ways of improving communication patterns; and
15. comments on nonverbal communication. [30]

Group Communication, Dynamics, and Process

Interpersonal or group communication can take the form of a dyad or group of more than one person, usually not larger than twenty persons, which engages in interpersonal communication for some purpose. Most of our focus in this text has been on the intrapersonal and the nurse-client relationship. Families, groups, and communities have been alluded to only briefly. As nursing experience, communication, and leadership skills improve, the holistic nurse will find more of his or her energy being devoted to group and community dynamics, development, and process.

The rules for communication with one other person apply to family and group communication patterns as well. Basically, a family or group should be able to:

1. complete transactions, check perceptions, and ask questions;
2. sense and interpret hostility;
3. see how others see them;
4. see how they see themselves;
5. tell each other how they express themselves verbally and nonverbally;
6. tell each other what they hope, fear, and expect from each other;
7. disagree;
8. make their own choices;
9. learn new information and skills through practice (trial and error);
10. free themselves from harmful effects of past models;
11. give a clear message and be congruent in their behavior, feelings, and verbal communication; and
12. limit hidden and double messages. [30, p. 176]

Every group has its own dynamics or complex interdependent forces. These forces involve the interactions in the group, the interpersonal relationships, the communication problems, and the way in which members make decisions. These dynamics go on in every group. In order for a group to function effectively certain roles and functions must be performed:

Task-Oriented Functions	Group Maintenance Functions
1. *Initiating*—tasks, goals, ideas, procedures	1. *Encouraging*—friendliness, responsive to ideas of others, giving recognition
2. *Information seeking*—requesting facts, ideas, opinions	2. *Expressing group feelings*—sensing and sharing with others, reconciling disagreements
3. *Information giving*—offering facts, stating beliefs	3. *Harmonizing*—exploring differences.
4. *Clarifying*—reflecting ideas, straightening out confusion	4. *Compromising*—admitting error, encouraging participation
5. *Summarizing*—pulling together related ideas; offering the decision for group to accept or reject	5. *Gate-keeping*—keeping communication open and facilitating discussion of group problems
6. *Consensus testing*—checking to see how much agreement has been reached	6. *Setting standards*—expressing and applying standards in evaluating group functioning and production

As summarized in Chapter 3, the interpersonal relationship is based on trust, and from Chapter 4 we know that basic trusting relationships are established in infancy. Being authentic, genuine, and open as a nurse, client, or group member involves a risk. Suppressing anger and hostility may appear to placate and smooth relationships, but actually such behavior decreases the amount of ourselves we are willing to disclose and as such is detrimental to interpersonal and group trust in the long term. Clients under stress often disclose parts of themselves unintentionally and feel self-conscious, betrayed, and later, angry. Group dynamics, psychotherapy, interpersonal relations, communications, and assertiveness courses attempt to help people through practice in groups to learn to express feelings and emotions clearly, to communicate support and understanding, and to identify strengths in others. Group process theory will be described in more detail in Chapter 10.

COMMUNITY COMMUNICATION

The purposes of communication center around the ability of sender and receiver to get in tune with one another so that ideas, information, and attitudes may be shared. This is difficult enough in a one-to-one or group relationship in which nonverbal messages can be exchanged, felt, and feedback exchanged. In larger groups or in situations in which the sender and receiver are separated by time, space, and circumstance, much more care must be taken to formulate a message that is in tune with the receiver's needs at that particular moment in time.

The nurse is in the unique position of being the interpreter of one type of language (medical) to the lay person. The nurse sifts through enormous quantities of data, selects what is important for clients to know, and then finds ways to transmit that information. When this process is carried out on the community level, public relations and information and health education personnel become involved. Mass media—which includes campaigns in newspapers, television, films, books, magazines, and journals—is one method used to spread health information.

In community communication, the questions, "Who are those target populations?" and "What are their value orientations?" become of utmost importance. For example, if an immunization campaign is planned, which group of parents is most in need of convincing, and how can they be most effectively reached? Social psychology is a field which predicts the kinds of stimuli which will affect certain groups of people. These and other resources are tapped to plan a community education program.

To stimulate behavior change in an individual or community, three areas must be triggered: (1) the cognitive thinking level, (2) the motivational and feeling level, and (3) the behavioral (action) level. All of the factors which influence interpersonal communication affect community communication, for example, the values, interests, concerns, and needs of an audience; their cultural assumptions about health and illness; their understanding of health jargon and their attitudes toward health-care personnel and people in "authority"; anxiety levels, and potential barriers to communication within the sender and receiver relative to values, motives, and so forth. More detail on communication for health education is included in Chapter 9.

Professionals communicate within their own communities through professional organizations, meetings and committees, symposia, conventions, journals, and books. (Further discussion of staying informed of developments within the profession will be discussed in Chapters 8 and 10.) It is essential, especially in holistic nursing, to communicate with others participating in the movement in order to keep abreast of new findings and techniques and to provide support and energy for the continued breaking of new ground. Mastery of effective communication techniques on the interpersonal, group, and community level is the key to any teaching, changing, or politicizing effort.

REFERENCES FOR CHAPTER 7

[1] Mary G. Almore, "Dyadic Communication," *AJN*, 79, no. 6 (June 1979), 1076–78.

[2] Donald B. Ardell, *High-Level Wellness* (Emmaus, Pa.: Rodale Press, 1977).

[3] George R. Bach and Peter Wyden, *The Intimate Enemy* (New York: Avon Books, 1968).

[4] Lewis Berstein, R. S. Dana, and Richard Dana, *Interviewing: A Guide for Health Professionals,* 2nd ed. (New York: Appleton-Century-Crofts, 1974).

[5] Fay Bower, *The Process of Planning Nursing Care* (St. Louis: C. V. Mosby Co., 1977).

[6] David Brandon, *Zen in the Art of Helping* (New York: Delta Books, 1976).

[7] Pamela Brink, ed., *Transcultural Nursing* (Englewood Cliffs, N.J.: Prentice-Hall, Inc., 1976).

[8] Fritjof Capra, *The Tao of Physics* (Boulder, Colo.: Shambhala Publishing, 1975).

[9] Arthur W. Combs and others, *Helping Relationships* (Boston: Allyn and Bacon, Inc., 1978).

[10] Victor Daniels and Lawrence Horowitz, *Being and Caring* (Palo Alto, Ca.: Mayfield Publishing Co., 1976).

[11] Gerard Egan, *You and Me* (Monterey, Ca.: Brooks/Cole Publishing Co., 1977).

[12] Jean Elder, *Transactional Analysis in Health Care* (Menlo Park, Ca.: Addison-Wesley Publishing Co., 1978).

[13] Thomas Gordon, *PET in Action* (New York: Wyden Books, 1976).

[14] Thomas Gordon, *Parent Effectiveness Training* (New York: David McKay, Co., Inc., 1970).

[15] Thomas A. Harris, M.D., *I'm OK— You're OK* (New York: Avon Books, 1969).

[16] Jack Hofer, *Total Massage* (New York: Grosset & Dunlap, 1976), pp. 167–70.

[17] Sidney Jourard, *The Transparent Self* (New York: Litton Educational Publishing, 1971).

[18] Lynne B. Jungham, "When Your Feelings Get in the Way," *AJN*, 79, no. 6 (June 1979), 1074–75.

[19] Andie L. Knutson, *The Individual, Society, and Health Behavior* (New York: Russell Sage Foundation, 1965).

[20] Frederick Leboyer, *Loving Hands* (New York: Alfred A. Knopf, 1976), p. 27.

[21] E. John Lilly, Mickey Jackson, and Kay Kniesel, eds., *Non-Verbal Communication in Nursing* (Costa Mesa, Ca.: Concept Media, 1975).

[22] Alexander Lowen, *Bioenergetics* (New York: Penguin Books, 1975).

[23] Ruth Beckmann Murray and Judith Proctor Zentner, *Nursing Concepts for Health Promotion* (Englewood Cliffs, N.J.: Prentice-Hall, Inc., 1979).

[24] Margaret Pluckham, *Human Communication* (New York: McGraw-Hill Book Company, 1978).

[25] Sister Mary James Ramaekers, "Communication Blocks Revisited," *AJN*, 79, no. 6 (June 1979), 1079–81.

[26] Sharon L. Roberts, *Behavioral Concepts and Nursing Throughout the Lifespan* (Englewood Cliffs, N.J.: Prentice-Hall, Inc., 1978).

[27] Carl Rogers, *On Becoming A Person* (Boston: Houghton-Mifflin, 1961).

[28] Jurgen Ruesch, *Therapeutic Communication* (New York: W. W. Norton & Co., 1961).

[29] Virginia Satir, *Peoplemaking* (Palo Alto, Ca.: Science and Behavior Books, 1972).

[30] Virginia Satir, *Conjoint Family Therapy* (Palo Alto, Ca.: Science and Behavior Books, 1967).

[31] William C. Schutz, *The Interpersonal Underworld* (Palo Alto, Ca.: Science and Behavior Books, 1966).

[32] Abbot Zenkei Shibayama, *A Flower Does Not Talk* (Rutland, Vt.: Charles E. Tuttle Co., 1975).

[33] Sandra Sundeen and others, *Nurse-Client Interaction* (St. Louis: C. V. Mosby Co., 1976).

[34] Paul Watzlawick, *Communication: The Language of Change* (New York: Basic Books, 1978).

[35] Paul Watzlawick and others, *Pragmatics of Human Communication* (New York: W. W. Norton & Co., 1967).

Chapter 8
problem solving

CHAPTER OUTLINE

F. Community, Cultural, and Societal Applications of Problem Solving
   1. Nonmedical Religious Healing Systems
      a. Navajo Indian Healing
      b. Black and Hispanic Healing
   2. Homeopathic Approaches to Healing
   3. Community Health Assessment and the Problem-Oriented Record
   4. The Canadian Health "Field Concept"

CHAPTER OBJECTIVES

1. Differentiate inductive reasoning from deductive reasoning and give one example of each.
2. Compare the steps of the problem-solving, nursing, and research processes.
3. Trace the development of the rational thought process from reductionism to systems theory. Describe how systems theory is used in nursing.
4. List the sources of information for the health assessment.
5. Describe four methods for arriving at a problem statement. Contrast a nursing problem with a medical problem, through example.
6. Critique six holistic data-gathering techniques according to the criteria presented in the text.
7. Define problem-oriented charting and list the components of the problem-oriented record.
8. List the commonalities which all secular and religious healing methods share.
9. Describe the Canadian "Health Field Concept" as a community problem-solving approach which promotes prevention and wellness.

OVERVIEW, BACKGROUND, AND DEFINITIONS

Problem solving is the systematic process through which decisions are made. It begins in early childhood and is a continuous, lifelong process of refining and perfecting. Problem solving has always been a pivotal concept in nursing, but it came into particular prominence in the late 1960s under the name Nursing Process. Yura and Walsh have defined the nursing process as an "orderly, systematic manner of *determining* the client's *problems, making plans* to solve them, *initiating the plan* or assigning others to implement it, and *evaluating* the extent to which the plan was effective in resolving the problems identified." [33] Although client participation in this process is not spoken to, the major steps of the problem-solving process in professional nursing are neatly summarized.

Nurses and clients have been using inductive and deductive reasoning to work through everyday personal problems, although they may not have examined their own problem-solving styles. Oftentimes a client or nursing problem may be one primarily of inadequate or inappropriate problem-solving techniques for the situation. Attitudes toward solving problems are extremely important in pursuing solutions. If a nurse or client has had difficulty solving certain kinds of problems in the past, they may be less than enthusiastic about approaching a similar problem situation. If a problem appears completely novel and different—new health problems are prime examples—a client may abandon usual, successful problem-solving methods in panic.

Chapter 8 will examine the use of inductive and deductive reasoning and intuition in the solution of problems, view systems theory as a way of organizing and analyzing data and actions in a deliberate, systematic fashion with holistic applications and ramifications. Problem solving, the nursing process, and the research process will be compared. High-level problem solving via nursing diagnosis and problem-oriented charting will be proposed as indicators of the expanding role and skills of professional nursing, with particular emphasis on health assessment.

Alternative methods of health assessment will be reviewed as adjuncts to more orthodox medical techniques and technologies. A brief overview of other cultural systems of healing problems will be presented. Innovative strategies for self-assessment, diagnosis, and treatment will be mentioned.

Interpersonal problem solving between nurse and client as well as community problem solving will be scanned with focus on decision trees and algorithms in interpersonal and community health planning. Nursing interventions will be classified as preventive, nurturative, and/or generative in selected situations.

Systems Theory, Problem Solving, and the Holistic View of Humanity

Problem solving and the nursing process are filled with new terminology which the student must grasp in order to proceed with the remainder of this chapter. Since most problem solving in nursing is based on systems theory as proposed by Ludwig Van Bertalanffy or Paul Weis, a basic understanding of the systems approach is a prerequisite to further study of decision making in nursing.

Reductionism and Atomism versus Holism and Relativism

Prior to systems theory, ways of processing information had been divided into two camps—atomistic, reductionistic, or mechanistic and holistic, relativistic, or gestalt. Reductionists did what their name implies, that is, they isolated everything and studied it in its smallest reducible form (for example, looking at the trees rather than the forest.) The holists, as we have seen, chose to view wholes, patterns, and relationships, and then analyze their interconnections (for example, looking at the forest rather than the trees.) Each of these ways of viewing the world and its problems has its assets and drawbacks. Systems theory attempts to bring elements of both views together, although many philosophical holists object to this. As usual, reductionism and holism represent another polar struggle—each theory looks at different aspects of the same issue.

Atomism, or *pars pro toto* (that is, viewing the world in pieces), was a philosophy based on Democritus' notion of causality:

$$\boxed{cause \longrightarrow effect}$$

Clearly, this causal theory is linear and unidimensional, and is still held to be one adequate explanation for the workings of the universe. It is useful in that a part can be singled out, examined in detail, compared, and experimented with. The problem with the method surfaces when a situation—especially in health and disease—is multifactorial (occurring on several or all levels of existence), and when a cause cannot be isolated (see Figure 8-1).

Holism, on the other hand, attempts to look at "continuous networks of dynamics with ordered units on a hierarchical scale of orders of magnitude." [27] Figure 8-2 illustrates a systems view of the universe, a disturbance in that universe, and the multivariate effects on subsystems in the hierarchy of systems. Note how the information flows from one level to another. As with any model, abstract ideas are not adequately conveyed.

A system is a set of interrelated parts; it may be either open or closed. In closed systems no input is received, nor is any output produced. They occur often in physics and mathematics; they do not exchange matter or energy with the environment.

An open system does exchange matter with the environment; such a system is constantly changing and moving toward order. Human beings operate as open systems; they have elaborate feedback systems that keep the organism in a steady

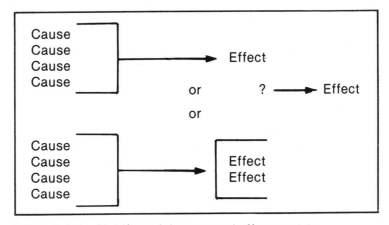

FIGURE 8-1 Multifactorial cause and effect models

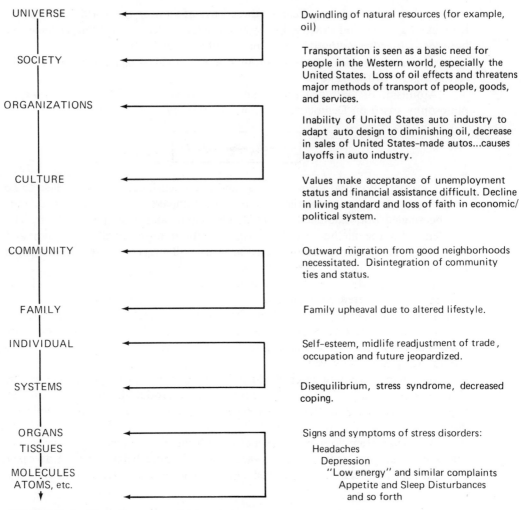

UNIVERSE	Dwindling of natural resources (for example, oil)
SOCIETY	Transportation is seen as a basic need for people in the Western world, especially the United States. Loss of oil effects and threatens major methods of transport of people, goods, and services.
ORGANIZATIONS	Inability of United States auto industry to adapt auto design to diminishing oil, decrease in sales of United States-made autos...causes layoffs in auto industry.
CULTURE	Values make acceptance of unemployment status and financial assistance difficult. Decline in living standard and loss of faith in economic/political system.
COMMUNITY	Outward migration from good neighborhoods necessitated. Disintegration of community ties and status.
FAMILY	Family upheaval due to altered lifestyle.
INDIVIDUAL	Self-esteem, midlife readjustment of trade, occupation and future jeopardized.
SYSTEMS	Disequilibrium, stress syndrome, decreased coping.
ORGANS TISSUES MOLECULES ATOMS, etc.	Signs and symptoms of stress disorders: Headaches Depression "Low energy" and similar complaints Appetite and Sleep Disturbances and so forth

FIGURE 8-2 The effect of upper-level changes on subsystems: The case of an unemployed auto worker

Adapted from Howard Brody, "The Systems View of Man: Implications for Medicine, Science, and Ethics," *Perspectives in Biology and Medicine* (Autumn 1973), 71-92.

state of equilibrium. Specific homeostatic mechanisms are described in Chapter 5, which explains inherent and acquired methods of adapting to stress.

General systems theory allows a view of humankind as an open system that is dynamically intertwined with an immensely diverse set of forces which possess the following four attributes:

1. Natural systems are wholes with irreducible properties.
2. Natural systems are self-regulating.

3. Natural systems create themselves in response to the challenge of the environment.

4. Natural systems are coordinating interfaces in nature's hierarchies. [4, p. 6]

Control, influence, and communication between systems rely on feedback. As mentioned in Chapter 5, positive feedback increases the deviation and disorder in the system while negative feedback causes it to return to balance. Feedback does not always follow a gradually increasing hierarchical communication. Sometimes it "leap-frogs" over one or more systems. Figure 8-2 demonstrates one person's development of a psychosomatic disorder that resulted from disturbances in a system far above his intrapersonal level.

In the words of Van Bertalanffy:

> General systems theory, then, is scientific exploration of "wholes" and "wholeness" which, not so long ago, were considered to be metaphysical notions transcending the boundaries of science. Hierarchic structure, stability, teleology, differentiation, approach to and maintenance of steady states, goal directedness—these are a few of such general systems properties. [27]

Later in this chapter, the components of systems theory will be applied to the nursing process, as it has been applied to communications theory, computer analysis, and many other disciplines.

Deduction, Induction, and Intuition in Science

Before we examine specific methods of thinking which are used by nurses and clients to define and solve problems, a review of the related functions of the two hemispheres of the brain is appropriate. Chapter 1 and Chapter 3 explain the left (masculine) and right (feminine) sides of the brain and their purported areas of dominance. In his treatise on the dialogue of Art versus Science or a subjective versus objective view of the world, Robert Pirsig differentiates between what he calls the *classic* and *romantic* world views:

Classic understanding: Proceeds by reason and laws;

                                    Masculine mode;

                                    Science, law, medicine;

                                    Making the unknown known;

                                    Bringing order out of chaos;

                                    Controlled and restrained.

Romantic understanding: Inspirational; imaginative; creative; intuitive;

                                      Feelings predominate; Esthetic conscience;

                                      Femininity;

                                      Free and natural style. [23]

These characteristics match the masculine and feminine principles, although different labels are used.

A problem arises when people function exclusively in one or the other mode of thinking, and hold stereotypical conclusions about the other mode (for example, "Classicists are dull, lack humor, and are uncaring."). No one is ever completely in one mode or the other, and the more balance that is developed, the richer the person becomes. Likewise, to judge another person to be of a type inconsistent with one's own cognitive style, oftentimes turns the relationship between the two people into an "I'm right, she's wrong" situation, thus creating a barrier in the relationship. In light of this, we are reminded of the Chinese saying "Things that oppose each other also complement each other." [11, p. 231]

Subjective and objective observations of reality have been a topic of discussion in physics for the past forty years. In atomic physics it is acknowledged in the quantum principle (Position of Particle = Mass x Velocity) that the scientist is not merely a detached objective observer but that he actually influences the properties of the observed objects. John Wheeler, the physicist, suggests replacing the word "observer" with "participant." This is a relatively new concept in physics, but Eastern mystics have always known that the subject and object are inseparable and even indistinguishable. [7]

Since physics is often viewed as the epitome of the rational sciences, other scientific areas are beginning to acknowledge that the observer is part of the experiment and vice versa. Nurses classify data as subjective and objective in the data-gathering process, but these are merely universally recognized labels for certain kinds of observations rather than a reflection of the truth.

Most students have been educated under the influence of Aristotelean logic, which divides reality into mutually exclusive categories. "If an observation has a certain characteristic, than it cannot at the same time have another characteristic," is a commonly-held belief, indeed, one that has helped students to develop "either-or" patterns of thought. This leads to statements such as, "He can't eat this way and still care about his health," or "He can't both love and hate his wife at the same time."

Jung (see Chapter 4), Fromm, and the Eastern mystics all refute this type of logic and offer paradoxical logic as an alternative. Paradoxical thought and language says that things that appear to be contradictory may at the same time also be true.

There are two types of rational ("classical") reasoning—*deductive* and *inductive*. Deductive reasoning starts with general knowledge or a principle and predicts specific observations. An example would be to see a client with "strep throat" and expect to observe redness and white spots in the throat, pain on swallowing, elevated temperature, a positive throat culture, and swollen parotid glands.

Inductive reasoning proceeds from specific observations to conclusions, as seen in the case of a young adult who presents himself with shortness of breath, elevated respirations, acute anxiety, numbness and tingling in the extremities, and tightness in the chest with no complaints of abdominal pain. Given the aforementioned observations, the nurse can reasonably initially conclude that the most common diagnosis would be the hyperventilation syndrome.

Most problems in nursing and the health sciences are too complicated to involve merely one type of reasoning or another. Pirsig states that the solution of problems too complicated for common sense to solve is achieved by long strings of mixed inductive and deductive inferences that weave back and forth between the observed machine (in his case, a motorcycle) and the mental hierarchy of the machine (as found in the manuals). The correct program for this interweaving is formalized as the *scientific method.*

All experimental research is based on the scientific method, which relies almost totally on rational thinking. Most researchers will acknowledge, however, that intuitive insights are what give them new creative directions and hypotheses to test via the scientific method. These insights often come during periods of relaxation or while their left hemisphere is preoccupied. Intuitive—sometimes called "lateral"—thinking is characterized by sudden bursts or flashes unrelated to other thoughts and scattered. Nurses need to reopen themselves to this complementary side of themselves, as well as to the rational thinking which we will now discuss in detail.

Problem Solving, the Nursing Process, and the Research Process

The problem-solving, nursing, and research processes are compared in Figure 8–3. The following section elaborates on the definition and use of these three processes in purposefully helping clients move themselves toward high-level wellness.

RESEARCH OR SCIENTIFIC METHOD	PROBLEM SOLVING	NURSING PROCESS	PROBLEM-ORIENTED SYSTEM
Identify General Problem Area Define Specific Problem	Identify Problem	Assessment	Observation Assessment
Review Related Information Propose Hypothesis	Plan	Planning	Planning
Test Hypothesis	Action	Implementation	Intervention
Analyze Test Results	Evaluation	Evaluation	Evaluation
Terminate or Modify Study	Revision	Revision	Plan Revision Total Reassessment

FIGURE 8-3 Problem-solving methods commonly used in nursing

NURSING DIAGNOSIS AND DECISION MAKING: HIGH-LEVEL PROBLEM SOLVING

Nursing process is seen by most nursing theorists as the core process by which the goals of nursing are accomplished. [33, p. 26] It encompasses other essential processes, such as nursing history, nursing assessment, nursing diagnosis, nursing care planning, nursing orders, and nursing evaluation. [3, p. 26] Nursing process forms the basis for a conceptual form of nursing practice rather than a technique, function-based type, as seen in nursing's earlier development. Nursing process aligns nursing with the other "hard" sciences (physics, chemistry, microbiology), as well as with the behavioral sciences (psychology, sociology, anthropology), since interpersonal skills are incorporated and deemed highly important.

Nursing process is a step toward formulating a knowledge base unique to nursing, but it is still largely reliant on the biologic and social sciences for its knowledge. How can *nursing* knowledge be generated? Primarily through nursing research, which has only formally been in existence for thirty years. Nursing research historically has focused on the development and evaluation of techniques, tools, technology, and teaching methods. This is all vital information for practitioners and students, but it has not stimulated new concepts or theories.

It is the feeling of this and other nurse educators that the nursing process, leadership process, and research process are all necessary ingredients in every nursing care situation. Every time a nurse defines a problem, researches it, draws conclusions and relationships, sets goals with clients, families, and colleagues, and systematically evaluates the effectiveness of the process, new learning *should* be generated, tested, and used to build nursing theory.

Beginning and practicing nurses usually find themselves involved in *applied research,* which seeks solutions to everyday nursing problems. This is most easily accomplished by a search through the literature. This is usually done by looking through such indexes as *American Journal of Nursing: Annual and Cumulative Indexes, Cumulative Index to Nursing Literature, Nursing Outlook: Annual and Cumulative Indexes* (since 1953), and *Nursing Research: Annual and Cumulative* (since 1952). [31, p. 27] Indexes refer researchers to specific topics in a variety of nursing journals.

Large university libraries and some specialized libraries will conduct computerized searches (usually for a fee) for those looking for all available information on a very specific topic. This type of review of the literature is usually used by master's and doctoral level nurses participating in or conducting their own research projects.

When nurses attempt to generate their own *new* knowledge it is termed *basic research*. This should be the focus of current and future nursing research, especially in holistic nursing areas in which research is desperately needed. Valid and reliable experimental studies usually require a background in statistical analysis and a familiarity with data collection and sampling methods. A basic knowledge of computer programming is another asset in organizing and analyzing data. Without a solid expanding research base, nursing cannot advance as a profession.

There is a popular trend in nursing to adopt "standardized" care plans for nursing care which incorporates tried and true problems and solutions for typical problems associated with certain medical and surgical diagnoses. An example of one, although illness-oriented, is exhibited in Figure 8–4. These protocols are the result of years of nursing experience and research. One drawback is that standardized care plans tend to give nurses a false sense of having covered all the potential problems before they have even assessed the client. There is the danger that the client becomes merely a problem and that individual needs are overlooked. An individual care plan must be designed for every client no matter how stereotypical or "classic textbook" he may appear. The other inherent drawback is that nurses who use standardized care plans already made for them may not feel the need to generate their own research to discover other areas unique to nursing that could be identified. Since standardized care plans are built upon the medical model of disease, there are few problems that are not medically based. An entire world of health-oriented needs awaits the motivated nurse practitioner/researcher.

Health Assessment: The Data Base

Health History: Nursing Interview

Health assessment involves the gathering, sorting, classifying, and interpreting of a variety of data to form a conclusion. Also, it requires a health history and health examination which demands observation and clinical evaluation. A demonstration of the components of a typical health assessment is shown in Figure 8–5.

Observation

The use of the interviewing and communication skills presented in Chapter 7 are essential in observation. Observation and clinical evaluation involve the use of the senses of sight, smell, touch (palpation, percussion, energy-field scanning), taste, and hearing (auscultation and percussion). Clinical laboratory data or further diagnostic studies, such as chest X-ray or electrocardiogram, are often ordered to substantiate this phase of health assessment.

Other Sources of Data

Part of the data-gathering process includes researching the client's own past health records, if any, and searching available or library literature for background information. Textbooks, and particularly journals, are extremely helpful sources for practitioners to gain additional up-to-date knowledge. Familiarity with a medical library is requisite knowledge for solving nursing problems.

Sorting, Classifying, Categorizing, and Analyzing

While data is being gathered, all sorts of cognitive processes of the inductive, deductive, and intuitive variety are occurring simultaneously. Part of the beauty of the systematic approach to solving problems is that it forces the nurse not to skip

FIGURE 8-4 A standardized nursing care plan

Excerpted from Marlene Mayers, *Standardized Nursing Care Plans* (Palo Alto, Ca.: K/P Company Medical Systems, 1974). Reprinted with permission of El Camino Hospital and the author.

CAST, PATIENT IN

DISCHARGE CRITERIA:
1. Verbalize understanding of and ability and willingness to follow M.D.'s outpatient regimen.

If still in cast when discharged:
1. Verbalize awareness of approximate time to return to hospital.
2. Demonstrate understanding of cast care and explain conditions of cast that need immediate attention.
3. Reiterate signs and symptoms of impaired circulation and pressure sores and verbalize understanding of need to report to M.D.

DATE	USUAL PROBLEMS	EXPECTED OUTCOMES	DEAD-LINES	NURSING ORDERS
	1. **Potential impaired circulation and/or nerve damage due to constricting cast**	1. Able to move toes or fingers Toes or fingers warm, pink and respond to stimuli No edema	√ q 8 hr	1. Check fingers or toes of affected extremity every hour for 4 hours (12-4-8) and report immediately: -cyanosis or pallor -swelling -coldness -numbness or loss of motion -lack of blanching sign (blood should return immediately after pressure released from toe or fingernails)
	2. **Potential development of pressure points due to cast not being thoroughly dry for 48 hours**	2. No development of pressure sores	48 hrs √ q 8 hr	2A. Keep cast exposed to air for 48 hrs (heat cradle and sunlight help to dry cast) B. Turn patient to unaffected side 4 times for 2 hours each to allow posterior side to dry C. If wet cast to be elevated, use rubber or plastic covered pillows
	3. **Potential pressure sores from contact with cast and immobility**	3. Observable skin clear and intact No musty odors No complaints of pressure or burning under chest	√ q 8 hr	3A. After cast dried, pull stockinette lining out over edges and secure with adhesive or plaster B. If spica or body cast, protect groin with waterproof material C. Turn at least every 4 hours (12-4-8) and encourage to lie on abdomen 4 hours a day (see that toes of casted leg do not dig into mattress while lying prone) D. Check daily for musty odor and report any complaints of burning or pressure especially over heel, ankle bones, iliac bones and dorsum of foot
	4. **Potential bleeding under cast**	4. Early detection of any bleeding	√ q 8 hr	4A. Circle any blood stain on cast with pencil. B. Check at least every hour for 4 hours for spread of area of bleeding
	5. **Potential development of complications when cast is removed due to fragility of bones and improper support**	5. No complications when cast is removed	Dis-charge √ q 8 hr	5A. Assist when using affected extremity for first time B. Provide adequate support for all joints that have been in a cast
	6. **Potential concern over home management (if still in cast at time of discharge)**	6. Reiterates conditions with cast that will need immediate attention Verbalize understanding of cast care Verbalize signs/symptoms to report immediately	Dis-charge √ daily	6A. Instruct that broken casts, casts worn threadbare or softened from secretions need immediate attention B. Instruct not to get cast wet C. Instruct in cast care including ways to relieve itching D. Describe signs of impared circulation and pressure sores and stress need to report immediately E. Instruct to elevate extremity to relieve swelling or throbbing

FIGURE 8-5 Health assessment. (Legend: ADLs—activities of daily living; ROM—range of motion; hg—hemoglobin; Crit.—hematocrit) (Continued on p. 322.)

Reprinted with permission from The National League for Nursing, *Problem Oriented Systems of Patient Care,"* (New York: National League for Nursing, 1974).

COMMUNICATION: *Language*—Dialect, vocabulary, grammar, quantity; *Voice*—pitch, volume, quality, *Patterns*—rate, articulation, frequency; *Organs of speech*—lips, teeth, tongue, palate, etc.; *Nonverbal*—vocalizations, gestures, posturing, expressions, writing, somatics; *Comprehension*—reading, calculating, highest level of school achievement, "fast eyes, slow ears, etc."

SENSORIUM: *Touch*—avoidance, hypersensitivity, numbness, dominance, use of; *Vision*—acuity, use of, dominance, glasses, aids, drops, motion sickness; *Hearing*—acuity, use of, dominance, aids, Otitis Media during infancy; *Taste and smell*—preferences, responses to, attention, seeking, avoidance; *Affect*—flattened, heightened; *Memory*—retention, recall, auditory, visual, motor, recognition span; *Balance*—head, sitting, kneeling, standing, running, turning, eyes closed; *Consciousness*—attention span, focus and control, perception, attitude seizures; *Kinesthetic awareness*—awareness of body parts, position in space; *Circadian rhythms*—cyclical swings of mood, control, activity, behavior, productivity, time sense, anniversary reactions.

LOCOMOTION—ACTIVITY: *Gross and fine motor*—ADLs, self-help skills, utilization of optimum potentials, pattern of rest, sleep, and exercises, residual reflexes; *Strength*—symmetrical, tissue turgor, voluntary use of *ROMs*—limitations of active ROM, limitations or abnormal joint movement, needed passive ROMs, orders for stretching; *Appliances*—aids for sleeping, alignment, ambulation, locomotion, ADLs; *Coordination*—voluntary control of eyes, limbs, head, eyes and hands, tremors or jerks; *Work, school, play*—type, place, productivity, response, level of achievement, regularity, attitude.

RESPIRATORY—CIRCULATORY: *Source of O_2*—Air, tank, croup tent, croupette, vaporizer, nebulizer, quality of air, smoke; *Ability to inhale and exhale*—expiratory grunt, inspiratory wheeze, mouth breathing, position of choice, patent airway, tracheotomy, labored breathing; *O_2—CO_2 exchange*—color of mucosa, nailbeds, circumoral duskiness, hg-Crit., shape of chest, chest sounds, x-ray report, sickle cells, lethargy, growth rate; *O_2—CO_2 transport*—characteristics of vital signs, fluid shifts, local color; *Cell utilization*—energy level, skin condition, bruises, healing, mental clarity, pain, shape of fingers, frequency of infections, inflammation, immunization status.

NUTRITION: *Physical appearance*—body build, height, weight, energy, hair, skin, etc.; *Eating patterns*—appetite, best meal, snacks, reaction to stress, seasons; *Position*—table, highchair, special seat, held, propped, standing, on the run; *Place*—dining room, desk, cafeteria, kitchen, alone, with family; *Type and amount*—offered, actually eaten, cultural influences, financial influences, likes and dislikes, diet characteristics; *Ability to ingest*—dental

FIGURE 8-5 (continued)

status, intactness of structures, tongue thrust, hyperactive gag, clenching, tongue chewing, grinding, incoordination of lip closure, bite, chew, suck, tongue movement, swallow and breathing; *Ability to digest*—adequate hydration and secretions, size of abdomen, unusual amount of diaphoresis, weakness, color of skin, Hg-Crit., nailbeds, location, timing and severity of body pain; *Ability to metabolize*—rate of healing, nervous and mental state, metabolic problems; *Aids*—bottles, nipples, feeders, built-up utensils, special utensils, dish anchors, gastrostomy or gavage tubes, medications; *Securing food*—financing, purchase and selection, planning diet, transporting; *Storing*—refrigeration, freedom from infestation; *Preparing*—washing, cooking and serving techniques.

ELIMINATION—HYGIENE: *Patterns and characteristics of external secretions*—nose, eyes, ears, perspiration, urine, stool, vaginal, draining wounds, colostomy, ileostomy; *Management of bodily discharges*—frequency, type and location of usual cleansing activities for catheter, drains, bags, diapers, dressings, frequency and type of baths, toileting routines, aids used; *Personal hygiene*—ADLs, self-help skills, menstrual care, bathing, dressing, selection of clothes, wash and comb hair, shave, use of deodorants, wash and purchase clothes and equipment, tooth brushing; *Degree of independence*—clothing, housing influences, housekeeping aids, other aids or techniques, level of developmental achievement.

PSYCHO–SEXUAL DEVELOPMENT: *Self-concept*—sexual roles, consistency of role model, role conflicts, body image, self-image, self-esteem, sense of belonging, shyness, attention seeking; *Relationship with family and others*—source of support, concern for others, caring, parenting, closest people, relationship with others outside home, school phobias, infringements on others; *Sexual concerns*—knowledge and understanding of sex and sexual development, menstruation, attitudes, safety, modesty, limitations; *Coping mechanisms*—problem-solving methods, risk taking, decision making, discipline, impulse control, masturbation, head banging, finger sucking, eating, drinking, drugs; *Life style*—organization of family, responsibility for direction of family, daily habits, goals, disturbing elements, parental concerns; *Developmental stage*—of individuals, of family; *Fertility*—family planning, prenatal and postpartum changes, menarche, mensis, menopause, potency, parity, abortions, unusual births, family tree.

OTHER: *Medical history*—sources of care, satisfaction with finances, problems, operations, hospitalizations, accidents, medications, understanding of releases obtained and sent; *Preventive measures*—current immunization status, teaching done, health guidance, safety, awareness of needs and value; *Follow-up*—physical and financial ability to follow advice, attitude, available association, thoughtful use of, blind obedience, multiple directions; *Diagnostic tests*—those desired, needed, or avoided, those other than through medical sources above, understanding of; *Allergies*—substances, type and severity of reaction, treatment; *Pattern of seeking care*—regular intervals, only when ill, constantly, procrastinates, avoids GP, specialist, clinic, private, ER.

any steps. If the nurse *does* jump to a conclusion, she can retrace steps later to get back on the track, although this usually requires extra work, and hence, frustration.

At times, the data-gathering, sorting, and interpreting processes can be likened to a Sherlock Holmes game, in which multitudes of intellectual tricks, blind alleys, and false clues abound. Keep in mind that problem solving in nursing is more than an intellectual exercise—especially to the client whose privacy is being invaded, whose bodily parts are being palpated, tapped, and touched, and whose body image is being shaken, if only temporarily.

It has been conservatively estimated that the relative importance of the three elements of the data base are as follows:

History (70 percent)
Health examination (20 percent)
Laboratory and other procedures (10 percent) [9, p. 10]

It is not uncommon for a medical student to spend as much as three to four hours in obtaining this historical and health examination data. It is not unreasonable, therefore, to expect that a beginning nurse will find this first step of the nursing process amazingly time-consuming. Without an adequate data base, however, the rest of the process is a sham. Sometimes a health problem will be so glaring (as stated in a chief complaint) that the temptation is to dive into solutions. This temptation should be resisted, however. Indeed, the client may push for quick solutions, but one of the chief reasons the nurse is being sought out is because of her unique knowledges and skills; therefore, they should be used. A computerized health history form should not be accepted unless it is reviewed with the client in a step-by-step fashion.

Some additional hints on history-taking are called for. Sometimes, oblique indirect methods of questioning are necessary. A client may be able to describe inability to climb the stairs to his apartment much more easily than he can respond to the direct question, "Do you have shortness of breath on exertion?" Get specific answers or probe for more information. If a person says he has "low blood," find out what he or she means by that. Be alert for changes in symptoms. When did the sputum change color? Is a symptom normal for that person even though it seems strange to you? Has the client always complained of gas following a meal consisting of certain vegetables? Is the person an accurate or reliable historian or do you need to seek help from others? Precision is difficult to maintain in history-taking, but it is little better in laboratory values. One of the differences between orthodox medicine and holistic approaches is the reliance of medicine on incredible varieties of technical diagnostic tests. Exotic tests should only support the practitioner's well thought out hunches and hypotheses.

The Problem Statement: Nursing Diagnosis

Assuming that the data base is relatively complete, the practitioner moves on to the next step—diagnosis. One way of expressing this very complex and variegated process is: Data Base + Information Base + Logic = Problem List or Diagnosis. [9, p. 26]

The data base is all the information gained from the client himself through history-taking (subjective data), plus the observations gained through examination and other methods (objective data). The information base is all the information the nurse has stored and gathered from her background, prerequisite courses, experience, and research. Logic entails the use of inductive, deductive, and intuitive processes, using those principles which lead to the proper conclusions.

Factored into logical thinking is certain demographic data which will immediately rule out certain problems—for example, age, sex, race, and location. In addition, three maxims have been formulated by Cutler:

1. Common problems occur commonly, or the rarest diagnosis should not be chosen first.
2. Uncommon manifestations of problems are more common than common manifestations of uncommon problems.
3. No problem is rare to the client who has it. [9, p. 27]

Above all, William Osler's comment should be carved in stone: "Variability is the law of life, and so, no two faces are the same, no two bodies are alike, and no two individuals react alike, and behave alike under abnormal conditions . . . " [9, Osler as quoted therein, p. 36]

Some other problem-solving methods work in certain health situations. Some are being used as "shortcuts" in primary care in which rapid diagnosis is needed. Some of these methods are being applied to the rapidly expanding fields of self-diagnostics and self-care.

The main concern with the previously mentioned "traditional" method of problem solving is the extreme time factor. Another popular method of arriving at conclusions from large amounts of data is called the Branching Technique, in which all diagnoses are viewed as a huge tree. As various clues begin leading to one of the many systems of branches, more questions related to that area or system are asked. If answers are negative, the practitioner backs up and tries the next most likely branch. After he or she finds and solves the main problem, the practitioner briefly reviews the rest of the branches and prunes any excess material. The Branching Technique is being used successfully in computer diagnostics and with flow charts.

Related to the Branching Technique is the dendrogram. In this problem-solving method, mechanisms such as flow charts, algorithms, and decision trees may be used to formulate some basic hypothesis. Sometimes the chief complaint and presenting clinical picture are enough to send the diagnostician up one particular branch of the tree as more substantiative data is gathered. The end of the branch should yield the problem. Figure 8-6 demonstrates a dendrogram used in a medical systems approach. Nurses need to determine which trees will help them in their own problem-finding and problem-solving process. [9]

Decision paths and flow charts have become very popular because they can save health examination and assessment time and require only *yes* or *no* answers as a conclusion becomes more and more obvious. The potential problems are easily imagined—using prefabricated, nonindividualized, rigid recipes which take the creativity out of health problem solving is one. The direct question approach does little to facilitate the caring relationship or to help the nurse gain personal

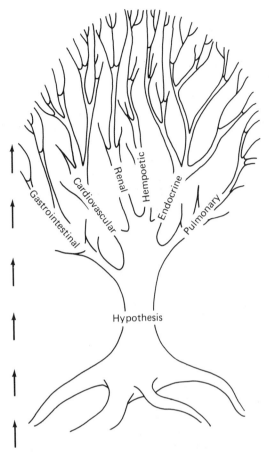

FIGURE 8-6 The diagnostic tree

knowledge of the client's problem from his point of view. Medicine may be becoming more efficient, but this only intensifies the need for more humanistic health care. [9, pp. 51-52]

Other complex mathematical concepts are helping the rational decision-making process in medicine by predicting probabilities of occurrence for certain clues that overlap or are common to several problems. What is the likelihood that a specific problem is occurring? Again, these are helpful tools, although not the panacea or replacement for good problem solving.

Another method of problem solving deserves description because it is based on a Gestalt view; it is called pattern recognition. It involves more than syndromes, triads, tetrads, or clusters of observations such as those everyone memorizes to pass a pathology or medical nursing examination. It is more than a hunch; it involves a series of clues coming together more quickly than the conscious mind can process them. Upon reflection, however, they are readily apparent.

Much time and mental effort go into any assessment. Defining the problem, by Western standards, is almost more important than a solution. This is, perhaps, good reason for this, since solutions to problems are often hit and miss—especially in psychosomatic disorders.

Of course, all these problem-solving techniques are medical problem oriented. One of the finest methods for recording and insuring that systematic problem solving occurs has been devised and will be described in a later section of this chapter as a multidisciplinary team approach to problem solving. Confusion occurs when nurses try to define what a *nursing* problem is as opposed to a *medical* problem. Several schemes that focus on basic human needs have been suggested by Abdellah, based on theories by Maslow (page 75). This appears to be the state of the art to date, thus we see nursing diagnoses incorporating: alterations in patterns of sexuality, self-concept, body image, disruptions in mobility, communication patterns, grieving, and so forth. It is also possible for a sign, symptom, or piece of data to be a nursing diagnosis. Pain is an example of a symptom that is also a problem, and its nursing diagnosis would be pain management.

Bower suggests that the nursing diagnosis be stated as a need or a problem which points the way to the nursing goal. [5] The need or problem is seen in a stress-response framework that is especially helpful for beginning nurses because it is simple and acknowledges the major role of stressors in the development of adaptive and maladaptive coping responses.

The Nursing Goal

There are many nursing process formats. They are often called nursing care plans by institutions. Care plans seem to skip steps at first glance, but it should be kept in mind that the practiced nurse can subsume, *not skip,* certain steps that need not be written down. The nursing goal is another step that is not always stated outright. All nursing goals should be clear, simple, and specific, and imply the nursing intent:

Problem: Mrs. G is unable to control the pain of her contractions.
Goal: To help Mrs. G regain control over her pain.

Action-Implementation

The nursing goal, in turn, points to the nursing actions necessary to achieve that goal. The actions should be listed in order of priority, for example:

1. Explain to Mrs. G three methods of pain relief (with pros and cons); for example, laying-on-of-hands by nurse (nurturative), progressive relaxation (generative), pain medication (protective and nurturative), or nothing.
2. Encourage choice and order of preference and perform or teach the method of choice.
3. Follow with other methods if the first fails; depending on the method selected, this could be protective, nurturative, and/or generative nursing action.

EVALUATION OF CLIENT CARE PROBLEM SOLVING

DIRECTIONS: Place a check in the column which is appropriate for your response. The goal is to have all questions answered with a *yes* response.

	Yes	No	Comments
1. Are the problems or needs a logical outcome of assessment data?	___	___	___
2. Do they reflect current theory applied to the individual patient?	___	___	___
3. Are high-priority problems indicated?	___	___	___
4. Are the goals appropriate to the problems identified?	___	___	___
5. Are both short- and long-term objectives stated?	___	___	___
6. Are evaluation criteria included with the objectives?	___	___	___
7. Is there evidence that physical needs were considered? mental? emotional? spiritual? social? environmental?	___	___	___
8. Do the nursing actions or orders indicate: What is to be done? When it is to be done? Specific hours? How it is adapted to the client? How to do it? For how long?	___	___	___
9. Do objectives pertain to prevention? therapy or palliation? rehabilitation?	___	___	___
10. Do the nursing actions represent a variety of nursing measures? nurturative-comforting? generative-teaching? preventive and nurturative-counseling? preventive and generative-referring? preventive-observing?	___	___	___
11. Do the nursing actions reflect application of current theory?	___	___	___
12. Is there a clear delineation of the responsibilities of the various members of the nursing team?	___	___	___
13. Does the plan indicate the client's dependency level and how nursing promoted independence?	___	___	___
14. Has the nursing care plan been updated?	___	___	___
15. Is there a discharge plan for continuity of care?	___	___	___

Adapted from Lucille Lewis, *Planning Patient Care* (Dubuque, Iowa: William Brown & Co., 1976), p. 196.

Evaluation Criteria

Once the actions have been listed, the criteria for evaluating effectiveness of the plan should be determined. The *actions* are not evaluated; the *results* of the actions are evaluated in terms of the goal. In other words, is the goal achieved and how do we know it has been achieved? Mager [15] offers three criteria for evaluating a goal:

1. Describe the specific behavior that is acceptable as evidence of the desired outcome.
   Example: Mrs. G will go through a complete contraction cycle without grimacing, holding her breath, gritting her teeth, or crying out.
2. Describe the important conditions under which the behavior will occur.
   Example: With the coaching of a nurse or her husband.
3. Describe the criterion of acceptable performance.
   Example: Eight out of ten contractions, or 80 percent of the time.

With all three criteria pulled together, the final Evaluation Criteria Statement becomes:

> *Example:* With the coaching of her husband or nurse, Mrs. G will go through a complete contraction cycle without gimacing, holding her breath, gritting her teeth, or crying out, in eight out of ten contractions.

The evaluation, then, answers the question of whether or not the criteria was satisfied. If the feedback is positive—the opposite of a biologic feedback mechanism—the process is terminated. If the evaluation is negative, adjustments need to be made somewhere in the process, which must then be begun again. All steps need to be checked and revised, if necessary.

Nurses need to look at their own problem-solving and nursing process styles and abilities. A self-questionnaire appears on p. 327. How does your nursing care planning measure up?

HOLISTIC DATA GATHERING AND PROBLEM-SOLVING TECHNIQUES IN HEALTH PROMOTION AND HEALING

The major orthodox methods of gathering information from and about self and clients have been mentioned. Holistic practitioners utilize many of these methods or refer clients to orthodox health-care facilities for further study if needed. Oftentimes, clients have already been subjected to batteries of diagnostic studies, many of which are of the laboratory variety, before they seek out holistic methods.

Assessment Methods

Inventories such as those included in Chapter 6 and the appendices are considered borderline or dual-purpose assessment techniques; that is, they have been adopted by many orthodox health care systems as well as by holistic systems. Some assessment strategies or questionnaires included in this category are the Wellness Inventory, the Health Risk Index, Stress Testing and Fitness, fat-muscle ratio measurement, and biofeedback assessment.

Hair analysis is gaining credibility in the health community, and is even being reimbursed by third-party payers (if it has been termed, in medical jargon, as a "toxic mineral test"). Another measurement of nutritional status is the diet feeling diary, a variation on dietary recall; it is used by many holistic clinics.

Self-inventories that assess feelings and self-recorded journals or diaries are both of great importance in the motivational and teaching/learning areas of holistic nursing. Standardized objective tests of psychological well-being, such as the California Psychological Inventory, are considered valuable by some and serve as a link to scientific research on the statistical value of the tool. Other tests utilized to evaluate personality, perception, anxiety, and stress are listed in Figure 8-7.

All the body therapies we have mentioned (such as the Alexander technique, bioenergetics, rolfing, and polarity) involve astute observational skills in order to analyze the purposes behind certain movements and body language before an attempt at treatment can be made.

Applied kinesiologists use muscle testing, as described in Chapter 6, to ascertain the strengths, weaknesses, and even allergies in the body's energy system. Reflexologists sense problem areas based on palpation and subjective feedback from the client. Nurses using Therapeutic Touch scan the energy field for "differences or blocks," while examining the symmetry of the body visually. Historical questions are incorporated throughout the assessment. Other laying-on-of-hands modalities assess as healing occurs.

Psychic reading is a major component of holistic assessment for those who desire it. Psychic reading can involve a specific traditional system, such as the Indian Chakra system, or it can be a self-system that works for the reader. The occult sciences use:

1. *Astrology*—using day of birth on the zodiac chart to determine dominant sign and moon sign to chart character traits and future events.

2. *Numerology*—using name and birthdate to sketch the person, events, areas of potential change and growth, numerical elements that are missing or too heavily stressed in the personality, relevant work to be done with numbers, and geometric shapes and structures.

3. *Tarot*—a pictorial representation of the archetypes and states of consciousness on a special deck of cards. It helps reveal the inner life of the individual and can be used in symbolic healing.

1. Tests of Personality: Directed toward the measurement of relatively enduring characteristics of the person

   a. Inventories focusing on "normal" traits and dimensions
      California Q—Set
      California Psychological Inventory
      Edwards Personal Preference Schedule
      Omnibus Personality Inventory
      Sixteen Personality Factor Questionnaire
      Thurstone Temperament Schedule

   b. Inventories focusing on "pathological" traits and dimensions
      Eysenck Personality Inventory
      Minnesota Multiphasic Personality Inventory
      Thirty-two Personality Factor Questionnaire

   c. Miscellaneous Personality Devices focussing on specific dimensions of behavior
      Firo-B and Firo-F (Interpersonal relations orientation-behavior and feeling)
      Holtzman Inkblot Technique
      Rotter Internal-External Scale (locus of control)
      Thematic Apperception Test

2. Perceptual Tests
   Bender Gestalt Test
   Benton Visual—Motor
   Pursuit Rotor
   Embedded Figures Test
   Rod and Frame Test

3. Anxiety Tests
   Cattell's IPAT Anxiety Scale Questionnaire
   Fenz-Epstein Anxiety Scale
   Life Change Inventory
   State-Trait Anxiety Inventory
   Taylor Manifest Anxiety Inventory

4. Physically Related Tests of Stress
   Cold Pressor Test
   Bicycle Ergometer
   Harrower Stress Tolerance Test
   Sustained Handgrip
   Treadmill and Step-Stress Tests

FIGURE 8–7 Varieties of personality and stress assessment tests

Adapted from Barbara B. Brown, *Stress and the Art of Biofeedback* (New York: Harper & Row, 1977), pp. 226–27.

4. *Chirognomy*—the study of the palm of the hand to determine personal characteristics and past and future events.

5. *Graphology*—the study of handwriting to determine areas of the personality, attitudes, values, and important formative experiences.

Since this particular area of diagnosis and therapy is so rarely documented in the United States (though Russia has conducted many experiments on parapsychological phenomena), and since psychic reading is subject to charlatanism, great caution must be exercised in evaluating the data obtained from psychic evaluations. No one diagnostic technique, orthodox or alternative, is used alone. Assessment is a multisensory modality process. The more noninvasive methods that can be tapped to help the nurse reach a valid conclusion the better. Criteria for selection of diagnostic tools should also include:

1. level of client participation,
2. cost,
3. level of discomfort and anxiety to client,
4. risk of contagion,
5. accuracy (false positives/negatives), and
6. level of complexity.

Despite the countless number of holistic assessment techniques, the number of fully developed philosophies of health and disease are still culturally and ethnically circumscribed within a small number. One of these cultural systems is Chinese medicine. Contrary to popular belief, it is not a whimsical, intuitive art, but a logical, consistent, and rational framework that is *complementary* to Western Medicine. [29, p. 111]

Sobel compares Western and Chinese medicine and finds that Western medicine is concerned with an analysis of "material phenomena," that is, with a system of measuring and comparing *quantitative* data (centimeters, grams, seconds). [29, p. 112] Chinese medicine, on the other hand, looks at *functional* relationships based on *energetic* qualities (yin and yang; and the five evolutive phases of earth, wood, water, fire, and metal). [29, p. 112]

Not that medicine wasn't concerned with relationships, as Hippocrates indicated in Epidemics 1, Chapter XXIII:

> The following were the circumstances attending the diseases, from which I framed my judgment, learning from the common nature of all and the particular nature of the individual, from the disease, the patient, the regimen prescribed and the prescriber—for these make a diagnosis more favourable or less; from the constitution, both as a whole and with respect to the parts, of the weather and of each region; from the custom, mode of life, practices and ages of each patient; from talk, manner, silence, thoughts, sleep or absence of sleep, the nature and time of dreams, pluckings, scratchings, tears; from the exacerbations, stools, urine, sputa, vomit, the antecedents and consequents of each member in the successions of diseases, and the abscessions to a fatal issue or a crisis, sweat, rigor, chill, cough, sneezes, hiccoughs, breathing, belchings, flatulence, silent or noisy, hemorrhages, and hemorrhoids. From these things must we consider what their consequents also will be. [29, Hippocrates as quoted therein by Jones, p. 196]

The Chinese system makes use of the life force energy (*chi*) which can be stimulated, balanced, and unblocked through acupuncture, acupressure, and moxibustion (burning a substance at the site of the acupuncture needle). The definitive work on Chinese medicine is the Yellow Emperor's Classic of Internal Medicine which reinforces the importance of *chi*, "nowadays [1500s A.D.] vitality and energy are considered the foundation of life." [29, p. 187]

One widely recognized practitioner of Chinese medicine for over thirty years is Naboru Muramoto. In a collection of his lectures and discussions, he summarizes some of the simpler diagnostic tools other than acupuncture or pulses. To look at someone's face and its features is likened to reading a book about that person's health—past, present, and future. Figure 8-8 depicts some facial characteristics and their possible meaning as clues to the diagnostician. Occasionally, a strong parallel to Western medical principles is seen.

FIGURE 8-8 Assessing facial features in Chinese medicine

Excerpted with permission of Michael Abehsera, ed., from Naboru Muramoto, *Healing Ourselves* (New York: Swan House Publishing Co., 1973).

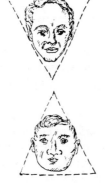

THE SHAPE OF THE FACE

Yin-shaped face

> The chin is pointed.
> The face forms a triangle with base up.
> Notice the large forehead.

Yang-shaped face

> The chin is somewhat flattened.
> The face forms a triangle
> with base down.

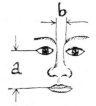

Contraction of facial features (Yang)

The distance between the eyes and mouth (a) is relatively short.
The distance between the inside corners of the eyes (b) is very narrow.
The nose is contracted and almost flat.
The eyes are small.

Expansion of facial features (Yin)

The distance between the eyes and mouth (a) is rather long.
The distance between the outside corners of the eyes (b) is rather wide.
The nose is long and expanded.
The eyes are large.

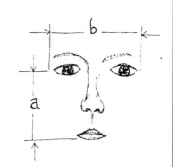

FIGURE 8-8 (continued)

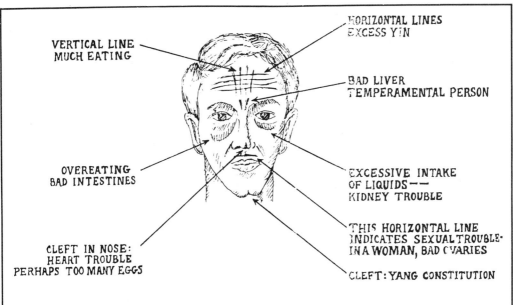

VERTICAL LINE
MUCH EATING

HORIZONTAL LINES
EXCESS YIN

BAD LIVER
TEMPERAMENTAL PERSON

OVEREATING
BAD INTESTINES

EXCESSIVE INTAKE
OF LIQUIDS —
KIDNEY TROUBLE

CLEFT IN NOSE:
HEART TROUBLE
PERHAPS TOO MANY EGGS

THIS HORIZONTAL LINE
INDICATES SEXUAL TROUBLE.
IN A WOMAN, BAD OVARIES

CLEFT: YANG CONSTITUTION

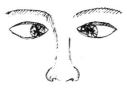

THE EYE

Iris turned toward the nose is a Yang sign.
It is in general a sign of blood
acidosis and high blood pressure.

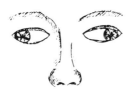

Iris turned toward the ears is a Yin sign.
Shows a condition of alkalosis in the
blood and a proclivity for cancer.

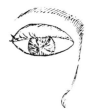

Swelling around the eyes, particularly a swelling of the upper eyelid, indicates gall bladder stones. When the stones
pass, the swelling drops immediately.

A dark brown color under the eyes indicates overly Yang
kidneys and trouble in the female organs.

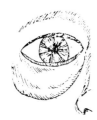

Swelling under the eyes indicates kidney stones. A formation of gall stones or blood stagnation may also be indicated.

Dark blue or violet under the eyes reveals blood stagnation,
probably caused by consumption of fruit, sugar and meat.

Bulging eyes indicate a Yin condition and thyroid trouble.

Pimples on the interior of the eyelid (sties) signify excess
protein. They usually appear and disappear relatively quickly.

An eyelid that is almost white signifies anemia. The inside
of the eyelid should be red. To examine, gently pinch the
eyelid and pull it away from the eye.

FIGURE 8-8 (continued)

EYEBROWS

A broad, thick eyebrow is Yang. A thin eyebrow is Yin.
Too much sweet food, especially sugar, makes the eyebrows
thinner and eventually causes them to disappear. People with
almost no eyebrows are prone to cancer.

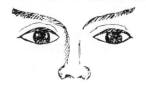

EYEBROWS UP :
LONG TIME MEAT-EATING

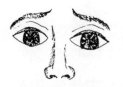

NOSE

An examination of the nose can tell much about the condition of the person being diagnosed. Reduce your intake of
food, and you will see your nose grow smaller.
A nose can save your life.

EYEBROWS DOWN:
VEGETARIAN, FRUITARIAN

A long nose starting high up on the face is Yin.
A short nose indicates a strong constitution.

YIN

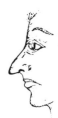

STRONG
CONSTITUTION
YANG

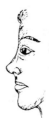

A small nose pointing upwards
is a sign of strong Yang.

The center of the nose indicates the condition of the heart. An
enlarged nose shows an enlarged heart (excess eating and
drinking). The nostrils show the condition of the lungs. The
larger the nostrils, the better. Small nostrils indicate weak
lungs. Well-developed nostrils are a sign of masculinity.

USUALLY
HEART TROUBLE

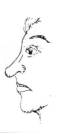

FIGURE 8-8 (continued)

STRONG LUNGS   WEAK LUNGS

A fat nose which is somewhat oily and sometimes shiny indicates overconsumption of animal protein. Red vessels on the tip of the nose are an indication of high blood pressure. Heart disease will follow.

THE MOUTH

A small mouth is Yang. A large mouth is Yin. A horizontal line between the mouth and nose shows a malfunctioning of the sexual organs.

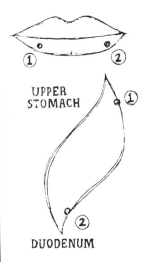

UPPER
STOMACH

DUODENUM

LIPS

The lips should be of equal thickness. In general, thick lips indicate a Yang constitution and thin lips a Yin constitution. The size of the upper lip shows the condition of the liver. If the lip is swollen, the liver is enlarged. The subject eats too much and is prone to mental disorders. The size of the lower lip indicates the condition of the large intestine. When the lower lip is swollen, there is a weakness, a looseness, in the intestines, and thus constipation. Epilepsy is a possibility when both lips are enlarged. This condition indicates that as a child the patient was given too much food.

Lips should usually be pink; however, they grow darker with age. A young person with dark lips has blood stagnation. The blood circulation is bad due to an excessive intake of animal protein and strong Yin foods. People with dark lips tend to develop cancer, pineal troubles, and diseases of the sexual organs.

The texture of the lips reveals the condition of the stomach.

(1) A cyst on the right side of the mouth indicates stomach trouble—acidity or the beginnings of an ulcer on the left side of the stomach.

(2) A cyst on the left side of the mouth indicates a problem in the right side of the stomach.

Urine, feces, any bodily discharge, and any body odor is indicative of any number of possible diseases or bad habits. Muramoto's comments on salt, urine, and the kidneys follow:

The urine of a healthy person is golden in color, like beer. Someone whose condition is too Yang, or who has taken too much salt, urinates less because his kidneys are contracted and release less liquid. His urine is usually brown, like dark beer. On the other hand, if excess Yin food is consumed, the kidneys become too relaxed and filter too much water. This causes frequent urination of a liquid that is pale or colorless, like water. [18, p. 33]

Salt feces and the intestines are likewise described:

If too much salt is consumed, the large intestines absorbs extra water and one's feces become shrunken and dry. On the other hand, if one's diet consists mostly of milk, fruits, and sugar, or if insufficient salt is consumed, there is more liquid needed by the intestines. In this case, the feces have no shape. [18, p. 33]

Experienced nurses have known for years the significance of "acetone breath" in a client who is slipping into a diabetic coma, for example, or the stench of gangrene or *escherichia coli* in a wound. But what are the smells of health? "Garlic breath" is present in clients who come from cultural backgrounds that use large amounts of garlic, and also in those who believe in its curative and preventive powers. Clients taking B-complex vitamins *smell* like those vitamins. Persons fasting in order to cleanse their systems may have "acetone breath" and experience a peculiar series of tastes and smells. Muramoto feels that heavy meat eaters have a bad smell. It behooves nurses to discover descriptive terminology for such observations.

Pulse diagnosis is based on careful palpation of the twelve pulses, six in each wrist. The Yellow Emperor writes:

One should feel whether the pulse is in motion or whether it is still and one should observe attentively and with skill. One should examine the five colors and the five viscera, whether they suffer from excess or whether they show an insufficiency, and one should examine the six bowels whether they are strong or weak. One should investigate the appearance of the body whether it is flourishing or deteriorating. One should use all these five examinations and combine their results, and then one will be able to decide upon the share of life and death. [29, as quoted therein, p. 180]

Iridology is a method of health evaluation that has been receiving much attention from medical and holistic practitioners. Iridology is the science of determining by iris readings, various information about the state of health of the client. Dr. Bernard Jensen has developed the chart shown in Figure 8–9 and has researched, written, and taught this novel approach for over forty-five years.

According to Dr. Jensen, iridology can point out structural defects, toxic substances, deposits, inherent weaknesses, glandular conditions, and chemical imbalances in a client, as well as estimate the individual's ability to self-heal. The color of the wedge sections shown on the iridology chart help the iridologist determine inflammation, the stage of inflammation, its cause, and the lifestyle changes required. Further evaluations are performed to measure progress or further deterioration.

Problem Statements

Whatever the series of assessments conducted, at some point the nurse formulates a calculated hunch using deductive and inductive reasoning as well as intuition. This *diagnosis* is usually stated in the form of a need (safety, security, self-esteem, nutrition, etc.) or a problem; in the case of a holistic diagnosis:

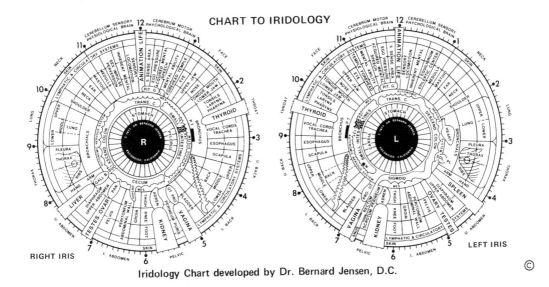

CHART TO IRIDOLOGY

Iridology Chart developed by Dr. Bernard Jensen, D.C.

FIGURE 8-9 Iridology chart

Reprinted with permission of Dr. Bernard Jensen, D.C., Route 1, Box 52, Escondido, Calif. 92025.

1. energy imbalance, congestion, blockage, excess or deficient yin or yang;
2. needs to reexperience or to get in touch with a particular feeling; and
3. needs to modify certain lifestyle abuses or needs to reduce health risk of coronary artery disease.

Goals

Following the problem statement or nursing diagnosis, an overall goal is stated which is implied in the problem, and therefore this step is often not repeated. Goals for problem (1) above might be to balance energy, reduce congestion, remove blockage, increase yin, and decrease yang.

Actions

The plan gets very specific in the next step—the implementation or action phase—in which any of the therapeutic methods or lifestyling modifications can be initiated. Would the interventions were *that* simple! In fact, the intervention would more accurately be: Teach concept of human lifestyling. That is a very global intervention, however, and might require subinterventions, such as:

1. respond to interest and questions regarding lifestyle changes;
2. provide resource materials;

3. set up question and answer time on new material;
4. design with client, or encourage client to design, own lifestyle modification program utilizing nurse feedback and reinforcement; and
5. involve support system.

Criteria For Evaluation

To evaluate whether the client is actually moving toward a stated goal of implementing one lifestyle modification of "choice," the nurse would determine via Mager's criteria whether this goal was achieved. Some examples follow:

1. The client will be given a baseline evaluation before the Lifestyle Modification program begins, be reevaluated in one month, and show a 20 percent improvement in resting pulse, percent of fat or carbohydrate in diet, etc.
2. The client will subjectively state satisfaction or motivation to continue program.

The evaluation, then, could be any of the following statements:

1. "Yes, the criteria were met; do not change, continue present program."
2. "No, the criteria were not met; reevaluate, change the entire program, or certain aspects of it."

The problem with many holistic methods is the lack of experimentally valid evaluation tools. Nursing needs to define measurable parameters of improvement for itself by researching, testing, and validating these methods.

INTRAPERSONAL PROBLEM SOLVING

As with any of the processes used in this book, it is strongly advised that the nurse perform a nursing process on herself. This means the nurse/client is expected to use some of the forms shown in this text or a preferred form of his or her own. Try to visualize yourself taking your own health history. Basically, your history should include one (or a *very few*) pressing complaints or problems you would like to work on. If you are already receiving advice for a problem, set it aside and choose a new one. Be honest with yourself. If you're tired and lethargic, and really believe you have mononucleosis, then state so. Don't play a game with yourself! You'll wish clients were as candid with you about their real fears and "self-diagnoses."

Sketching the history of your present problem is important. When did it start? Can you describe it using all your senses? Include any items that might have influenced the development of your problem. This could include anything from changes in important social relationships to substances being ingested, and so forth. Have there been any memorable changes in your life pattern?

The past history is important background information and should include family history, illnesses, hospitalizations, surgeries, and allergies. These questions are usually direct or short answer. It is important to probe what the client means by "allergic," for example, "breaking out in pimples," or "difficulty breathing," and so on.

A review of systems is performed with a complete health exam, and any gaps that may have been missed are filled in. The review of systems proceeds from head to toe, according to the particular system. Usually, a social history is also performed with a complete exam and, for nursing, is often the most important area to assess for lifestyle, habits, and personal problems.

A self-observant nurse can provide other valuable pieces of data for herself. The self-care movement mentioned earlier in this book advocates self-diagnostics as a step in the self-care process.

Self-Health Assessment, Self-Diagnostics

All nurses should know how to take their own temperature and basal body temperature (which helps to assess ovarian and thyroid function), pulses (carotid, femoral, pedal, radial, apical, etc.), respirations (these may change if you take your own), blood pressure, and be able to examine their own lymph glands.

More and more women are examining their own breasts, doing their own vaginal exams and early pregnancy tests (EPT), as well as controlling conception through basal temperature and examining their cervical mucous. Women are also experimenting with self-screening for gonorrhea, doing their own urine cultures, and diagnosing vaginal infections.

Home throat cultures and self occult-blood-in-the-stool tests are becoming more commonplace. Urine sugar and acetone level testing has been performed by diabetics and has been advocated as an adjunct to certain low carbohydrate diets. A more accurate test—a fingerstick blood sugar test—is now being evaluated as a self-diagnostic technique.

These discrete methods of data gathering, plus the other self-help inventories and practices advocated in this text, can help the nurse get a fairly clear picture of what the possible problem and appropriate interventions are. Self-help manuals, such as Vickery and Fries' *Take Care of Yourself,* offer algorithms or decision trees to take the nurse/client through a series of problem-solving steps to rule out other possibilities and arrive at a reasonable conclusion involving self-help or referral to a professional. A typical stressed student with a headache can apply the algorithm offered by Vickery and Fries, as shown in Figure 8–10.

Assessing Own Problem-Solving Style—
A Transactional Approach

What about problem-solving style in nursing? Jean Elder offers a Transactional Analysis (TA) approach to evaluating the way people look at and solve problems. Although logical, systematic problem solving is important, the extralogical human dimensions of past experience, feelings, and creativity are also valuable for the nurse to integrate. Each ego state (Parent, Adult, and Child) exists in every person and has both positive and negative qualities. When the negative characteristics of

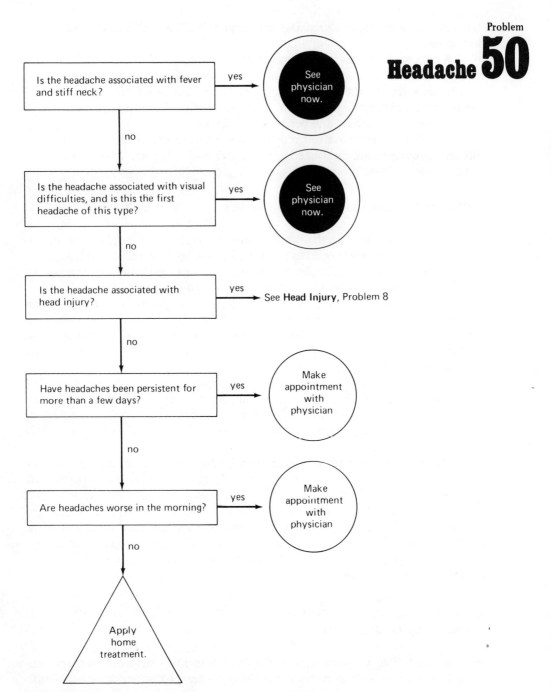

FIGURE 8-10 Self-diagnosis using an algorithm for headache

Reprinted from *Take Care of Yourself* by Donald M. Vickery, M.D. and James F. Fries, M.D., copyright ©
1976, by permission of Addison-Wesley Publishing Co., Reading, Mass.

one state infiltrate those of another, "contamination" is said to occur. When these are communicated in the problem-solving process, the real problem becomes clouded and other problems predominate.

The nursing goal is to develop an integrated problem-solving style which incorporates the creativity of the Child, the clear thinking of the Adult, and the wealth of experience of the Parent.

One of the major tasks of problem-solving from a TA point of view is to identify the problem and then to determine who "owns" the problem. It is important that the problem statement be made in clear terms that both the members of the health team and the client can understand. The problem statement must be based on accurate and pertinent information or the conclusion will be deduced and/or induced from insufficient evidence.

Owning an intrapersonal problem should be easy if the nurse is honest with herself and can separate herself from negative feelings about a situation.

EXAMPLE

    Problem: I am obese. (*based on substantiating data*)

      Goal: I need to reduce my intake and increase my activity.

If a problem is mutual, for example, if a personality conflict with a client exists, then each person's point of view needs to be examined and a mutual problem statement agreed upon.

EXAMPLE

    Problem: Client is rejecting nursing care and support. Client is highly independent; nurse is mothering.

      Goal: Nurse needs to refrain from trying to overpower client and client needs to articulate things he needs help with.

The advantage of identifying ownership of a problem and articulating it is that the nurse does not have to struggle to change things that are not her problem. For example, a nurse cannot stop a client with a drinking problem from drinking. Likewise, she cannot make decisions for other people that are not hers to make.

The problem statement must reflect ownership. For example, a student nurse's care is refused by a client. The problem statement reads: "Client hostile—refuses care." This is true in one sense, but not in another. Is the problem that *all* care is refused, or only the student's? Isn't it really the dreadful, rejected feeling on the part of the student that is the real problem which needs to be worked out? Maybe she can work it out with the client—maybe not. In any case, the student controls whether she wishes to dwell on rejection as a statement on her entire professional career or whether she chooses to accept that *this* client, at *this* moment, did not want her care.

TA also advocates brainstorming as a creative way to stimulate ideas for innovative-generative interventions. This is best done in a group. Each idea is recorded and examined and requires good group process skills. Evaluation is performed objectively and systematically, working through the criteria versus the observed performance, noting discrepancies without blame or criticism. This is an essential part of the process and is best done by the Adult Ego state.

INTERPERSONAL PROBLEM SOLVING AMONG THE NURSE, CLIENT, AND HEALTH TEAM

Nurses help clients and families to generate alternatives to problems:

1. for which they have been unable to find a solution given their current problem-solving abilities;
2. for which no foreseeable solution exists;
3. for which there are several confusing or conflicting ways of solving the problem; and
4. for which other methods have been tried and have failed.

Nurses help clients to help themselves through the caring relationship described in Chapter 3. Problem solving in nursing from a holistic perspective acknowledges the clients' own power to create health or illness. It recognizes the psychosomatic components of all health/illness states and the inseparability of the body/mind/spirit's influence on these states. If a client is "stuck" for one of the above reasons, one of the first suggestions (after establishing trust) that the nurse makes is that the client step back from the problem—for example, by using a relaxation exercise.

The result of achieving this meditative state involves removing oneself from past influences, future expectations, and present distractions. Goleman describes these activities which relate directly to improving problem-solving capabilities:

1. The merging of action and awareness in sustained, nondistractible concentration on the task at hand;
2. the focusing of attention on a limited stimulus field, excluding intruding stimuli from awareness in a pure involvement devoid of concern with outcome;
3. self-forgetfulness with heightened awareness of functions and body states related to the involving activity;
4. skills adequate to meet the environmental demand; and
5. clarity regarding situational cues and appropriate response. [22, Goleman as quoted therein, p. 206]

Since the client in a holistic interpersonal relationship in a wellness-oriented situation is the master of his own health, the nurse's role is that of well-informed colleague, observer, active listener-counselor, and humanistic teacher. In a transitory stressful situation the nurse assists the client to mobilize his own coping mechanisms and problem-solving abilities. Helping the client to stand back and look at his state of "arousal" is important. Exploration, sometimes guided by the nurse, of precipitating stressful intrapersonal and environmental events and cues are labeled cognitively and rationally, even if incorrectly. Engaging in the rational problem-solving process activity in itself often triggers understanding and a subjective feeling of regaining control.

In an illness setting, the client is helped to find purpose and meaning in illness, the secondary gains he is getting from the disease, and reasons why he might actually want or need the disease. Change involves changing an entire self-being structure. Relating to the experiment and the observer, as mentioned earlier in this chapter, the observer creates the experiment according to his world view. The way the client chooses to view his situation is how that situation will develop. This is sometimes called a "self-fulfilling prophecy."

The preventive, protective aspects of problem-solving involve a much more in-depth evaluation of the person's lifestyle, his relationship with the environment (socioeconomic, political), family, peers, work, living situation, and self-concept than is now being conducted in most health assessments. (Some of the health inventories shown in the appendices begin to accomplish this task.)

Holistic nurses need to keep in constant touch with an enormous amount of research by drawing relationships between lifestyle factors, disease prevention, and health promotion. This knowledge base, the nurse's unique assessment of the client, coupled with her interpersonal and problem-solving skills, make the nurse particularly qualified to be a partner and consultant in the client's path to self-care.

Several innovative interpersonal problem-solving techniques have developed during the past ten years, namely problem-oriented records, contracts, and algorithms for decision making in health.

Comprehensive Problem Solving With The Problem-Oriented Medical Record (POMR)

Perhaps the most well-known medical problem-solving technique is the Problem-Oriented Medical Record (POMR) first developed by Laurence Weed in 1970. According to Berne and Readey, the purpose of the problem-oriented medical record is to construct a detailed model of health care problem solving and recording that, once implemented, will be improved on and expanded by all health care personnel—a model that is a behavioral analysis system engineered to become a health care audit. [3, p. 3]

POMR utilizes the scientific method and complements the nursing process, with the exception that it focuses on medical problems which may or may not be the clients' or the nursing problems. The following outline summarizes the POMR:

1. Data Base
   Problem List
   Initial Plans or Orders
   DX/Assessment

2. Therapeutic Plans

3. Client Education

Progress Notes:

1. Narrative
   a. Subjective findings
   b. Objective findings
   c. Assessment—Problem Statement
   d. Plans
2. Flow sheets—daily follow-up of SOAP
3. Discharge Summary

Yura and Walsh suggest adding IER (Implementation, Evaluation, Reassessment) to the SOAP acronym to insure implementation, evaluation, and reassessment of client's needs. [33, p. 35]

Advantages of the POMR include its serving as a multidisciplinary approach to client problems in that any member of the health team may write on the SOAP chart, add problems, and update progress notes. SOAP charting forces nurses and others to make accurate assessments. Nursing notes stating "up and about" or "good day" add very little to the objective data base.

SOAP charting is performed every day, shift, or clinic visit. The standard form is as follows:

Date, Time, Problem Number, and Title.		Problem #1: Puncture wound on sole of foot.
Subjective: What the client or family tells you.	S	"I was out cutting the grass in my sneakers and I stepped on a nail." "I haven't has a tetanus shot in 10 years."
Objective: Information gathered from any other source.	O	Puncture wound is clean, uninfected, no foreign bodies, no nerve or muscle damage.
Assessment: What you think is happening based on subjective and objective findings. Patient reaction to treatment or diagnosis.	A	Shallow puncture wound needs watching and client needs a tetanus booster.
Plan:	P	
1. *Diagnostic*: What is being done to solve the problem?		1. Clean and bandage wound; apply antibiotic ointment.
2. *Therapeutic*: How the problem is being treated—client's reaction to treatment.		2. Administer tetanus booster. Answer questions.
3. *Education*: What the client and family are being told regarding the problem.		3. Explain rationale behind tetanus booster and signs to watch for an indication of infection or blood poisoning; explain daily care of wound.

One of the other advantages of SOAPing is that continuity of care from one shift, one unit, one facility or clinic to another is made possible. In addition to the

SOAP charting, flow sheets monitoring blood pressure, pulse, blood sugars and laboratory results or any other routinely recurring variable, such as weight or activity, can be monitored in a graphic fashion. At a glance, any health team member can follow a client's progress. This type of data lends itself to clinical research. When health team members see how demystified the recordkeeping really is, they begin to see their work as a contribution to research and to the development of a new knowledge base.

Algorithms

Closely related to the POMR is the clinical algorithm, which is not unlike a standardized care plan for certain predictable types of problems. Algorithms are similar to protocols, except that they afford choices to the decision maker on the basis of certain assessments which may change the direction of the care. Algorithms are being successfully used in self-care as has already been indicated (see Figure 8–10). The same book [32] is being used in a Northern California Blue Cross/Blue Shield-controlled pilot study to determine if such a manual can decrease utilization of health care facilities, especially emergency rooms.

The Kaiser-Permanente Health Maintenance Organization uses telephone "advice nurses" who respond to calls, elicit information, make assessments, and, in effect, decide if a visit to the Health Maintenance Organization is necessary. Recommendations for home remedies and health education are then given. Clinical algorithms have been a great aid to rapid decision making, particularly in primary care settings.

Contracts

Contracts, as discussed in Chapters 2 and 3, are another example of interpersonal problem solving in action. A contract has a clearly and mutually defined goal—in this case, between a nurse and a client. There must be time for both parties to consider the contract. Both parties are to get something out of the contract. Each person must be competent to fulfill his part of the contract. Nurse and client must agree to the means of reaching the goal. The nurse or the client should not make promises that can't be kept. Through experience, the nurse learns what she can *realistically* hope to fulfill in terms of her part of the contract. She cannot also be responsible for the client's part of the bargain. In crisis or illness situations, clients may not be capable of negotiating or fulfilling contracts.

COMMUNITY, CULTURAL, AND SOCIETAL APPLICATIONS OF PROBLEM SOLVING

Several cultural approaches to problem solving have been cited in the text. In order to obtain a fuller overview of the variety of cultural healing systems actively functioning as preprimary health care agents, several prototypical healing systems, religious and secular, will be scanned. The commonalities of most nonmedical healing will be highlighted. The position that the social network or community may be as important, or sometimes *more* vital than the individual's own healing abilities, will be proposed. This position does not indicate a contradiction of the self-responsibility, self-healing principle; it merely suggests that the social network has an essential role, and indeed, a dominant one in some cultures. Nurses need to assess and support clients who express unfailing faith in a power outside themselves to heal them. It is for researchers to discover whether or not the self-healing mechanisms activated by such beliefs are similar to self-healing rituals and practices.

Nonmedical Religious Healing Systems

Navajo Indian Healing

Navajo Indian practices center around what Gardner describes as "symbolic healing," that is, a manipulation of culturally accepted symbols which act directly on the client's unconscious. These symbols may consist of such things as charts, sand painting, and prayers, all of which contain four basic theme patterns that bespeak modern psychotherapeutic theory—especially as theorized by Jung. They are (1) a return to the origins; (2) management of evil; (3) death and rebirth; and (4) restoration of a stable universe. [29, p. 134]

Unlike laying-on-of-hands psychic healing, Navajo Indians' healing requires belief on the part of the client. The result may in fact be physical healing or tolerance of inescapable suffering. [29, p. 142]

Many properties of healing rituals in primitive societies show resemblances to naturalistic psychotherapeutic methods. [29, p. 233] It is believed in these religiously-oriented societies that illness can be caused and cured by the intervention of supernatural forces. [29, p. 233] Religious healing tends to exist side by side *with* naturalistic treatment by medicines, manipulations, and surgery. With the development of a highly technical and scientific approach to health-illness, however, this cooperative relationship becomes an adversary one.

Every society has its own theory or theories about illness and healing and the most effective methods for dealing with ill health. These are part of an individual's belief and value system. Imagine prescribing radiation therapy for a Navajo client. Think of the attitude leap that client would have to make to accept such a proposition. It is always good practice in an initial interview to have the client describe his or her notions about health and illness—causative factors, acceptable healing methods, healers, the role of science and technology, religion, etc. A theory of health and illness is necessary in every culture in order to help an individual make sense out of his or her "chaotic, mysterious feelings, and suggest a plan of action, thus helping him to gain a sense of direction and mastery and to resolve his inner conflicts." [29, p. 248]

Another example of nonmedical religious healing occurs in Lourdes, France, where the grotto is attributed by Catholics and non-Catholics alike with miraculous healing powers. Christian Scientists combine religion and healing, as do many Fundamentalist groups.

Secular therapies range from homeopathy to more medically accepted ones, such as chiropractic and osteopathy. In 1965, Inglis cited an estimated 35 million clients of chiropractors in the United States. [Inglis, as quoted in 29, p. 259] Healing cults are appearing every day and are nearly impossible to count since many keep their activities secret.

Black and Hispanic Healing

Several other cultural healing systems bear mention since they influence the belief systems of a large number of black and Hispanic peoples. Although experiential reports of healing are numerous, controlled studies proving efficacy of these systems are lacking. Alternative cultural healing systems have time and tradition to speak for them, that is, they continue to exist and effect cures for problems that modern medicine doesn't seem to touch—for example, psychosomatic, psychiatric, family, and marital problems.

Black healing in the United States can be traced to the era of slavery, although it originated in Africa. The basis of belief is spiritual. Illness and disease result from not living according to God's plan. Certain healers are singled out by God and recognized by the community as having healing powers or powers of voodoo or vodoon. Some healers have a special knowledge of herbs, and/or use charms, amulets, prayers, chants, and other methods to cause healing to occur.

Hispanic healing systems involve three major subsystems—Curanderismo, Santeria, and Espiritismo, the last two of which will be briefly described. Santeria is an African cult whose followers live primarily in Cuba, Puerto Rico, New York, Florida, and California. The language spoken is a ritual language having Nigerian and Spanish influences. Most of the people who believe in Santeria also function within traditional Catholicism. Rituals and "Saints" are sincretised or tied to Catholic patrons and are responsible for certain aspects of daily living. The "Santero" is the contact who brings advice from the particular saints to the client. Beads, colors, shells, candles, oils, and waters are all used to promote healing, which invariably involves changing one or more aspects of life.

Espiritismo is a healing system seen in Puerto Rico, the Mediterranean, and the Philippines. It was adapted from Hinduism and subscribes to reincarnation and the spirit world (spiritism). Spirits from all ages in time and all places can cause illness and must be contacted, appeased, or gotten rid of. Often a person who has undergone a healing will become a self-appointed healer. Espiritismo also makes use of herbs, prayers, candles, incense, other paraphernalia, and dramatic rituals. Sometimes the aura is worked with and often laying-on-of-hands is used.

Common to the Hispanic healing systems is the reinforcement of traditional values and the belief that illness comes from outside the person and is beyond his control, thus creating no guilt feelings. Self-responsibility enters the picture when the healer gives the prescription to the client and tells him what he must do to get better.

Some similarities among secular and religious healing are:

1. methods that arouse hope, bolster self-esteem, emotionally affect and strengthen ties with a social network;
2. healers who represent or project hope, who personally project certain attributes (confidence, caring, etc.), and who have been designated the healing role;
3. methods prescribe sets of activities, for example, confessions, purification or atonement rituals, and mutual service for others which cements the bond with the community;
4. the "healee" is transformed intrapersonally. If the illness is not healed, the healee at least feels more virtuous and is highly regarded by the community and often changes his or her lifestyle. [29, pp. 262–63; Frank as quoted therein]

Homeopathic Approaches to Healing

Since the concern of this book is not illness, but health, homeopathy will not be examined except in relation to orthodox medical notions of *health* and disease. Homeopathy in the United States was closely aligned with medicine until the nineteenth century when it was legislated as illegal on the basis of philosophical beliefs of homeopathists which can be summarized as follows:

> The processes of health and disease are based on the Hippocratic idea of vital forces in which the body reacts to external stimuli. The expression of this reaction takes the form of symptoms, which are a sign of the homeopathic curative process in action. To suppress, change, or terminate this process means shutting off the body's own healing processes. Any medicine given by a homeopathic physician is one which supports and stimulates the organism's own healing efforts. It may, in fact, contain more of the allergen, toxin, called moribific agent. The view of the body as an active participant in fending off external assault is reinforced by homeopathists. [28]

Samuel Hahneman, the father of homeopathy, presented three rules for practicing homeopathic physicians:

1. Prescription of the drug according to the Law of Similars—treating the symptoms peculiar to that client, not the disease.
2. The minimum dose—so minimal that allopathic doctors accuse it of being a placebo.
3. The single remedy—one remedy at a time which is carefully observed. [29, p. 300]

Community Health Assessment and the Problem-Oriented Record

Community health nursing has always been in the vanguard of wellness-oriented assessments and innovative problem-solving strategies (such as POMR) with clients, families, and communities. Community assessment (see Figure 8–11) typifies the kinds of information nurses should assess about their communities. Problem solving is as an important a process for the community system as it is for an individual. How communities solve their problems tells the nurse much about how supportive an environment she has in order to help clients, families, and communities make changes.

Figure 8–5 shows the kind of information community health nurses gather on individuals in their homes. Note the combination physiologic systems (neurologic-sensorium circulatory-respiratory, community process, lifestyle, nutrition, activity, self-care and hygiene practices, stress reduction, coping and psychosexual development, human development) and beginning holistic process health assessment format. Such a data base could easily be organized around a holistic nursing framework applied to the client, that is, all of the life processes that holistic nurses use are applicable and can be applied to the client.

---

a. The historical development and physical description.
b. Political philosophy.
c. Community power structure.
d. Health status of the community—environmental, socioeconomic, and behavioral conditions.
   (1) Statistical characteristics (vital)
   (2) Specific causes of death
   (3) Prevalence of presymptomatic illness
   (4) Number of special-risk groups
   (5) Environmental health status indicators
      (a) Physical environment (purity of H_2O, adequacy of housing)
      (b) Social environment—accessibility and workability of community organizations and communication networks, crowding, quality of neighborhoods, recreation facilities
e. Health-related personnel—roles, values, relationships
f. Health-related policies and priorities
g. Health-related capabilities
   (1) Economic, human, and institutional resources, organization, and distribution of them (e.g., education, welfare, etc.)
h. Health action potential—how does this community deal with common problems?
   (1) Who does what, who talks to whom?
   (2) How are decisions made and who makes them? (Is there a group or just 1 or 2)?
   (3) Where do people go when sick or in trouble? (appropriate community resources, or friends, neighbors, and folk remedies)
   (4) Where do health and education stand in relation to other community concerns?
   (5) How does the community view change?

FIGURE 8-11 Assessing a community, its health status indicators, and its health problem-solving potential

Some professional political community incentives have stimulated creative use of problem solving in nursing with the establishment of in-house Nursing Audit Committees and external Peer Standards Review Organizations (PSROs) to evaluate quality of care within hospitals. PSROs have been legislatively authorized and funded to monitor workable medical and nursing audit systems.

The Canadian Health "Field Concept"

Other countries, Canada, for example, have proposed bold, broad changes in viewing health and health care delivery problems. One of the most innovative health planning problem-solving documents of the 1970s was the Task Force working paper "On the Health of the Canadians," published in 1974. This document proposes a "Health Field Concept" for looking at health problems that is truly holistic in nature and attempts to pull health problems out of the province or jurisdiction of the medical and/or bureaucratic organizational structure.

Briefly, the document outlines the limitations of traditional views of analyzing the past to determine influences on states of health and illness and of looking at current statistics to ascertain underlying causes of disease. The results of both these methods lead to a few conclusions which form the basis for a conceptual framework which incorporates improving the environment, moderating self-imposed risks, and adding to present knowledge of human biology. From this triad the Canadian government has developed the Health Field Concept which includes human biology, environment, lifestyle, and health care organization as contributing to the health or illness of the population of Canada.

What this framework tries to do is cut across traditional boundaries to view health problems in a holistic fashion so that a stated problem of traffic mortalities can be analyzed, for example, as being due to risks taken by individuals, with a lesser importance given to the design of cars and roads, and to the availability and quality of emergency treatment, with human biology bearing little significance on the problem. Thus, program planners could roughly attribute causes of traffic deaths, for example, to lifestyle (75 percent), environment (20 percent), and health-care organizations (5 percent). This would give planners, legislators, and department heads a basis for planning programs and allocating resources. It doesn't take much imagination to envision the controversy this would stir up in the health care organizations and for practitioners who specialize in emergency medical units and who lobby for health care dollars.

As in any systems approach, the first category, lifestyle, may be subdivided into impaired driving (alcohol, blindness), carelessness, failure to wear seat belts, and speeding. The task force feels that this holistic health field concept brings fragments together into a whole, allows recognition of all factions, and delegates responsibility to appropriate agencies.

With all of the previous information in mind, the government of Canada has established two broad health objectives:

1. To reduce mental and physical health hazards for those parts of the Canadian population whose risks are high; and

2. To improve the accessibility of good mental and physical health care for those whose present access is unsatisfactory. [14, p. 67]

From these objectives are created courses of action, some of which are spelled out here:

The development for the general public of educational programs on nutrition.

The enlistment of the help of the food and restaurant industries in making known the caloric value and nutritional content of the food they sell.

Educational campaigns to increase awareness of the gravity and underlying causes of traffic accidents, deaths, and injuries.

Information to increase awareness of the hazards of self-medication.

Further information campaigns to increase public awareness of health problems due to the abuse of alcohol, drugs, tobacco, and venereal disease.

Encouragement among employers of programs designed to ease the transition from employment to retirement.

Reinforcement of successful programs for making life more interesting for the aged.

Promotion and coordination of school and adult health education programs, particularly by health professionals and school teachers.

Direct awareness activities tailored to the responsibilities of specific sectors for the reduction of self-imposed and environmental health risks including business, trade unions, governments, voluntary associations and action groups, communities, professions, parents, and teachers.

Continued and expanded marketing programs for promoting increased physical activity by Canadians.

Enlistment of the support of the educational system in increasing opportunities for mass physical recreation in primary and secondary schools, in community colleges, and in universities.

Promotion of the development of simple intensive-use facilities for more physical recreation including fitness trails, nature trails, ski trails, facilities for court games, playing fields, bicycle paths, and skating rinks.

Continued pressing for full community use of present outdoor and indoor recreation facilities, including gymnasia, pools, playing fields, and arenas.

Continued and reinforced support for sports programs involving large numbers of Canadians.

Encouragement of private sports clubs to accept more social responsibility for extending the use of their facilities to less-privileged segments of the Canadian population.

Extension of present support for special programs of physical activity for native peoples, the handicapped, the aged, and the economically deprived.

Enlistment of the support of women's movements in getting more mass physical recreation programs for females, including school children, young adults, housewives, and employees.

Enlistment of the support of employers of sedentary workers in the establishment of employee exercise programs.

Enlistment of the support of trade unions representing sendentary workers in obtaining employee exercise programs.

Increase in the awareness of health professionals of factors affecting physical fitness.

Completion of the development of a home fitness test to enable Canadians to evaluate their fitness level. [14, pp. 68–69]

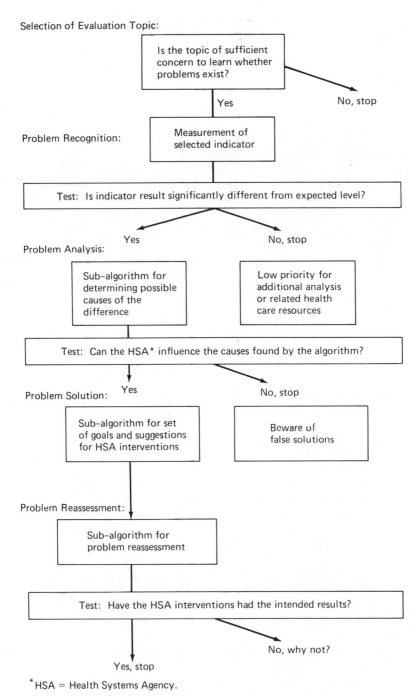

Selection of Evaluation Topic:

Is the topic of sufficient concern to learn whether problems exist?

Yes

No, stop

Problem Recognition:

Measurement of selected indicator

Test: Is indicator result significantly different from expected level?

Yes

No, stop

Problem Analysis:

Sub-algorithm for determining possible causes of the difference

Low priority for additional analysis or related health care resources

Test: Can the HSA* influence the causes found by the algorithm?

Yes

No, stop

Problem Solution:

Sub-algorithm for set of goals and suggestions for HSA interventions

Beware of false solutions

Problem Reassessment:

Sub-algorithm for problem reassessment

Test: Have the HSA interventions had the intended results?

Yes, stop

No, why not?

*HSA = Health Systems Agency.

FIGURE 8–12 Outline of algorithm approach to outcome-based health planning

Excerpted with permission from "Algorithms for Health Planners," vols. I, IV, and VI (Santa Monica, Ca.: The Rand Corporation, 1977).

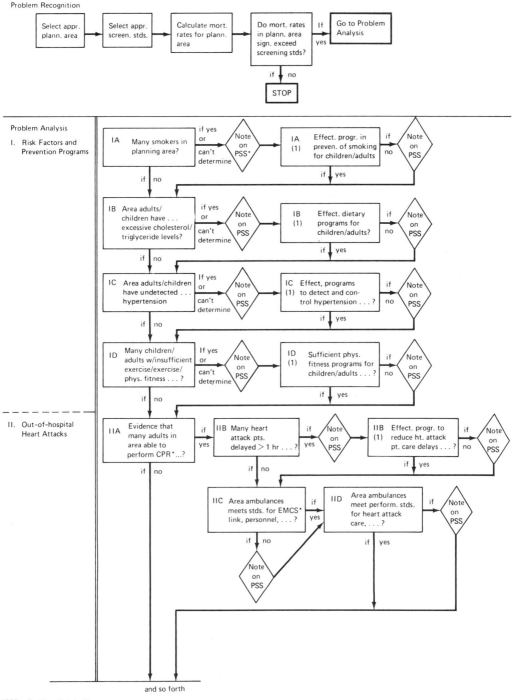

FIGURE 8-13 Health planning algorithm for hypertension

Excerpted with permission from "Algorithms for Health Planners," vols. I, IV, and VI (Santa Monica, Ca.: The Rand Corporation, 1977).

In summary, the Canadian Plan is problem solving in health on the governmental political community level. A systematic approach has been used to stimulate some creative wellness-oriented programs and policies.

Community health planning is an area that nurses do not often associate with their role and functions. It is essential that holistic nurses help determine the community health planning for the future. Specific change theories and methods will be discussed in Chapter 10; however, the use of the problem-solving process in health planning will be briefly demonstrated. Health planners are using the algorithm approach (see Figure 8–12) to help solve multifactorial problems such as hypertension (as demonstrated in Figure 8–13).

There is no doubt that creative problem-solving techniques are generating some exciting ways of viewing health problems. Holistic nurses have the background and experience in problem solving to contribute to this generative process on the intrapersonal, interpersonal, and community levels.

REFERENCES FOR CHAPTER 8

[1] Donald B. Ardell, *High-Level Wellness* (Emmaus, Pa.: Rodale Press, 1977), pp. 207–12.

[2] Loretta S. Bermosk and Sarah E. Porter, *Women's Health and Human Wholeness* (New York: Appleton-Century-Crofts, 1979).

[3] Rosemarian Berne and Helen Readey, *Problem-Oriented Medical Record Implementation* (St. Louis: C. V. Mosby Co., 1978).

[4] Henrik Blum, "National Health Policy," *AJHP,* 1, no. 1 (July 1976), 4–22.

[5] Fay Bower, *The Process of Planning Nursing Care* (St. Louis: C. V. Mosby Co., 1977).

[6] Marjorie L. Byrne and Lida F. Thompson, *Key Concepts for the Study and Practice of Nursing* (St. Louis: C. V. Mosby Co., 1978), pp. 45–46.

[7] Fritjof Capra, *The Tao of Physics* (Boulder, Colo.: Shambhala Publishing, 1975).

[8] Jane E. Chapman and Harry H. Chapman, *Behavior and Health Care* (St. Louis: C. V. Mosby Co., 1975).

[9] Paul Cutler, *Problem Solving in Clinical Medicine* (Baltimore: The Williams & Wilkins Company, 1979).

[10] Joanne M. Dalton and others, "Nursing Diagnosis," *Nursing Clinics of North America,* 14, no. 3 (September 1979), 497–569.

[11] Victor Daniels and Lawrence Horowitz, *Being and Caring* (Palo Alto, Ca.: Mayfield Publishing Co., 1976).

[12] G. E. Alan Dever, *Community Health Analysis: A Holistic Approach* (Germantown, Md.: Aspen Systems Corporation, 1980).

[13] Jean Elder, *Transactional Analysis in Health Care* (Menlo Park, Ca.: Addison-Wesley Publishing Co., 1978).

[14] Marc Lalonde, *A New Perspective on the Health of the Canadians* (Ottawa, Canada: The Ministry of Health, 1974).

[15] Robert Mager, *Preparing Instructional Objectives* (Belmont, Ca.: Lear-Siegler, Inc./Fearon Publishers, 1972).

[16] Ann Marriner, *The Nursing Process* (St. Louis: C. V. Mosby Co., 1975).

[17] P. B. Medawar, *Induction and Intuition in Scientific Thought* (London: Methment Co., Ltd., 1969).

[18] Naboru Muramoto, in Michael Abehsera, ed., *Healing Ourselves* (New York: Swan House Publishing Co., 1973).

[19] Ruth Beckman Murray and Judith Proctor Zentner, *Nursing Concepts for Health Promotion* (Englewood Cliffs, N.J.: Prentice-Hall, Inc., 1979).

[20] The National League for Nursing, *Problem-Oriented Systems of Patient Care* (New York: National League for Nursing, 1974).

[21] Lucille E. Notter, *Essentials of Nursing Research* (New York: Springer Publishing Co., 1974).

[22] Kenneth R. Pelletier, *Toward a Science of Consciousness* (New York: Dell Publishing Co., 1978).

[23] Robert M. Pirsig, *Zen and the Art of Motorcycle Maintenance* (New York: Bantam Books, 1974).

[24] Sharon L. Roberts, *Behavioral Concepts and Nursing Throughout the Lifespan* (Englewood Cliffs, N.J.: Prentice-Hall, Inc., 1978).

[25] Mike Samuels and Hall Bennett, *The Well Body Book* (New York and Berkeley, Ca.: Random House/Bookworks, 1975).

[26] Karl E. Schaefer and others, *Individuation Process and Biographical Aspects of Disease* (Mount Kisco, N.Y.: Futura Publishing Co., 1979).

[27] Karl E. Schaefer and others, *Toward a Man-Centered Medical Science* (Mount Kisco, N.Y.: Futura Publishing Co., 1979).

[28] Abbot Zenkei Shibayana, *A Flower Does Not Talk* (Rutland, Vt.: Charles E. Tuttle Co., 1975).

[29] David S. Sobel, *Ways of Health* (New York: Harcourt Brace Jovanovich, 1979).

[30] University of California, Berkeley, *Student Health Service Manual* (Berkeley, Ca.: The Regents of the University of California, 1977).

[31] Phyllis J. Verhonick and Catherine C. Seaman, *Research Methods for Undergraduate Students in Nursing* (New York: Appleton-Century-Crofts, 1978).

[32] Donald M. Vickery, M.D. and James F. Fries, M.D., *Take Care of Yourself* (Reading, Mass.: Addison-Wesley Publishing Co., 1976).

[33] Helen Yura and Mary B. Walsh, *The Nursing Process,* 3rd ed. (New York: Appleton-Century-Crofts, 1978).

Chapter 9
teaching/learning

CHAPTER OUTLINE

3. A Private/Public Multidisciplinary Preventive Education Program
4. Self-Care Education

CHAPTER OBJECTIVES

1. List the three kinds of learning and give two examples of learning activities for each kind.
2. Describe the three pivotal theories of learning and their principal theorists, noting similarities and differences.
3. Identify the components of the teaching/learning process and relate them to the nursing process.
4. Explain the importance of developmental tasks to teaching/learning and education.
5. Assess your own teaching/learning style, including strengths and weaknesses.
6. Define process teaching, independent learning, and self-learning modules.
7. Review eight holistic affective educational models, and their responsible theorists, naming the primary life processes and their rationales as incorporated in each model.
8. Describe three community health education areas, pointing out two learning principles and two learning methods or activities that operate in each.

INTRODUCTION AND THEORETICAL BACKGROUND

Learning has been defined as a change of behavior resulting from practice and experience. *Teaching*, then, includes the plan of action designed to bring about learning or that which allows it to occur. Nurses and health professionals find themselves continually involved in health teaching. With so much time devoted to health education, one would expect to find more health promotive behavior in operation. Perhaps Galileo summarized the teaching/learning dilemma best by stating, "You can not teach man anything; you can only help him to find it within himself." Unless teaching is geared to the learner's cultural value and belief system, very little learning can be expected.

Education is an institutionalized system created by the dominant culture to impart its values and to prepare individuals to assume designated social roles. If the educational system only prepares a person to accept the status quo and to understand the world only as it presently exists, the individual will be unprepared for rapid change, revolution, ambiguity, conflicting values, cultures, and the unknown.

Institutionalized teaching and learning in the United States is accused by Third-World peoples and conservative taxpayers alike of perpetuating itself rather than of preparing learners to think critically, make responsible decisions, and evaluate alternatives that often appear confusing and conflicting.

Health education is a formalized program for facilitating attitudes and behaviors which optimize high-level wellness. *Health teaching* includes those methods designed to encourage behavior and communicate information and values directed toward optimizing health. *Patient education* or teaching actually refers to care for clients within an institutional framework such as a hospital, clinic, public health department, or private practice and involves teaching self-care for a diagnosed disease or propensity toward it.

Does the holistic approach incorporate values that apply to the educational process? How can this approach be used to help nurses and clients learn in a manner that will foster self-direction, self-growth, and creative thinking? Recall the basic processes of holistic nursing: self-responsibility, humanistic caring, communication, problem solving, lifestyling, and human development. All the theories and knowledge incorporated in these processes are inseparable from the teaching/learning process. Many of the theories and ideas supported by this chapter will appear familiar because they have been proposed elsewhere in this text from a developmental, self-identity or other point of view. They all contribute to or stem from the teaching/learning process.

Teaching and learning cannot be seen as separate activities. Teachers and students come together to engage in a teaching/learning process. Thus, when references to this interactive process as it relates to teacher and student or nurse and client are made, the terminology "teaching/learning" will be used. [10, p. 8]

This chapter explores just what it is that promotes, nurtures, and generates learning and creativity in the nurse and client. What stimulates this process will vary from individual to individual. The excitement of a true learning activity or experience is universal, whether it be a nurse learning to lead a prenatal nutrition discussion or a client learning to monitor accurately his own maximal intensity pulse level.

Are there certain universal learning triggers or are there too many cultural, societal, economic, and developmental variables to stereotype this complex activity? This chapter attempts to search out the commonalities, theories, and principles that may facilitate learning in nursing and in health. Specific applications are scattered thoughout to help the practitioner make the intellectual leap from theory to practice. Most examples have a wellness orientation and try to bring together many of the holistic theories and practices mentioned throughout the text.

Teaching/Learning and Problem Solving

The teaching process is almost identical to the problem-solving, nursing, and research processes described in the preceding chapter:

1. *assessing* a learning *need* and readiness of the learner;
2. *setting goals* and behavioral objectives;
3. *implementing* various *strategies* to convey content, attitudes, and behaviors; and
4. *evaluating* and *reassessing,* if necessary.

The learning process is similar to teaching in that the learner performs all the aforementioned steps either independently or with support. Any teaching/learning plan or curriculum takes into account the knowledge to be communicated, the learner, and the setting in which the learning is to occur or be used. In order to teach a family how to provide continuing care for a hospitalized relative in the home setting, for example, a plan must be adapted to suit the resources and constraints of that home situation. Ideally, teaching is done in the setting in which it is intended to occur. When this is impossible, a simulated situation is devised that takes into account as many of the variables of the home setting as possible.

Developmental Tasks, Teaching, and Learning

It has been shown that the problem solving and teaching/learning processes are dynamically interrelated. Human development and learning are also inseparable life processes. This is best demonstrated in Havighurst's concept of developmental tasks, which were defined in Chapter 4. Learning a developmental task assumes an *active* learner interacting with an *active* social environment to meet maturational dictates, cultural demands, and individual desires. [19]

A clear understanding of human developmental tasks is essential to any individual or group health education plan. Defining developmental tasks is one way of predicting age- and stage-related interests in well populations. What are the tasks that human beings are concerned with at particular ages and stages? An example of inferring health education content from developmental characteristics follows:

Age Level	Developmental Task and Characteristics
Upper elementary, ages 9–11	Children learn the difference between sexes; some are maturing sexually.

Related Health Education Content

1. Anatomic and physiologic differences (growth and development)
2. Sex education:
   a. sex characteristics (primary-secondary)
   b. sex roles (changing)
3. Related health needs

Changes in Education

When students learn the basics of active listening and other communication techniques, they are often role played with other students in simulated settings with simulated roles. A great deal of teaching is transmitted in an institutionalized setting (for example, in a school or university) far removed from the real world. It is no wonder learners suffer from "reality shock" upon encountering the actual setting in which they are to utilize their new knowledges and skills. [25]

Critics of formal education as it exists today advocate deestablishing the considerable educational bureaucracy and returning to apprenticeships and peer teaching in the community. Some secondary levels of education are beginning to respond with internship programs. True learning appears to take place in an informal noncognitive manner, that is, changes in behavior are largely due to right-hemisphere-dominated affective teaching and learning. This is not surprising to educators with a holistic humanistic orientation.

Other changes in education are being stimulated by education research. It has been demonstrated that self-directed learners need plans of learning that are self-appropriated and relevant to their concerns and learning goals. New relationships between teachers and learners are being established that emphasize goal-referenced instruction and evaluation. [18, p. 8] Learning objectives are behaviorally oriented and very specific, and success or failure is easily measured by both teacher and learner at frequent intervals. Contracting for grades—an offshoot of criterion-referenced learning—is instituted as teacher and learner become partners in the educational endeavor (see Chapter 2).

Directly related to responsible education and evaluation is teacher/learner accountability. Just who is accountable for material to be mastered? A clearly stated objective leaves little doubt about the answer. The Student Bill of Rights (presented in Appendix G) includes very clear references to objectives that are concrete, understandable, and mutually acceptable in terms of responsibility and accountability. In Figure 9–1 Dalis and Strasser suggest a strategy checklist for evaluating teacher and student behaviors aimed at achieving specific goals.

Motivation and Learning: Maslow's Needs Theory

This section contains a brief review of learning and motivation. *Motivation* has been defined as the process by which behavior is initiated in response to a need. [23, p. 7]

One of the most well-known holistically-oriented motivation theorists was Abraham Maslow, whose needs theory formed the foundation of humanistic psychology. Figure 9–2 reviews his hierarchy of needs. Maslow's theory of human behavior is based on these universal needs which serve as primary influences on behavior. As a need arises, tension—either pleasant or unpleasant—develops,

Tally Each Occurrence	Teaching Behavior	Goal
_____	Tuning In To Process	• Helping the students become aware of the processes they or others use during a discussion.
_____	Probe for Rationale and Inferring Value	• Helping the students recognize that the decisions they make are based in part on the values they hold.
		• Helping the students become aware of some of the values they hold.
		• Developing the students' ability to more systematically explicate their own values and infer the values of others.
_____	Probe for Prediction	• Developing the students' ability to weigh possible/probable consequences before implementing a course of action.
_____	Probe for Data	• Helping the students become aware of the role of data in decision making.
_____	Probe for Data Source	• Developing the students' ability to analyze the source of data as one way of judging the validity of that data.
_____	Probe for Conditions	• Developing the students' ability to explicate the conditions that affect (1) the successful implementation of a course of action or (2) the prioritization of one's values.
		• Sensitizing the students to the role of conditions in decision making.
_____	Focus Setting	• Developing the students' ability to recognize when they or others are shifting the topic of the discussion.
_____	Probe for Values	• Helping the students recognize that the decisions they make are based in part on the values they hold.
		• Developing the students' ability to more systematically explicate their own values and the values of others.

FIGURE 9-1A Teaching behavior/goals checklist

Reprinted with permission from Gus T. Dalis and Ben B. Strasser, *Teaching Strategies for Values Awareness and Decision Making in Health Education* (Thorofare, N.J.: Charles B. Slack, Inc., 1977), p. 162.

Tally Each Occurrence	Goal
_____	• Awareness that the decisions they make are based in part on the values they hold.
_____	• Awareness of the role of data in decision making.
_____	• Awareness of the processes they or others use during a discussion and the effects of those processes on others.
_____	• Awareness of some of the values they hold.
_____	• Ability to systematically explicate their own values.
_____	• Ability to systematically infer the values of others.
_____	• Ability to analyze the source of data as one way of judging the validity of that data.
_____	• Ability to weigh possible/probable consequences before implementing a course of action.
_____	• Ability to recognize when they or others in a discussion are shifting topics.
_____	• Ability to use language patterns that enable them to disagree with others while maintaining open lines of communication.
_____	• Ability to interact effectively with others whose values differ.
_____	• Ability to communicate their feelings, opinions and attitudes effectively.
_____	• Ability to explicate the conditions that affect (1) the successful implementation of a course of action or (2) the prioritization of one's values.
_____	• Awareness of the role of conditions in decision making.

FIGURE 9-1B Student behavior/goals checklist

Reprinted with permission from Gus T. Dalis and Ben B. Strasser, *Teaching Strategies for Values Awareness and Decision Making in Health Education* (Thorofare, N.J.: Charles B. Slack, Inc., 1977), p. 163.

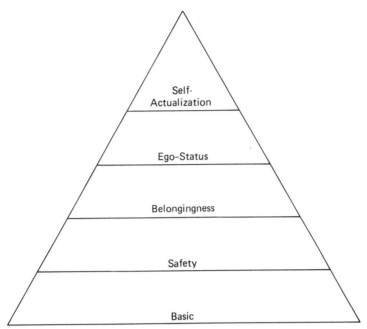

FIGURE 9-2 Maslow's hierarchy of needs

which motivates behavior. The goal of the behavior, which will be appropriate for satisfying the particular need, is to reduce the tension. Thus, an infant in need of food will experience hunger, cry, and usually, be satisfied with food as the need is met. Each level need must be partially met in order for an individual to move up to higher level needs. According to Maslow's theory, it would be inappropriate to introduce self-growth strategies to someone struggling to achieve the more basic need for security. [41]

Acute and long-term care nurses have found Maslow's hierarchy particularly useful in defining nursing problems and in organizing nursing care. Persons experiencing an illness, either chronic or episodic, may find themselves, often for the first time, needing help with very basic needs which they had once taken for granted (for example, nutrition, elimination, oxygenation, and so forth). Since needs are hierarchical and interdependent, deficits on one level affect other levels. Being forced to return to these basic need levels has tremendous psychosocial implications and greatly affects safety, love, and belongingness as well as ego, self-esteem, and higher-order needs.

Human beings determine what behavior is appropriate to meet a goal or to satisfy a need through the inherent and acquired learning processes or systems everyone is equipped with and capable of developing. Figure 9-3 summarizes the entire learning process as it will be discussed in the next section.

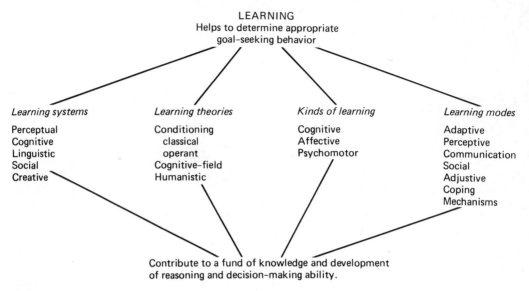

FIGURE 9-3 The complex systems, theories, and styles that contribute to high-level wellness

Kinds of Learning—Cognitive, Affective, and Psychomotor

Learning begins—as does communication—with the perceptive systems, the reasoning and cognitive faculties, feelings, linguistic expression, and other creative processes. The material to be learned to function effectively in any society is described as *cognitive* (facts, ideas, information), *affective* (feelings, beliefs, attitudes), and *psychomotor* (behaviors and skills). Obviously, all three kinds overlap and can contribute to any total learning outcome.

It is important to consider which domain of learning is being focused upon because there are specific teaching strategies and learning activities geared to each category. Bloom and associates developed such an approach to organizing content and learning objectives and experiences, and it has remained a classic in education. [7]

The learning objective reflects the level and the domain to be achieved. For example, in a client situation, the mutually defined objective is: "Suzanne will tabulate and summarize the results of her Wellness Inventory." This objective aims at two levels of cognitive learning—the knowledge level and the higher synthesis level in which she is asked to make some creative conclusions from her raw data.

In another situation, a client is asked to: "Consider your rights as a client and act in a self-assertive manner in a nurse-client contract negotiation." Again, two levels of affective learning are included in the objective—one low and one high.

When a nurse is formulating an objective for herself or for a client the choice of the kind of learning and the level expected is critical. Expectation of high-level performance without acquisition of prerequisite learning is an unfair expectation.

In planning learning activities the nurse must also take learning domains into consideration (cognitive, affective, and psychomotor).

The area of most concern to beginning practitioners is probably psychomotor learning because it is into this domain that most nursing skills fall. A nurse beginning to perform a blood pressure assessment with a client is first concerned with the cognitive aspects of blood pressure measurement—anatomy, physiology, ranges of normal, instrumentation, and proper procedure. Interconnected with this learning are all the affective aspects of the task—attitudes about blood pressure as an accurate assessment indicator, memories and feelings associated with past experiences with blood pressure measurements, concern about the client's feelings and reactions, fears about own competency, and so forth. Finally, there is the problem of manually learning a new motor visual skill—how to handle, manage, and adapt equipment to the situation competently. Putting all three domains together comfortably and competently constitutes the overall goal, which requires some fairly intricate learning experiences.

Whenever the nurse prepares a teaching/learning plan, she should break down the overall learning objectives into component learning domains and examine the prerequisite knowledge, attitudes, and skills inherent in the task. Easy integration of a new skill for either nurses or clients is a complex, time-consuming matter requiring both planning and patience.

People learn in various ways, but it is the three theories of learning that form the conceptual framework for this text which is the point of focus here. Every teaching/learning situation the nurse will encounter contains principles derived from one or more of these theories, and two of the theories—cognitive-field and humanistic—strongly resemble each other and are particularly holistic in nature. The third—stimulus-response learning—although rather narrow in its original conception, has broadened and is being effectively used in holistic health care today. Clinical applications of each theory will be demonstrated in later sections of this chapter.

Three Theories of Learning

Stimulus Response—Operant Conditioning

Stimulus-response learning theory began in the 1920s with animal training experiments which relied on stimulating reflex responses with a stimulus unrelated to the needs of the animal (for example, a bell, word, or signal) and reinforcing or rewarding the appropriate behavior. This was termed *classical conditioning*. Intent or motivation is of much less value in this type of learning than in cognitive-field or humanistic learning theories.

Operant conditioning, pioneered by B. F. Skinner, greeted the era of neobehaviorism and was based on classical conditioning. Operant conditioning involved animals acting on their environments; it did not involve insight into the learning or behavior, however. Positive and negative reinforcements, spaced irregularly, were shown to make the behavior more permanent.

Operant conditioning has formed the basis for "programmed instruction" learning, which provides students with small units or modules of learning and provides immediate feedback about correct or incorrect choices. In this type of program, goals must be very specific, parts of the task sequentially ordered, and all potential questions or problems analyzed and answered. This system works particularly well within the cognitive domain.

Another example of operant conditioning is behavior-modification techniques, which may take the form of aversion control—that is, presenting a real or imagined noxious stimulus which is associated with a habit to be extinguished. This has been attempted with alcoholics, for example, by maintaining them on a substance called "antabuse" which causes extreme nausea if alcohol is ingested.

Other less primitive forms of behavior modification include some self-monitoring methods, such as logs and diaries, which point out certain feelings, symptoms, behaviors, and habits. Such a log is shown for a women's health research project (Figure 9–4).

Much of the early biofeedback work developed from operant-conditioning theory. The biofeedback monitor is used to reward correct behavior. The biofeedback signal is given when a particular physiologic activity changes to a previously agreed upon level. The level can then be changed to approach more closely the desired goal. A sample of a typical headache and pain log used by a client undergoing biofeedback is shown in Figure 9–5.

Low arousal, hypnotic, or meditative states have conditioning origins. The results of using this "twilight state" to learn are fascinating:

1. Learning is intuitive, left-hemisphere-dominated, and often, very creative.
2. Material that the student has formerly thought of as unlearnable can be absorbed.
3. Positive mental sets and attitude changes can be stimulated.
4. Retrieval or exploration of less-conscious mental processes and information may be possible. [9, pp. 378–79]

The moral and ethical implications of this kind of research need further investigation.

Cognitive-Field—Gestalt Learning Theory

In 1942 Kurt Lewin proposed his cognitive-field theory of learning. This theory, more than either the (S-R) stimulus response or humanistic theories, touches Smuts' original idea of holism in that the person perceives his world or situation as it comes together to form a total picture, pattern, or Gestalt. In his theory, Lewin includes an existential aspect to the world which exists as the individual chooses to perceive it.

Cognitive-field psychologists find the clue to the meaning of learning in the aspects of a situation within which a person and his psychological environment come together in a psychological field or "life space." Life space contains the person, his psychological environment, the goals he is seeking as well as the negative "goals" he is trying to avoid, the barriers between himself and his goals which restrict his psychological movement toward them, and the potential and actual paths to his goal.

Cognitive-field psychology integrates biologic and social factors and treats respective persons as interacting with them. A person is neither dependent upon nor independent of his environment. Likewise, a person's environment is neither made by him nor independent of him.

According to the cognitive-field position, the only reality a person can ever know or work with is his own interpretation of what is real. Thus, for an individual, reality is what he gains through his five-plus senses and his manner of sizing it up.

Cognitive structure means the way in which a person perceives the psychological aspects of the personal, physical, and social world. Such a world includes a person and all of his facts, concepts, beliefs, memory traces, and expectations.

Cognitive-field psychology is a purposive psychology; it assumes that a person, at whatever his level of understanding, does the best he knows how for whatever he thinks he is. Hence, intellectual processes are deeply affected by an individual's goals; learning activity, including habit formation, is goal-directed. Accordingly, goal or purpose is central to cognitive-field learning theory. [6, pp. 204–10]

Humanistic Learning Theory

Humanism as a philosophy was described in detail in Chapter 3. Carl Rogers was its foremost proponent, and he incorporated it into the field of education. Humanists accept cognitive-field theory, for the most part, but place more value on the self-evaluation and self-growth of the learner. Humanists deal largely with the affective (emotional) aspects of human behavior. They are interested in explaining man's relationship to his world and to other people and in learning how an individual feels about things. [27]

The following are some of the beliefs of humanistic learning theorists:

Human beings have a natural potentiality for learning. Significant learning takes place when the subject matter is perceived by the student as having relevance for his own purposes.

Learning which involves a change in self-organization—in the perception of oneself—is threatening and tends to be resisted. Those types of learning which are threatening to the self are more easily perceived and assimilated when external threats are at a minimum. When threat to the self is low, experience can be perceived in a differentiated fashion and learning can proceed.

Much significant learning is acquired through doing. Learning is facilitated when the student participates responsibly in the learning process. Self-initiated learning which involves the whole person, feelings as well as intellect, is the most lasting and pervasive.

Independence, creativity, and self-reliance are all facilitated when self-criticism and self-evaluation are basic and evaluation by others are of secondary importance.

The most socially useful learning in the modern world is the learning of the process of learning, a continuing openness to experience and incorporation into oneself of the process of change. [37]

In humanistic learning theory, then, man is seen as a whole person who lives with purpose and intent, and for whom the meaningfulness of his own experience is of the essence. [22, p. 176]

```
                              DAILY LOG

Code: _____    Date: _____    Weight: _____    Temp: _____    Hrs./sleep: _____

AWAKENING DIARY:

Waking Time: _____              Breathing through:  Nose: ____  Mouth: ____
Alarm Time: _____               If through nose, which nostril is predominant:
     Circle one for each item:      Right: ____  Left: ____  Neither: ____

Sleep quality:          Poor  Fair  Mod  Good  VGood    Intercourse: Yes ____  No ____
Amount of dreaming:     VLow  Low   Mod  High  VHigh    Pain w/intercourse: Yes ____  No ____
Dream experiences:      Bad   Fair  Mod  Good  VGood    Orgasm w/ intercourse: Yes ____  No ____
Energy on waking:       VLow  Low   Mod  High  VHigh    Orgasm w/o intercourse: Yes ____  No ____
Expectations for today: VLow  Low   Mod  High  VHigh    Method of birth control: _____
```

BEDTIME DIARY: Diary Time: _____		

```
Breathing through:  Nose: ____  Mouth: ____
If through nose, which nostril is predomi-
nant:  Right: ____  Left: ____  Neither: ___

Weather today (CHECK AS MANY AS APPROPRIATE):

Comfortable: ____    Hot: ____    Cold: ____
Humid: ____   Cloudy: ____   Windy: ____
Rain: ____   Fog: ____   Other: _____

Activities (CHECK AS MANY AS APPROPRIATE):

Work day: ____    Leisure day: ____
At school: ____   Vacation: ____
Non-routine day: ____   Away from home: ____
On diet: ____    Sick: ____
Saw doctor: ____    In hospital: ____
Late party: ____   Late date: ____
Air travel: ____   Other: _____

Stress Levels:
```

```
KEY:  VH: Very High   L: Low
      H: High
      M: Moderate     VL: Very Low
```

(CHECK ONE FOR EACH ITEM)

	VH	H	M	L	VL
Tiredness during day					
Work pressure today					
Physical activity today					
Mental activity today					
Influence of weather					
Personal happiness					
Punctuality					
Fun activities					
Feeling of being rushed					
Guilty feelings					
Anger expressed today					
Anger held in today					
Criticism of others					
Sexual thoughts					
Depressed feelings					
Sense of time today					

```
KEY:  E: Extreme    S: Slight
      G: Great      N: None
      M: Moderate
```

	E	G	M	S	N
Irritability					
Nausea					
Heavy Feeling					
Backache					
Leg ache					
Inner sides of thighs ache					
Breasts sore and tender					
Headache					
Dizziness					
Weakness					
Crying					
Abdominal fullness					
Allergies					
Indigestion					
Cough					
Sneezing					
Thirst					
Urination					
Cramps					
Blemishes					
Gas					
Belching					
Smoking					
Drugs					
Caffeine					
Alcohol					
Snacks					
Appetite					
Annoyances					

```
Bowel movements:
   Number: 0 ____  1 ____  2 ____  3 ____  More ____
   Type: Liquid: ____  Loose: ____  Normal: ____
              Constipated: ____  None: ____

Vomiting:  Yes ____    No ____

Other symptoms important to you: _____
_____
```

(continued on other side)

77-741P

FIGURE 9-4 Women's health research project daily log

Reprinted with permission of Erik Peper, The San Francisco State University Women's Health Study, 1978, and Dr. Charles F. Stroebel, from Dr. Charles F. Stroebel, Dr. Bernard C. Glueck, and Cay Luce, *Psychophysiological Diary,* Institute of Living, 1973.

Other symptoms (continued): _____
_____
_____
_____
_____

Vaginal/Genital symptoms:

	N	S	M	G	E
Vaginal discharge ____					
Vaginal itching ____					
Genital swelling ____					
Burning when urinating					
If discharge, color:					
odor:					

Other vaginal/genital symptoms (i.e.,
vaginal warts, herpes, etc.):
_____
_____
_____

Did you do anything to alleviate vaginitis
symptoms? Yes_____ No_____
If yes, what did you do? _____
_____
_____
_____
_____

Was it successful? Yes_____ No_____
Did you douche? Yes_____ No_____
If yes, with what? _____
_____

Underwear:
   None _____ Nylon _____ Cotton _____

Slacks/pants/nylons: Loose_____ Tight_____

Bathing: Shower_____ Bath_____ None_____

   Water temperature: Cool _____ Lukewarm_____
                      Warm_____ Hot_____

If doctor seen, diagnosis: _____
_____
_____
_____

Medications for vaginitis? Yes_____ No_____
If yes, what type:_____
   Dosage/Frequency:_____
   Oral or vaginal: _____

Other medications (i.e., aspirin, laxatives,
   tranquilizers, birth control pill, anti-
   biotics, etc.)
   Type: _____
   Frequency: _____
   Type: _____
   Frequency:_____

      (continued in next column)

Other medications (continued)
   Type: _____
   Frequency: _____
   Type: _____
   Frequency: _____

Day of menstrual cycle: _____
   (Day 1 = 1st day of menstruation)

If menstruating: tampon/pad/other_____

   Flow: Scanty_____ Light_____
         Moderate_____ Heavy_____
         Very heavy _____

   Menstrual cramps? Yes _____ No _____
   If yes, rate pain/discomfort:
      Slight_____ Moderate_____
      Great_____ Extreme_____

   Did you do anything to alleviate menstrual
   discomfort? Yes_____ No_____
   If yes, what did you do? _____
   _____
   _____
   _____
   _____
   _____

   Was it successful? Yes_____ No_____
_____
Please jot down any additional observations.

FIGURE 9-4 (continued)

HEADACHE LOG

Date	Time AM/PM		Intensity*	Medication		Type of headache	Location of headache
	Began	Subsided		Name	Dose		

PAIN LOG

Date	Time AM/PM		Intensity*	Medication		Type of pain	Specific location of pain
	Began	Subsided		Name	Dose		

FEEL GOOD (PEAK EXPERIENCE) LOG

Date	Time	Duration in hours	Cause or Reason	Medication if any	Intensity*	Comments

* Rate on a scale of 1 to 10 with 10 as best feeling state.

Post-Treatment Questionnaire

1. Do you feel you are better able to relax quickly?
2. Do you feel you can relax more deeply?
3. Do you feel you have a better understanding of relaxation?
4. Do you feel the biofeedback helped you to relax?
5. Did you like the biofeedback training?

Subjective Units of Tension (SUT scores)

The client estimates his subjective feelings of tension on a scale of 0 to 10 both before and after relaxation exercises.

Insomnia—Sleep Record

1. Time to fall asleep
2. Number of hours slept
3. Number of nightly awakenings
4. How felt in morning (scale 1 to 5)

FIGURE 9-5 Logs used to evaluate effects of biofeedback training

Adapted from Barbara Brown, *Stress and the Art of Biofeedback* (New York: Harper & Row, 1977), pp. 210–11.

These aforementioned major humanistic premises lead Jenny to suggest three principles of humanistic teaching and learning:

1. That which governs the behavior of a person is his unique perception of himself and the world in which he lives and the meanings that this relationship has for him. Thus all behavior is a function of the person's perceptions, and not the physical environment, except as it comes to be represented in the mind of the behaving individual. The initial task of the teacher is to help the learner to perceive a reality which is consonant with the actual situation, since this is the basis of the teacher's instructions.

2. All behavior is directed towards achieving increased personal adequacy and ability to cope with life. Thus the second teaching challenge is to assist the learner to perceive that he is capable of coping and to substantiate his feeling of adequacy for the learning tasks ahead of him. People learn early in life to avoid situations for which they feel inadequate.

3. Those needs perceived as immediate receive the person's attention before any future oriented problems. Thus, the concerns uppermost in the learner's mind must be satisfied before he will attend to distant eventualities. [22]

What all this means is that the values of the client are paramount. Imposing the values of the health professional on the client is a useless exercise. The nurse should be prepared to negotiate new values which the client can see as worthwhile, and contributory to healthier living.

All of these three learning theories are employed in the holistic teaching/ learning process. All the principles which nurses use automatically to teach clients, themselves, and each other are derived from one or more of these theories.

Teaching/Learning Principles Derived from Theory

From stimulus-response, cognitive-field, and humanistic learning theory some working principles of teaching/learning can be drawn. Thus, when a nurse develops a teaching/learning plan, goals, activities, and methodology are supported by sound learning theory.

Stimulus-response theory offers some principles which can be utilized in almost any new learning situation, but particularly in the acquisition of new psychomotor skills, for example:

The learner should be active, not merely a passive recipient of data. The more a person can learn by doing, the better.

Repetition is an important part of mastering any skill. Overlearning can guarantee retention in both cognitive and skills areas.

Reinforcement is essential. When a new learning is repeated successfully, it should be rewarded. Although success in itself can be viewed as a reward, and indeed, is more predictably motivating than failure, an additional incentive or reward should be structured into the learning activity.

Generalization as well as discrimination should be encouraged so that new learning can be broadened to include new situations.

Cognitive-field theory contains particularly useful principles for situations that require intellectual development, discussion, synthesis, and critique. Information is not only memorized, but also seen as an element in the entire scheme, concept, theory, etc., and hence, as a step toward some desired goal. Cognitive-field theory holds the following beliefs:

the perceptual features of a learning situation are important conditions of learning. Therefore, a combination of sense experiences (sight, sound, touch, smell, taste), along with dialogue, discussion, and reading, should be included where possible to develop an idea or concept.

The organization of information should be an important concern of any teacher. Direction of learning should move from simple to complex, from concrete to abstract, and from part to whole. It is the teacher's function to help students or clients see the relationships between facts and concepts and their connectedness to rules, principles, and generalizations. Facts are not enough. The meaning of those facts to the whole and to the learner is important.

Learning with understanding is more lasting and can be transferred more easily to new situations than can rote learning.

Cognitive feedback confirms correct knowledge and corrects faulty information. It can also serve as reinforcement.

Goal setting by the learner serves as motivation for learning. Success is a motivator and helps determine how the learner sees himself and how he sets future goals.

Thinking which diverges from the status quo but leads to inventive and creative solutions should be encouraged and supported. Clarification of such thinking can be sought by asking the learner to restate an idea in his own words or by giving examples.

Humanistic learning theory incorporates Maslow's theory of motivation and various other theories of personality and human development. Some overlap with stimulus-response and cognitive-field theory is inevitable. Humanistic learning theory is not so concerned with the what or how of learning itself, but with the nature of the learner, that is, with all of what he or she brings to any learning situation. The uniqueness of that person and how to shape the learning to suit those special abilities, needs, wants, and fears is a goal of the teacher. The attitude of the learner toward the learning is as important as the learning itself. Certainly, this learning theory lends itself to affective learning, for example, to the development of values, ethics, and caring behaviors. Humanistic learning theory proponents believe the following:

The learner's abilities are important and the learning plan should provide for slower as well as gifted learners. If learning steps are too easy, motivation lags; if they are too difficult, the learner feels overwhelmed, discouraged, and frustrated. For example, a less mature learner needs concepts presented in more concrete ways with examples close to his own experience.

Although prenatal influences and genetic endowment are important, postnatal development is as powerful a determinant of ability and interest. The teacher should look at and take into consideration those influences.

Learning is culturally relative and determines meaningfulness of material. Assessment of subcultures of learners as well as contemporary cultural demands helps the teacher design learning that has connections to the person's life experience.

Anxiety level of the learner may add or detract from the learning. High-anxiety learners perform better if not constantly reinforced, whereas low-anxiety learners need frequent evaluation and encouragement.

All learners are not motivated by the same learning situation. Learning is more effective when the learner is "ready" in terms of attitudes, skills, and knowledges.

The organization of motives within the individual is important. Long-range goals, such as nursing, can help students survive prerequisite courses they might otherwise see as irrelevant.

The learning atmosphere (structured and rigid, or open and democratic) will affect satisfaction as well as the product of learning. Different types of learners respond to different environments, for example, competitive versus cooperative. [20, pp. 562–64]

INTRAPERSONAL APPLICATIONS OF TEACHING/LEARNING

Developing a Philosophy of Continuing Teaching/Learning for Holistic Nursing Practice

The kind of holistic teaching/learning philosophy that can be synthesized from the preceding theories should incorporate values and beliefs about the nature of human beings, how they learn most effectively and with optimal satisfaction, and how this learning affects and is affected by states of health. The purpose of education is to help individuals to maximize their creative potential, to examine and critique relevant issues and problems, and to live productively in their own unique way, making contributions to the advancement of society.

All learning has cognitive, affective, and psychomotor components which are integrated and goal-directed. Teaching is any activity which facilitates and stimulates the learning potential of the person. Teacher and learner come together in a safe environment to set learning goals and create opportunities for self-learning and self-evaluation. The teacher serves as a resource person who respects and enhances each learner's unique cultural background, belief system, and life experiences.

The goal of health teaching is to enable practitioner and client to enter each other's worlds, recognize mutual health values, and learn more about each other and themselves. Humanistic concerns are shared and mutual learning goals are agreed upon. Learning is acknowledged as a lifelong search for truth.

As persons and as nurses we could not have developed our present potentials without conditioning, with cognitive and humanistic teaching/learning processes affecting that growth. Much of what we think and do is unconsciously "programmed"—either by ourselves, parents, or significant others. How much of it have we merely accepted? How many habits would be worth changing? There's nothing wrong with conditioning as long as it is a pattern of behavior we choose or accept. When a person decides to become self-aware and responsible, he or she takes time to evaluate everyday habits and make desired changes.

Assessing Own Teaching/Learning Style

Daniels and Horowitz suggest a technique used by Fritz Perls to break into the cycle of automatic responses and to evaluate resistance to change:

> Notice some of your habits—the way you dress, the way you brush your teeth, the way you open or close a door . . . . If . . .some alternative seems just as good and has the advantage of offering variety, try to change . . . . Do you take pleasure in learning the new way? Or do you encounter strong resistances? . . .What happens if you watch someone perform a task similar to one of your own? Do you get annoyed, irritated, indignant at small variations from your own procedure? [14, p. 93]

Intrapersonal Applications of a Holistic Teaching/Learning Philosophy

In the next activity some principles of operant conditioning can be applied to self. Choose a habit you would like to extinguish. Assess for yourself how ingrained this habit is. How many times a day does it occur and under what circumstances? Is the habit used to alleviate stress? If so, it will take more than just removing the habit to solve the whole problem. Substitution of another habit which alleviates or reduces the stress may be necessary. How long has the activity been a habit? Extinguishing it may take considerable time and some failed attempts. Do you really want to change this habit? Are the rewards worth it? Are you doing this for yourself or for someone else in order to win his or her approval?

Once these questions have been answered some simple principles of conditioning can be applied. Keep in mind that:

1. Any act that brings a reward tends to happen more often. This can be in the form of supportive verbal feedback from a friend who knows what you're trying to achieve; or it can be a monetary reward or just being good to yourself by doing something pleasurable that you rarely do. Reward can also be achieving a desired goal related to extinction of the habit, such as experiencing fewer headaches by drinking less coffee and eating fewer refined carbohydrates.

2. Any act that no longer brings the rewards it used to bring tends to happen less often and eventually leads to extinction. If one peer group reinforced a smoking habit and you interacted with a new group that did not reinforce the smoking behavior, it would help you to stop smoking.

3. Any act that is punished tends to be suppressed, often temporarily, but the potential to act in the original manner is still present. If you punish yourself for failing a test by not going out all weekend and making yourself miserable, you probably will not change the behavior that caused you to fail the test.

Think of all the weight loss and smoking cessation programs based on the preceding principles. Some methods also include aversion or negative reinforcement. The long-term extinction rates of these methods do not support reliance on aversion therapy except as a last resort. Punishment of children is a prime example of negative reinforcement and is a heavily debated issue among parents, teachers, and psychologists.

In addition to applying principles of operant conditioning in changing a behavior or learning new information, attitudes, or skills, principles of Gestalt and humanistic learning theory are simultaneously operating. Your goals and feelings are essential in any behavior change. Much of the success of acquiring a new behavior will be based on your past experiences and attitudes about such behavior and your aspirations about what this behavior will mean to you and/or others. If your objective is to better your active listening techniques to improve your relationships with clients, acquiring these sometimes difficult behaviors will be viewed as relevant and important to your development as a sensitive, caring person and professional.

Self-assessment of teaching/learning style includes looking at your own teaching/learning strengths and weaknesses. Begin with the way you learn and ask yourself questions such as:

1. Do I like being an *active* learner?
2. Do I like to set my own learning goals?
3. Do I like contracting for grades?
4. Do I like authoritarian teaching situations in which the student is a passive recipient of information?
5. Do I like straight-lecture, discussion, or seminar learning?
6. Would I like a completely programmed course?
7. Do I value feedback from teachers and others?
8. Do I prefer an assignment which requires memorization and regurgitation of information?
9. Do I like comparing and critiquing ideas rather than rote memorization?
10. Do I like expressing myself in writing?
11. Do I prefer learning by doing rather than by reading and writing?
12. Do I prefer a learning situation in which my opinion is important?
13. Do I like a teacher who is a resource, not a dictator?

These are a few examples of the kinds of self-evaluative questions learners should ask themselves. No answer is considered right or wrong, and knowing your own learning strengths, weaknesses, favorite learning methods, content, and so on, will help you formulate your own teaching/learning philosophy and goals. Recognizing your own learning style will help you in teaching others. Not all theories and methods will suit you or the client. Recognition of teaching/learning philosophies and of characteristics of teacher and learner is an essential step in the health education process.

Independent Learning

An application of self-learning that has been utilized for years in high-school, college, and graduate school courses is termed independent study. Again, if this method is to be used with clients, it should be carefully piloted, researched, and evaluated. It can be used effectively in school health education courses in which students are enrolled, followed closely, and given credit or some other type of reward.

The characteristics of a learner able to assume responsibility for independent learning include the ability to:

1. perceive worthwhile things to do;
2. personalize learning;
3. exercise self-discipline;
4. make use of material and human resources;
5. produce results; and
6. strive for improvement. [3]

Independent learners should be able to write their own learning objectives as is considered appropriate by both teacher and learner. The learning experience should be one that best suits these objectives. If a learner wants to apply principles of human lifestyling to himself, then reading a book is not a sufficient learning activity for that objective. A learner's level of knowledge or skill acquistion can be ascertained through pretests so that motivation isn't dampened by unstimulating material.

Another important element for self-learning is the achievability of the learning task. The student should have frequent self-measurement and external feedback on progress and deficiencies. It also serves as a motivator. Verbal praise, extra credit, recognition, and released time all can serve as motivators. Without motivation, any learning system will fail. Evaluation is related to motivation and is required almost as frequently. If learners, students, or clients are keeping logs or diaries or using self-recording devices, they need feedback on their progress, their interpretations, and their conclusions. Ideally, feedback should occur within days—not weeks—after a progress check. As practitioners learn in leadership theory, some delegation of tasks can allow more frequent feedback, as long as the teaching/learning assistant has clear guidelines.

Finally, independent learning activities should relate to universal theories, principles, and processes the student can apply to other areas of life. The more "transferable" the knowledges and skills, the better the student will like the experience. All these prerequisites of independent learning apply to any type of teaching/learning situation.

All the self-assessments supplied and referred to in this text are self-learning materials. Many of them encourage practice with supervision and evaluation. A nurse or client has already reached a high level of independent thinking and self-responsibility in order to use them. Self-initiated learning is a goal, not usually a starting point, in most health care interactions. Assuming self-learning on the part of the client may be as false an assumption as ignoring the self-learning potential in that person.

Self-Learning Modules

One of the greatest innovations in self-teaching/learning has been the development of the self-learning module or SLM. Self-learning modules are discrete units of study complete with performance objectives which establish guidelines for satisfactory student completion. [11] A modularized course is one "in which a number of these units are combined sequentially to provide an overview of a particular area of interest of a specific body of information." [11]

The basic format of any module should include the following:

1. introduction and directions;
2. general goal;
3. pretest;
4. prerequisite knowledge and skills;
5. specific learning objectives;
6. learning resources;
7. learning activities; and
8. posttest.

Modularization lends itself to the learning of prerequisite information—cognitive and psychomotor—for the performance of a skill, such as proper toothbrushing technique in a busy dental clinic, or some one of the other numerous skills nurses need to learn. The role of the evaluator is crucial, especially when the final learning activity involves demonstration by the teacher, practice supervision, and return demonstration by the learner. With proper time for question-and-answer, discussion, supervised practice, and frequent checkpoints for evaluation, modularization can be a successful strategy that encourages self-pacing.

Evaluating Self as a Teacher/Learner

As a beginning teacher/learner in nursing, in interpersonal relationships and groups, some questions might be asked of self to evaluate the internalization and integration of a gestaltist-humanistic philosophy of education. The questions could be asked of a client involved in a health education program, with an emphasis on self-awareness and self-growth [33, pp. 172–73]:

Can I function effectively in a group?

Do I hinder or facilitate the group process?

Do I give and openly receive feedback?

Do I make personal value decisions and do I commit myself to those decisions?

Do I support other students' efforts to make responsible decisions?

Am I able to communicate empathy, regard, and genuineness?

In what ways am I moving toward becoming a fully functioning person? in what ways am I not?

Am I becoming more centered and calm?

Am I developing my Higher Self? How?

Am I disidentifying from personality models that are restrictive to my development?

In what ways am I more creative and imaginative? In what areas can I improve my imagination and creativity?

What values are central to my sense of self? Do I act consistently on those values? What values would I like to develop and realize?

What are my principal concerns? How do these concerns relate to my sense of identity? In what ways can I deal with these concerns in order to realize a positive identity?

Am I living in the here and now? Am I able to relate my thoughts to my feelings? Do I see things holistically or in segments?

Am I committed to growth and development? Am I willing to take risks or do I avoid opportunities for growth?

Do I facilitate another person's growth and development? If so, how? If not, why not?

INTERPERSONAL TEACHING/LEARNING: HOLISTIC APPROACHES TO HEALTH EDUCATION

First, the practitioner develops a personal and professional philosophy of education and health education, applies that philosophy to her own teaching/learning style, then moves into the interpersonal world of health education. The holistic practitioner recognizes the holistic humanistic nature of learning and without disregarding all that has been said about stimulus-response and gestalt learning, focuses on the affective domain. It is within this domain that the gap between health information and health practices is bridged.

Rosenstock has observed that a decision to take health action is influenced by the person's state of readiness, by his socially and individually determined beliefs about the efficacy of alternative actions, by psychological barriers to actions, by interpersonal influences, and by one or more critical cues or accidents which serve to trigger a response. [22] Nurses are all too familiar with the incredible openness a hospitalized client may evidence to health teaching after an illness episode. Holistic practitioners call this a "healing crisis." Havighurst calls these sensitive or critical periods in which the human organism is especially able to learn quickly through certain kinds of experience, the "teachable moment." [19, pp. 6–7]

Readiness can occur naturally if the client perceives a health problem as threatening or a potential problem as having a high probability of occurrence; sometimes this reaction is referred to as "foxhole religion." The health information media has taken great advantage of this fact by creating "readiness" through convincing scare tactics—especially in the areas of venereal disease and drug abuse prevention. If the threat disappears, is not periodically reinforced, or is not perceived as real, then the individual's motivation may lag. Again, negative reinforcement is not as affective as a positive reward.

Applying Problem Solving to Teaching/Learning

Incorporated in the client's "readiness" to learn are observations of the client's present physical level of comfort, anxiety, restlessness, distraction, depression, fear, disbelief, denial, anger, or any other barriers to effective listening and interacting. The client may be blocking input due to pressing problems regarding time, money, inconvenience, distance, new skills to be learned, alteration in normal body functioning, change in body image, fear of forgetting, complexity of the regime, or undesirable side effects, especially of medications. [20, p. 179] Any of these factors can seem overwhelming to a client—especially to one under stress.

The holistic practitioner in a wellness-oriented interaction with a client applies the problem-solving process to preparing an educational plan of care by:

1. assessing the needs or problems of the individual or group;
2. stating learning objectives that are measurable, feasible, and able to be accomplished in a stated period of time;
3. determining content based on assessment of needs and objectives;
4. selecting teaching strategies that are appropriate to the ages, educational and cultural backgrounds, and problems and concerns of the individual or group; and
5. evaluating the progress of a learning plan at stated periods in order to review, continue, and make changes in program design. [31, p. 252]

Some practical hints to remember for nurses involved in behavior change are:

1. Information is often not enough to cause or enable a person to improve his lifestyle.
2. The benefits of a positive lifestyle change may be delayed or not directly experienced.
3. It is always sound to provide a positive alternative.

Another important point about values is that information which is inconsistent with a particular value or belief system will be ignored. Assessment of the client's beliefs about health, illness, and lifestyle habits and values is prerequisite to any health education plan.

The Health Belief Model

Becker and others have supported Rosenstock's proposed simplified but interesting model for predicting preventive health behavior in Figure 9-6. Research on the applicability of this Health Belief Model to health education is forthcoming, although a few results have been published on its use. Compliance is a paternalistic term referring to the extent to which the patient's behavior coincides with a therapeutic or preventive regimen. The Rosenstock model suggests four perceptions or beliefs which contribute to the likelihood that a recommended diet or other lifestyle modification will be followed:

1. perceived susceptibility or the client's perception of probability of experiencing an illness and/or complications;
2. perceived severity by the client of the potential illness and impact of it on his life;
3. perceived benefits of the preventive action in actually reducing susceptibility or the severity of the potential threat;
4. costs of the health action in money, time, convenience, effort, and side effects. [28, p. 242]

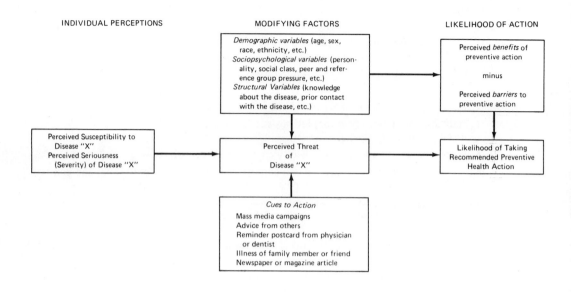

INDIVIDUAL PERCEPTIONS · MODIFYING FACTORS · LIKELIHOOD OF ACTION

Demographic variables (age, sex, race, ethnicity, etc.)
Sociopsychological variables (personality, social class, peer and reference group pressure, etc.)
Structural Variables (knowledge about the disease, prior contact with the disease, etc.)

Perceived *benefits* of preventive action

minus

Perceived *barriers* to preventive action

Perceived Susceptibility to Disease "X"
Perceived Seriousness (Severity) of Disease "X"

Perceived Threat of Disease "X"

Likelihood of Taking Recommended Preventive Health Action

Cues to Action
Mass media campaigns
Advice from others
Reminder postcard from physician or dentist
Illness of family member or friend
Newspaper or magazine article

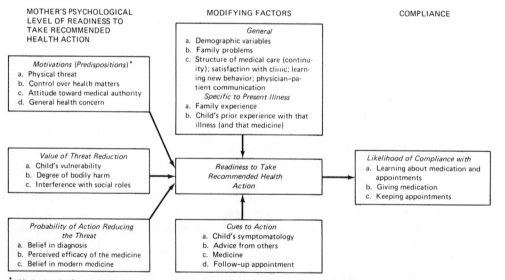

MOTHER'S PSYCHOLOGICAL LEVEL OF READINESS TO TAKE RECOMMENDED HEALTH ACTION · MODIFYING FACTORS · COMPLIANCE

General
a. Demographic variables
b. Family problems
c. Structure of medical care (continuity); satisfaction with clinic; learning new behavior; physician–patient communication
Specific to Present Illness
a. Family experience
b. Child's prior experience with that illness (and that medicine)

Motivations (Predispositions) *
a. Physical threat
b. Control over health matters
c. Attitude toward medical authority
d. General health concern

Value of Threat Reduction
a. Child's vulnerability
b. Degree of bodily harm
c. Interference with social roles

Readiness to Take Recommended Health Action

Likelihood of Compliance with
a. Learning about medication and appointments
b. Giving medication
c. Keeping appointments

Probability of Action Reducing the Threat
a. Belief in diagnosis
b. Perceived efficacy of the medicine
c. Belief in modern medicine

Cues to Action
a. Child's symptomatology
b. Advice from others
c. Medicine
d. Follow-up appointment

* "Motivations" refers to differential emotional arousal in individuals caused by some given class of stimuli (e.g., health matters).

FIGURE 9-6 The health belief model: a pediatric application

Reprinted with permission from Marshall H. Becker, Robert H. Drachman, and John P. Kirscht, "A New Approach to Explaining Sick-Role Behavior in Low Income Populations," *American Journal of Public Health,* 64, no. 3 (March 1974), 206–07.

Loustau has formulated a series of interview questions which can encourage the client to articulate his perceptions of these four areas:

1. Susceptibility and general beliefs about health and illness.
   a. What kinds of things cause you to become ill?
   b. When you have become sick, what do you think has most frequently been the cause?
   c. How would you rate your health—poor, average, or good?
   d. In comparison to others your age, how would you rate your health? about the same or better?
   e. How much do you worry about getting sick?
2. Severity of the potential problem.
   a. How serious do you think your present health problem is?
   b. How would you compare your potential problem with cancer, heart disease, stroke, pneumonia, venereal disease, diabetes, or tooth decay?
   c. Could it cause other problems? such as what?
   d. If you were to get sick, what would the effects be on your job, household, significant others? on your self-esteem?
3. Belief in the health practitioner and the effects of the proposed health action.
   a. To what extent do you think this lifestyle change will affect your potential health problem?
   b. How safe is this new health action?
   c. How likely are the health professionals to handle your potential problem or complications stemming from it?
4. Costs of treatment.
   a. In terms of transportation, how difficult is it for you to make it to your appointments?
   b. Do you have to take time off from work to see the health practitioner? Do you lose pay?
   c. How long did you have to wait to see us? Is that a long time for you?
   d. How much does this lifestyle modification interfere with your usual routine?
   e. Did you have to give up something you like in order to do it?
   f. Is your insurance reimbursing you for this?
   g. Are you having any other side effects from this new health program? [28, pp. 243–44]

Affective Education

Along with the trend toward humanistic health care, humanistic education has developed, as typified by Carl Rogers' nondirective approach. Some of the methods and philosophies have been incorporated in Chapters 2, 3, 6, 7, 8, and 9 of this text. Many more models of affective teaching are being tried and researched. They can be easily applied to health education which, like our traditional teaching/learning system, has focused primarily on cognitive skills. It is no surprise, then, that between 15 percent and 93 percent of all prescriptions are never filled, or that the incidence of high-school dropouts is ever on the increase. Students and clients alike are alienated, but certainly not by the quality of information nor by dramatically improving data systems.

Affective education attempts to reduce learner alienation and facilitate personal integration. Personal integration is the developmental process of becoming whole through risk taking, conflict, and crisis resolution. An integrated person is self-determined, can define and act on a set of values, and has a clear sense of self-identity. Integrated people can exercise intuitive and imaginative faculties as well as rational capabilities, and they can maintain a balance and unity among body, mind, and spirit. [33, p. 5]

Interpersonally, integrated persons are sensitive to the needs of others, feel a common bond with others, can communicate empathy and caring, and can function effectively in a group. [33, p. 5] The models summarized in Figure 9-7 are organized into four major categories—developmental, self-concept, sensitivity, and group orientation and consciousness expansion. Holistic life processes particularly emphasized by each category are listed along with the primary theorists, major goals of each model, and potential application of the approaches to individual and group health teaching situations and topics. Affective educational models offer some hope to holistic health educators.

Wellness Education: A Model in Action

Since this text focuses on wellness, an example of a wellness education program will be described. Dr. John Travis states that the first attitude that is questioned in this approach is the relationship between doctor and patient, in which the doctor is seen as the "pill fairy" who will take charge of the health/illness of the person. Through reading, audio-visual materials, referral files, dialogue, role-playing, individual and group discussion, clients are taught self-responsibility and how to care for themselves physically, emotionally, and spiritually. The lifestyle elements are examined for needed changes.

The objectives of wellness education are stated as helping the client to:

know what his real needs are and how to get them;

act assertively, not passively or aggressively;

relate to troublesome physical symptoms in ways that improve the condition as well as increase knowledge about self, patterns, and "signals" the body gives;

trust that his own personal resources are his greatest strengths for living and growing; and

experience himself as a wonderful person and learn to love himself.

Travis' Wellness Resource Center provides a variety of holistic health practices and five programs which focus on the following:

1. The wellness evaluation—wellness inventory, HHA, biofeedback, and other lifestyle assessments.
2. Body awareness.
3. Taking care of the body.
4. Taking charge of the mind.
5. Communicating needs—lifestyle evolution group.

In Figure 9-9 (p. 393) Travis illustrates his idea of wellness education and the focus of orthodox and alternative health disciplines, contracting healer-oriented, client/healer-oriented, and client-oriented systems. Judging from the diagram,

FIGURE 9-7 Applying humanistic holistic theories to health teaching

CATEGORY	LIFE PROCESSES EMPHASIZED	NAME OF MODEL AND THEORISTS	MAJOR GOALS	METHODS—ACTIVITIES	POTENTIAL HEALTH TEACHING TOPICS
Developmental	Stress Lifestyling Human Development Teaching/ Learning Self-Responsibility Caring Communication	Ego Development Erikson—Eight Stages of Man[1]	1. To successfully master each crisis and more as a more mature person. 2. To expose learner to basic concepts of human development.	Creating conditions conducive to crisis-resolution in an open *nurturing environment.*	1. Life crisis resolution. 2. Crisis Intervention. 3. Life Transition Counseling and Groups. 4. Parent Education—Ages and Stages.

		Psychosocial Mosher & Sprinthall[2]	1. To listen to people, their ideas and feelings, and respond.
			2. To understand self and express feelings.
			3. To be spontaneous and creative.
			4. To relate to others and have more complex, profound Interpersonal Relationships.
			5. To act on values.
			6. To perceive and articulate life goals.
			7. To develop a personal philosophy.
				1. Filmmaking—generative creative.
				2. Volunteer work and teaching.
				3. Student-initiated action projects, community service.
				4. Communication.
				5. Group process—T-groups—Self-analytic.
				6. Counseling—simulated and experiential.
					1. Teenage groups encouraging
					  a. Feeling expression and articulation—sexuality, intimacy, competition, etc.
					  b. Improving Communication & interpersonal relationships.
					  c. Formulation of goals.
					  d. Identity-crisis resolution.
					2. Young adult and youth
					  a. Career goal groups.
					  b. Creative lifestyle choices and education.
					  c. Community health service and activism.

[1] Erik Erikson, *Childhood and Society* (New York: W. W. Norton & Co., 1950).
[2] Ralph Mosher and Norman Sprinthall, "Psychological Education in the Secondary Schools," *American Psychologist*, 25 (1970), 911–24.

(continued)

FIGURE 9-7 (continued)

CATEGORY	LIFE PROCESSES EMPHASIZED	NAME OF MODEL AND THEORISTS	MAJOR GOALS	METHODS—ACTIVITIES	POTENTIAL HEALTH TEACHING TOPICS
		Moral Development Kohlberg[3]	1. Avoid stage retardation. 2. Stimulate attainment of post-conventional reasoning.	1. Identify stage of Moral development (nurturant). 2. Present moral dilemmas. 3. In discussion present reasoning one stage higher than student's. 4. Facilitate working through reasoning and probe inadequate reasoning in a nurturing nonauthoritarian manner.	1. Ethics & health. 2. Death & dying class. 3. Lifestyle modification and lifestyle abuses (drugs, ETOH, nicotine, etc.) 4. Contraception, pregnancy, abortion, right to life. 5. Medical technical advances and alternatives & the right to die—euthanasia. 6. The politics of health care, the Third World & the disenfranchised. 7. Unorthodox healing practices and the consumer. 8. Malpractice and client rights.
Self-Concept	Self-Responsibility Human Development Teaching/Learning	Values Clarification Simon et al.[4]	1. Clarify own value system through choosing freely. 2. Choosing some alternatives. 3. Choosing after considering consequences. 4. Prizing and cherishing own values. 5. Expressing and sharing values. 6. Acting upon choices. 7. Repeating—Consistency.	1. Simulated situations which cause revelation of own values & those acquired from others. 2. Discussion of each person's responses in open-nurturative-nonjudgmental atmosphere.	1. Health belief systems. 2. Cultural values and health. 3. Health—Eastern and Western perspective. 4. Exploring attitudes & behaviors regarding health, illness, chronic disease (general and specific), death, abortion, sex, loss, VD, contraception.

| Identity Education Fantini & Weinstein[5] | 1. To establish a positive identity, self-image. 2. Establish positive identity relatedness to others. 3. Establish self-determination. 4. Learning skills. | 1. Use of student articulated concerns. 2. Learning skills such as problem solving, forming concepts and ideas. 3. Learning basic skills. 4. Media. 5. Field excursions. 6. Self-awareness exercises. | 1. Health Beliefs—where they come from; the value of, and the use of. 2. Your community as a health resource. 3. Solving problems in health. 4. Learning to control your autonomic bodily processes. 5. How to reach your unconscious mind. 6. A visit to the doctor, clinic, hospital, etc., and how you can help. 7. Cultural health problems. 8. Health Career Options. 9. Caring for someone who is sick, depressed, anxious. |

(continued)

[3] Lawrence Kohlberg, "The Claim to Moral Adequacy of a Highest Stage of Moral Judgment," *Journal of Philosophy*, LXX, no. 18 (October 1973), 631–32.

[4] Sidney Simon, Leland Howe and Howard Kirschenbaum, *Values Clarification: A Handbook of Practical Strategies* (New York: Hart, 1972).

[5] Gerald Weinstein and Mario Fantini, *Toward Humanistic Education: A Curriculum of Affect* (New York: Praeger, 1970).

FIGURE 9-7 (continued)

CATEGORY	LIFE PROCESSES EMPHASIZED	NAME OF MODEL AND THEORISTS	MAJOR GOALS	TEACHING ACTIVITIES	POTENTIAL HEALTH TEACHING TOPICS
Sensitivity and Group Process	Communication Caring and Self-responsibility	Communication Training— Carkhuff[6]	To develop skills in empathy, genuineness, respect, specificity, confrontation, immediacy and self-disclosure.	1. Group Participation. 2. Role playing. 3. Critique by trainer. 4. Group members rate interaction according to goals. 5. Some lecture to set up session.	1. PET 2. Effective caring relationships. 3. Self-disclosure and mental health. 4. Self-assertive communication in health interactions. 5. Between parents and teenagers. 6. Mothers and daughters.
		Sensitivity— Consideration McPhail[7]	To develop sensitivity to another person's needs and feelings.	Films and field experiences with expression of feelings in group discussion.	Dealing with people in stress: Physical handicaps. Mental retardation. Who are different. Who are elderly. Sensory difficulties.
	Communication Caring Teaching/ Learning Human Development	Transactional Analysis— Harris, Berne, Ernst[8, 9, 10]	1. Open communication and personal growth. 2. Knowledge of ego states and games people play.	1. Same without critique and with discussion and drawing of generalizations. 1. Games are role played. 2. Transactions are diagrammed and diagnosed by group. 3. Role players are given positive strokes for *not* playing destructive games.	1. Successful interactions with others. 2. How to play the health care system game. 3. Using TA to better your life. 4. Taking responsibility through TA.

Consciousness Expansion	Self-Responsibility Problem solving	Human Relations Training or T-groups (No theorist)	1. To develop group process skills. 2. Develop openness to changing roles. 3. Learn how to learn. 4. Learn to cope with change. 5. Develop sensitivity and empathy.	1. Group process feedback. 2. Group exercises, critique and discussion. 3. Safe groups but with a certain amount of anxiety to facilitate new learning.	1. How to become effective in a group. 2. Helping your work group, school, living, function better. 3. Coping with stress and change. 4. Enhancing your sensitivity. 5. Human relations.
	Caring Communication Stress Lifestyling Problem solving Human Development Self-Responsibility Teaching/Learning	Meditation Ornstein[11]	To increase awareness, centeredness.	1. Explanation, demonstration. 2. Practice, return demonstration. 3. Discussion.	1. Meditation. 2. Human lifestyling. 3. Coping with stress. 4. Mind Body Interactions. 5. The Hemispheres of the Brain—New findings. 6. PSI phenomena—other realities.

[6] R. R. Carkhuff, *Helping and Human Relations*, vols. 1 and 2 (New York: Holt, Rinehart & Winston, 1969).

[7] Peter McPhail, *In Other People's Shoes* (London: Longmans, 1972).

[8] Thomas A. Harris, *I'm OK—You're OK: A Practical Guide to Transactional Analysis* (New York: Harper & Row, 1969).

[9] Eric Berne, *Games People Play: The Psychology of Human Relations* (New York: Grove Press, 1964).

[10] Ken Ernst, *Games Students Play* (Millbrae, CA: Celestial Arts Publishing, 1972).

[11] Robert Ornstein, *The Psychology of Consciousness* (New York: Viking Press, 1972).

(continued)

FIGURE 9-7 (continued)

CATEGORY	LIFE PROCESSES EMPHASIZED	NAME OF MODEL AND THEORISTS	MAJOR GOALS	METHODS—ACTIVITIES	POTENTIAL HEALTH TEACHING TOPICS
		Synectics Gordon[12]	1. To develop creative and imaginative capacities. 2. To develop an understanding of specified subject areas.	1. Lecture and Discussion. 2. Expose to situations requiring right-hemisphere thought.	1. Any of the holistic approaches or techniques. 2. Art and poetry therapy and wellness. 3. Learning how to learn —the influence of the right-hemisphere.
		Confluent Education Castillo, Brown[13, 14]	1. To facilitate integration. 2. To develop holistic perception. 3. Self-responsibility.	Body/mind integration through exercises in sensory awareness, imagination, space, art.	1. Holistic techniques. 2. Self-awareness. 3. Dance and movement. 4. Art—color therapy. 5. Body therapies. 6. Massage. 7. Psychosomatic health and medicine. 8. Self-care and assessment.
		Psychosynthesis Assagioli[15]	1. To develop centeredness. 2. To integrate conflicting aspects of consciousness.	Technique (see Chapter 4) to facilitate integration and group discussion.	Human growth—holistic theories.

[12] W. J. J. Gordon, *Synectics* (New York: Harper & Row, 1961).
[13] Gloria Castillo, *Left-Handed Teaching* (New York: Praeger, 1974).
[14] George Brown, *Human Teaching for Human Learning* (New York: Viking Press, 1971).
[15] Roberto Assagioli, *Psychosynthesis* (New York: Viking Press, 1971).

HEALTH EDUCATION

Anatomy and physiology of the female body (ages 18–40)

Stages of growth and development of women

Reproduction: menstruation, conception, pregnancy, childbirth, birth and child care, breast feeding, natural childbirth (Lamaze; Leboyer), prematurity, genetic counseling

Contraception: unwanted pregnancies, abortion

Family planning

Lifestyle alternatives

Divorce and separation

Creative parenting

Sex education: growing up female, Women-men relationships, women-women relationships, orgasm, masturbation

Common health concerns of women: venereal disease, stress and anxiety, dysmenorrhea, amenorrhea, cystitis, vaginal infections

Addictions: drug, alcohol, tobacco

HEALTH CARE CLASSES

Biofeedback	Aerobic dance	Creative movement
Hypnosis	Healing self and	Yoga
Rolfing	family	Tai-chi
Massage	Healing touch	Self-care
Polarity therapy	Women's Self-Help	Everyday acu-
Meditation	Relaxation; imagery	pressure

FIGURE 9-8 Suggested content areas for self-care classes for young adult women

wellness education is client-, holistic-, and wellness-oriented, even though it incorporates self-development practices that could be viewed as piecemeal and atomistic if considered separately. Most of the client/healer-oriented holistic practices can either be self-applied with practice or can be used as steps toward self-control and determination. The Travis model is by no means the only one, but it is certainly one of the first that attempts to bring together in a mutually interdependent and harmonious fashion some diverse and often polarized approaches.

An Eastern Approach to Health Teaching/Learning

The Oriental approach to traditional medical education typifies an attitude toward health and education. For over 3,000 years, five levels of doctors have existed. They are classified from most highly respected to lowest:

1. The Sage.
2. The Food Doctor.
3. The Surgeon.
4. The Doctor of General Medicine.
5. The Animal Doctor.

The Sage is a philosopher-doctor who focuses on teaching about the harmonious order of man and his world. [34, p. 3] Illnesses or symptoms are not seen as conditions to be destroyed or eliminated as quickly as possible. The teaching of the Sage stresses that destroying something does not cure it—removing a part cannot help but effect the whole person. Traditional Chinese medicine believes that every person can learn the yin-yang principle easily and then apply self-healing methods. The medicine that the people practice speaks the language of man and does not involve complex rules. [34, p. 4]

The goal of traditional Chinese medicine is freedom—not reliance on another person's judgment, which only perpetuates fear and dependence. Besides oral tradition, the Chinese have relied on several written classics, such as the Nei Ching, the Canon of Medicine, Lu Cheh Ch'an Ch'iu (the Annals of Spring and Autumn, 250 B.C.) to communicate the teachings of the Sages.

The doctor or paramedical worker and the client in both traditional and modern Chinese medicine have a collegial relationship which is based on mutual respect. The client is kept informed of any developments and considerable time is spent in explaining health problems or preventive regimens. This cooperative relationship has been enhanced since the Communist takeover of China in 1949, in which elitist relationships are frowned upon.

COMMUNITY HEALTH EDUCATION

Holistic nurses apply teaching/learning theories and principles in illness-oriented institutions where the process is usually called *health teaching*. Health teaching begins when a client is admitted to an unfamiliar unit with many new interpersonal contacts and relationships to cope with. Every interaction and skill that a nurse performs with and on behalf of the client requires explanation, with time for questions and feedback. Teaching/learning principles are operating continuously in any nurse-client interchange.

Teaching and learning in the well community system involve a broad spectrum of possibilities—ranging from the health instruction of an individual and/or family in a home setting to arranging a health fair for a school or community. Nurses develop, organize, and participate in community clinics and health centers, extended-care facilities, voluntary and official health agencies, and school and occupational health education programs, depending on their positions. Knowledge of group process and education skills is especially important in the community.

A few specific innovative holistically-oriented health education programs will be cited as examples of the increasing concern for holistic and humanistic educational practices.

Voluntary Organizations

Voluntary health organizations, such as the American Heart, Lung, and Diabetic Associations, The American Cancer Society, and others, have always had a strong public education and information focus. They all have volunteer programs that encourage one-to-one outreach programs and speaker's bureaus. Ex-smokers conduct Quit Smoking Clinics; others instruct high-risk groups in "Do It Yourself" Guaic Tests to detect blood in the stool. Nurses are teaching self-breast examinations. Educational programs for kindergarten and elementary-school teachers and their students emphasize an "Early Start to Good Health" program. Such programs are free and are conducted not only in the schools, but also in neighborhoods, clubs, places of employment, and at meetings and conventions. The American Cancer Society alone estimated it reached 22.5 million people in 1977 in two-way communication. Countless others may have been reached through mass media, films, film strips, posters, and pamphlets.

All voluntary organizations have public education committees composed of doctors, nurses, and paraprofessionals. Nurses have a definitive role to play in this kind of community health education.

Many senior citizen centers and housing projects have ongoing educational programs that center around common concerns. One of the most pressing is health. Nurses are a welcome addition and holistic health is becoming a topic of great interest, especially since the impact of SAGE (see Chapter 6) and other self-actualization programs for seniors. Convalescent and extended-care facilities house enormous numbers of clients interested in maximizing their widely diverse levels of wellness, decreasing their reliance on drugs, and increasing their activity levels and mobility, which are some beginning steps toward autonomy and integrity.

Federally Supported Health Education Initiatives and Education Programs (PL 93-641)

Along with local community attempts at establishing wellness-oriented preventive health education programs, the Federal Government has mandated "the development of effective methods of educating the general public" through local, state, and federal Health Systems Agencies (HSAs) and comprehensive Health Planning Agencies (CHPs) in passing PL 93-641.

Ardell suggests some possible approaches tied to this legislation. The Health Systems Agencies should:

1. set objectives for an education program;
2. sponsor or collaborate with other organizations in staging wellness "fairs," conferences, workshops, and/or seminars;
3. publicize the evidence linking lifestyle and disease and self-help information;
4. emphasize wellness objectives in written communications such as special reports, newsletters, articles, and other informational material to the public; and
5. undertake special studies of the wellness implications of major issues, for example,

Hospital Cost Control, health insurance premiums, elderly population, and institutionalization. [1, pp. 27–28]

Laws such as PL 93-641 are essential if public policy is to stimulate incentives for health education that is health promotive. More research needs to be conducted on client "compliance" with health prescriptions. Perhaps the use of such terminology indicates the kind of education that is being performed. Up until very recently no incentives were provided for health education by third-party payers, Medicare, or Medicaid. Health maintenance organizations such as Kaiser Permanente support health education as an effective means of reducing costs and unnecessary hospitalizations.

A Private/Public Multidisciplinary Preventive Education Program

A multidisciplinary effort at combining health education and research for health promotion was initiated at UCLA in 1978. The Center for Health Enhancement Education and Research is a combined health team approach by the Schools of Medicine, Public Health, and Nursing, and by the Department of Kinesiology (the science and physiology of exercise) dedicated to:

1. teaching "wellness";
2. teaching people to take responsibility for their own health;
3. focusing on the reduction and prevention of hypertension (high blood pressure), obesity, blood fats, smoking, and diabetes mellitus which contribute so greatly to coronary or atherosclerotic heart disease and other diseases of the blood vessels, including those that lead to stroke, and to chronic lung, liver, eye, and kidney disease.
4. helping people adopt new health habits and lifestyles;
5. Offering long-term follow-up support for participants, their spouses, and their families. *

The program is described as a four-week residential intensive course in wellness, health enhancement, and lifestyle change. The program begins with a complete health profile, some data of which has been previously gathered from referring health practitioners. Many of the laboratory and physical assessments are repeated weekly as a prescribed program of diet, exercise, and stress reduction is followed. The program offers lectures, workshops, and discussions on sound nutritional practices, weight control, stress reduction and relaxation, smoking cessation, the theory and practice of health enhancement, and group and individual counseling.

A major drawback of the program is that it is supported by the clients and by private donors, thus excluding an entire segment of high-risk, lower-income, and Third-World people. The Federal Government has not had the foresight to fund wellness research. It is relying on the capitalist system to subsidize projects (which

* Adapted from the Informational Packet for the University of California, Los Angeles, Resident Program at the Center for Health Enhancement Education and Research, 1979.

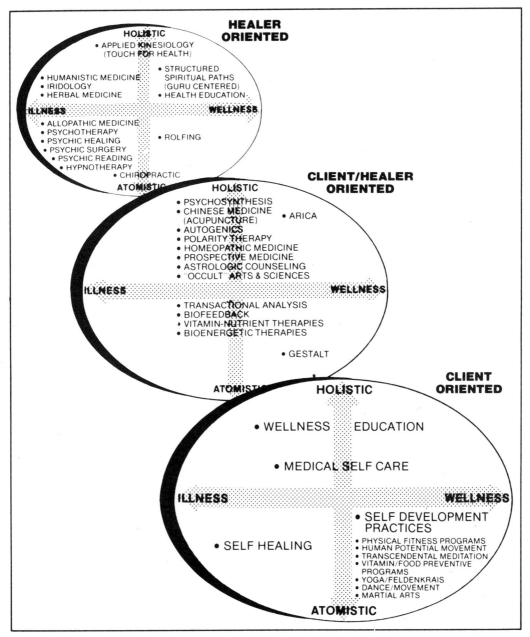

FIGURE 9-9 How traditional and alternative health disciplines relate to wellness education

Reprinted with permission from John W. Travis, ''The Wellness Workbook for Health Professionals,'' Copyright 1977; published by Wellness Associates, 42 Miller Avenue, Mill Valley, CA 94941.

will conceivably save the government money). The Blue Cross/Blue Shield Research Self-Care Project in Northern California (see Ch. 8) is another such example.

Self-Care Education

Once again, education in self-care practices warrants mention. Self-care skills can be learned by anyone, at any age. A look at a typical school health program yields the standard content that has been taught for the last three decades—hygiene, first aid, venereal disease and sex education information (limited according to community mores), and dental health. All of this content is important, but nowhere are attitudes toward self-care in health decision making or self-control in health care addressed. Socialization occurs in these early years, and if values of dependence on and fear of the medical care system are being incorporated, it will take years to change these beliefs.

Folk medicine and home remedies are often passed off as unscientific, quaint, and ineffective instead of as drawing on the rich cultural heritage of some learners. Self-care education in the schools cannot occur without parental, community, and health practitioner support and input. Social health education is one major frontier. Self-care classes are appearing at the grass roots level, as well as being offered in maintenance organizations, at alternative healing centers, women's health centers, and alternative universities. Occupational and industrial health settings are organizing self-care classes for their employees. Class topics include being your own paramedic, birthing, dying and grieving, the elderly, exercise, health consumerism, creative parenting, men's health, midlife transitions, sexuality, stress, therapy and growth, and women's health.

Self-care education is a burgeoning area for nurses with teaching/learning backgrounds. Figure 9–8 (p. 389) demonstrates suggested content areas for self-care classes. Classes can be included as part of any institutional setting, and can be offered privately or through adult education systems. The climate is conducive and the client is ready. Is nursing prepared to grasp the teachable moment?

REFERENCES FOR CHAPTER 9

[1] Donald B. Ardell, "From Omnibus Tinkering to High-Level Wellness: The Movement Toward Holistic Health Planning," *AJHP*, 1, no. 2 (October 1976), 15–33.

[2] Marshall H. Becker and others, "A New Approach to Explaining Sick-Role Behavior in Low Income Populations," *AJHP*, 64, no. 3 (March 1974), 205–15.

[3] D. W. Beggs and E. C. Buffie, eds., *Independent Study: Bold New Venture* (Bloomington, Ind.: Indiana University Press, 1965), p. 196.

[4] Loretta S. Bermosk and Sarah E. Porter, *Women's Health and Human Wholeness* (New York: Appleton-Century-Crofts, 1979), p. 191.

[5] Em Olivia Bevis, *Curriculum Building in Nursing* (St. Louis: C. V. Mosby Co., 1973), pp. 40–48.

[6] Morris L. Bigge, *Learning Theories for Teachers* (New York: Harper & Row, 1971).

[7] Benjamin S. Bloom and others, *Taxonomy of Educational Objectives* (New York: McKay, 1956).

[8] Barbara B. Brown, *Stress and the Art of Biofeedback* (New York: Harper & Row, 1977), p. 17.

[9] Thomas H. Budzynski, "Biofeedback and the Twilight States of Consciousness," in Gary Schwartz and David Shapiro, eds., *Con-*

sciousness and Self-Regulation, vol. 1 (New York: Plenum Press, 1976), pp. 378–79.

[10] P. S. Byrne and B. E. L. Long, Learning to Care, 2nd ed. (New York: Churchill Livingstone, 1975).

[11] California State University Colleges, Chancellor's Newsletter, "Future Talk," no. 2 (Winter 1973).

[12] Jane E. Chapman and Harry H. Chapman, Behavior and Health Care (St. Louis: C. V. Mosby Co., 1975).

[13] Gus T. Dalis and Ben B. Strasser, Teaching Strategies for Values Awareness and Decision Making in Health Education (Thorofare, N.J.: Charles B. Slack, Inc., 1977).

[14] Victor Daniels and Lawrence Horowitz, Being and Caring (Palo Alto, Ca.: Mayfield Publishing Co., 1976), pp. 91–95.

[15] The Faculty of the Department of Nursing, "The Conceptual Framework," (San Francisco State University, 1977).

[16] John T. Fodor and Gus T. Dalis, Health Instruction (Philadelphia: Lea and Febiger, 1971).

[17] Robert M. Gagné, The Conditions of Learning (New York: Holt, Rinehart & Winston, 1965).

[18] Kathleen N. Guinée, Teaching and Learning in Nursing (New York: Macmillan, 1978).

[19] Robert J. Havighurst, Developmental Tasks and Education, 3rd ed. (New York: David McKay, 1976).

[20] Ernest R. Hilgard and Gordon H. Bower, Theories of Learning, 4th ed. (Englewood Cliffs, N.J.: Prentice-Hall, Inc., 1975).

[21] Ivan Illich, Deschooling Society (New York: Harper & Row, 1971).

[22] Jean Jenny, "Humanistic Strategy for Patient Teaching," Health Values: Achieving High-Level Wellness, 3, no. 3 (May/June 1979), 175–80.

[23] George Kaluger and Meriem Fair Kaluger, Human Development (St. Louis: C. V. Mosby Co., 1974).

[24] Andie L. Knutson, The Individual Society and Health Behavior (New York: Russell Sage Foundation, 1965).

[25] Marlene Kramer, Reality Shock (St. Louis: C. V. Mosby Co., 1974).

[26] Larry Laufman and Joshua Weinstein, "Values and Prevention," Health Values: Achieving High-Level Wellness, 2, no. 5 (September/October 1978), 271–73.

[27] Guy R. Lefrancois, Psychology for Teaching (Belmont, Ca.: Wadsworth Publishing Co., 1975), p. 8.

[28] Anne Loustau, "Using the Health Belief Model to Predict Patient Compliance," Health Values: Achieving High-Level Wellness, 3, no. 5 (September/October 1979), 241–45.

[29] Robert F. Mager, Preparing Instructional Objectives (Belmont, Ca.: Lear-Siegler, Inc./Fearon Publishers, 1972), p. vii.

[30] Robert F. Mager, Goal Analysis (Belmont, Ca.: Lear-Siegler, Inc./Fearon Publishers, 1972).

[31] Kathleen Mahan, "A Sensible Approach to the Obese Patient," Nursing Clinics of North America, 14, no. 2 (June 1979), 252.

[32] Abraham Maslow, Motivation and Personality (New York: Harper & Row, 1954), pp. 80–106.

[33] John P. Miller, Humanizing the Classroom (New York: Praeger Publishers, 1976).

[34] Naboru Muramoto, Michael Abehsera (ed.) Healing Ourselves (New York: Swan House Publishing Co., 1973), pp. 3–5.

[35] Neil Postman and Charles Weingartner, Teaching as a Subversive Activity (New York: Dell Publishing Co., 1969).

[36] Barbara Klug Redman, Patient Teaching in Nursing, 3rd ed. (St. Louis: C. V. Mosby Co., 1976).

[37] Carl Rogers, Freedom to Learn (Columbus, Oh.: Charles Merrick Publishers, 1969), pp. 157–64.

[38] Carl Rogers, On Becoming A Person (Columbus, Oh.: Charles Merrick Publishers, 1961), pp. 286–90.

[39] Brewster Smith, "Humanism and Behaviorism in Psychology: Theory and Practice," Journal of Humanistic Psychology, 18, no. 1 (Winter 1978), 27–36.

[40] John W. Travis, "Wellness Education and Holistic Health—How They're Related," Journal of Holistic Health, II (1977), 25–32.

[41] Louise Trygstad and Sylvia Jasmin, Humanistic Concepts and Approaches (Long Beach, Ca.: California State University), pp. 6–9.

Chapter 10
leadership and change

CHAPTER OUTLINE

D. Leadership, Change, the Holistic Health Movement, and Holistic Nursing
  1. Self-Responsibility—Bane or Boon?
  2. East West Academy of Healing Arts
  3. "Self-Determination": Holistic Politics
  4. The Committee for Integrated Health
  5. Well-Being Centers: An Idea Whose Time Has Come
  6. Legal Considerations
  7. Toward a Holistic Paradigm

CHAPTER OBJECTIVES

1. Sketch the parallel development of women and nurses in Western society, listing two left-hemisphere-dominated and two right-hemisphere-dominated traits. State a use for these characteristics in leadership and change in nursing.
2. Differentiate leadership, management, and administration.
3. Trace the phases of the nurse-client relationship and group process.
4. List two change theorists and describe the stages of their theories.
5. State six areas to assess for motivation and/or resistance to change in a group or organization.
6. List five guidelines for helping a group work toward planned change.
7. Choose a health "demand" of interest and trace the required steps for bringing it to a policymaker's attention in government.
8. Describe two major issues paralyzing nurses, including symptoms and coping methods.
9. Utilizing available knowledge about leadership and change, critique one individual or group attempting to incorporate holistic philosophy and approaches into the existing health care and/or political system.

THE CLIMATE FOR CHANGE IN NURSING

Nursing has experienced a long history fraught with crises and change, and has struggled to produce strong leadership capable of challenging established practices, improving care, supporting client rights, persisting in the face of destructive forces, and asserting itself as a profession. Names such as Florence Nightingale, Lillian Wald, and Margaret Sanger represent the thousands of nurses who have dedicated themselves to social change and to the betterment of the human condition.

Today nursing has broadened and subspecialized to an unbelievable degree. Complex, interdependent decision making is an essential skill, not an abstract quality attributed only to high-level nursing administrators. The new graduate is expected to be able to comprehend and manage multivariate, constantly changing, and subtle individual, family, group, and community situations.

The Role of Women and Nurses in Western Society

Although the intrapersonal aspects of leadership and change will be examined, the larger issues of change in the health care system and the role of holistic nurses in the political process will be emphasized. Paring down the enormity of the crises in health care to some basic, manageable issues that holistic nursing can do something specific about is one goal of this chapter.

Nurses continue to define numerous issues, but the majority center around basic perceptions about the role of women and nurses in society. Nursing is still a woman-dominated profession, and it has undergone radical role redefinitions and conflict. Women- and nursing-assertiveness training workshops have been only one of several attempts to facilitate this shift in roles. Expectations of the resocialization of an entire society—*and* for a change in the complementary role of men, physicians, etc.—are often unrealistic and lead to disillusionment and disappointment. Physicians and administrators have found themselves in conflict with a group of people who could always be depended on to work long hours for little pay without "making waves." This is no longer the case in nursing.

Nurses are becoming more self-aware as women and professionals. They are beginning to express their feelings, assessments, and opinions. They are developing confidence in their decision-making ability. They are demanding their rights as women and as professionals. The process of change on an intrapersonal or group level is not a comfortable one. It is stressful and requires strong social support systems. Nurses must rise above intragroup divisiveness and disagreement to nurture themselves and each other as they have done for their clients throughout history.

In Western civilization women have been linked with healing since the Middle Ages. The art of healing, wisdom, nurturing, compassion, and skill were considered to be inherent to the nature of women. Although midwives represented the majority of healers, general practitioners, herbalists, and counselors were also found in their ranks. These wise women—they were called witches—used a variety of remedies, many of them magical, which had been tested through years of experience, but *not* by the scientific method. One of the best early compendia of natural healing methods was written by St. Hildegarde of Bingen (1098–1178). The book lists 213 varieties of plants, fifty-five trees, and numerous mineral and animal remedies. [18, p. 32]

University-trained physicians saw the "witches" as a threat to their practice, although they obtained most of their early knowledge from them, as stated by Paracellsus (the father of modern medicine). [18, p. 33] Witch hunts were an attempt to eliminate an alternative health care system which threatened to undermine the economic and formal educational bases of medicine. The systematic elimination of healers announced the beginning of modern medicine as a commodity—a far cry from the healing described by Ehrenreich and English:

> Healing cannot be made discrete and tangible; it involves too many little kindnesses, encouragements, and stored-up data about patients' fears and strengths . . . . It cannot be quantified: the midwife does not count the number of times she wiped the parturient woman's forehead or squeezed her hand. Above all, it cannot be plucked out—as a thing apart—from the web of human relationships which connect the healer and those she helps. [18, p. 40]

While women have traditionally set themselves up as the model for protecting, nurturing, and supporting the development of others, this exclusive role has made incorporation of other masculine, left-hemisphere-dominated traits such as assertiveness and leadership qualities all the more difficult. Thus, until very recently, we have women assigned to the socially essential professions of social work, teaching, and nursing, which do not foster these qualities.

Even if it can be assumed that only truly motivated individuals choose these professions for the right reasons, not because they have been conditioned toward them, what kind of power and leadership can we expect to find in these helping professions? Potential leaders will probably find their input limited to individual problem assessment and resolution—a very important but narrow application of the leadership and change processes.

As long as nursing remains tied to a particular client or group of client problems and caught up in the endless details of that worthwhile endeavor, system-wide or social changes will be viewed as issues beyond nursing's control and out of their sphere of influence. Is it possible that nursing, just as a client in midlife crisis, will wake up one morning and ask, "Where am I, what have I been doing, and where am I going?"

Nursing needs to preserve feminine archetypical Yin qualities that make it holistic. It also needs to use these invaluable traits to further itself professionally. Intrapersonally, and as professionals, nurses must perceive themselves as a distinct and powerful entity. They must value their own goals and be ready to articulate them even if it means not catering to someone's immediate "need"—a plea nursing has always answered before it has met its own legitimate needs.

Two feminine characteristics that are invaluable to the leadership and change processes are flexibility of operation and intuitive awareness of personal and social phenomena. [23, p. 571] Since women traditionally had to change their needs and goals to suit others, they have developed an amazing ability to shift plans when an opportunity presents itself. Women are particularly able to understand disappointing events and to rework old ideas; in short, they adapt to change. This flexibility is essential in a time of rapid social change.

Another quality, the intuitive aspect developed in many women, contributes to rapid assessment in crisis situations; they can see through garbled data and allow the right hemisphere to offer guidance. This psychic sense is a great asset, particularly in complex group interaction. Obviously, stereotyping attributes to any group is a haphazard exercise at best, but right hemisphere feminine qualities, be they inherent or consciously adopted, are traits worth cultivating in any leadership situation.

Two masculine traits that nurses must come to accept and feel comfortable with are the constructive use of conflict and confrontation. Both are part of the change process and can be used to a leader's benefit to stimulate change. Constructive conflict and confrontation strategies need to be developed. Both are being taught in management training seminars across the country as useful tools for change.

Trends in the Preparation of Nurses

Still to be resolved issues in nursing are:

1. *Upgrading nursing as a profession,* which means incorporating much more research into its body of knowledge and building theory based on valid studies. This means research should be stressed not only at the doctoral level, but also included in the basic preparation of every nurse. More doctoral programs in nursing are needed to stimulate and manage this huge task. Determining the best educational preparation for a nurse is another issue.

2. *Expanding the nurse role.* This is a major area of debate in nursing.

The advent of the nurse practitioner and clinical specialist has put nursing in the forefront of primary care. Are these professionals merely "physician extenders" who are being exploited for the benefit of others? Does this movement imply that the regular professional nurse is not capable of high-level health assessment and problem solving? In effect, is it removing some of the nursing activities such as a client education that nursing has traditionally assumed and bestowing it on specialists? Are all these subspecialties chipping away at the core of nursing? Where does the physician's assistant (P.A.) fit in? Is the P.A. in competition with nursing and in danger of phasing it out? All these questions point to the major question: "Just what is nursing?" What makes it unique and different from any of the other health professions? These questions have yet to be answered.

There are currently three ways in which a nurse may obtain a registered nursing (R.N.) license—through a baccalaureate (B.S.) degree in nursing associated with a university experience, through a diploma degree hospital-based school of nursing (usually, a three-year experience which is now rapidly being phased out), or through a two-year associate degree program from a junior college. There are other programs enabling RN's to return to the university for their B.S. while working; these are called external degree programs, and they are still being evaluated.

Nurse Practitioner programs vary in length from six months to two years and grant a certificate in an area of specialization in ambulatory care such as pediatrics, family practice, adult health, and geriatrics. Prerequisites vary from a registered nursing license to a Master of Science degree.

Nurse Clinician and Clinical Nurse specialist is usually a university-formalized program of study which grants a master's degree for a hospital clinical specialty such as pediatrics, thoracic nursing, etc.; it requires one-and-one-half to two years of master's preparation. Sometimes a hospital-based program will grant a clearly delineated institutional permission to function in an expanded role—for example, grant a title of kidney transplant nurse—but this is not universally recognized.

Physician's Assistant is a title describing a physician "extender" who is licensed, but who cannot prescribe independently; he or she has a clearly delineated sphere of technical expertise but no distinct body of knowledge apart from medicine. A registered nursing license is not a part or prerequisite of this training.

Many leaders in nursing are correct to question the validity of the nurse practitioner movement as it moves closer and closer to a medical model as definitive areas of practice are specialized and perfected. This movement may be valid, but is it keeping nursing from addressing the real issues of defining nursing knowledge and a nursing power base?

It is commonly acknowledged that advanced preparation is required in the special areas just mentioned. The issue appears to cloud when it is broadened to include all primary care. *Primary health care* is generally defined as the individual's first contact with a health care system or provider that leads to a decision of what must be done to help the individual maintain his optimum level of health. It places on the nurse the responsibility for assessing, planning, and initiating a total care approach to the client. This responsibility includes communicating and coordinating all aspects of care with the rest of the health care team, for example, social worker, nutritionist, physical or occupational therapist, kinesiologist, psychologist, and other health agency staff.

The setting may be an institution or clinic, but more often it is a group practice, health maintenance organization (HMO), or a private or group nursing practice. Nurses are licensed by most nurse practice acts to systematically conduct health and developmental assessments, discriminate between normal and abnormal findings, perform nursing (not medical) diagnoses, evaluate actions, and provide guidance and health education to clients and groups. None of these knowledges and skills is beyond the scope of baccalaureate-level education. Figure 10–1 outlines some modest expectations of primary care nurses in the community and prerequisite knowledges and skills. [36, p. 34]

The key to primary health care is not only autonomy, but also collaboration with others. Where and how does a nurse *learn* to be autonomous and form collaborative relationships? It begins with initial nursing learning experiences and, as always, with self-evaluation. Every piece of nursing content and process must be utilized and reinforced or it becomes extinct.

If a practitioner has all kinds of innovative ideas but cannot communicate or implement them in a manner acceptable to a client, administrator, or supervisor, he or she is at a standstill and frustrated. Knowledge and confident application of leadership and change strategies can assist the nurse in planning the demise of an outdated approach or system, in piloting a radical idea, or in pursuing an unorthodox goal.

The primary functions for which many nurses are now prepared and for which others could be prepared include:

Routine assessment of the health status of individuals and families.

Institution of care during normal pregnancies and normal deliveries, provision of family planning services, and supervision of health care of normal children.

Management of care for selected clients within protocols mutually agreed upon by nursing and medical personnel, including prescribing and providing care and making referrals as appropriate.

Screening clients having problems requiring differential medical diagnosis and medical therapy. The recommendation resulting from such screening activities is based on data gathered and evaluated jointly by physicians and nurses.

Consultation and collaboration with physicians, other health professionals, and the public in planning and instituting health care programs.

The assumption of these responsibilities requires that the nurse have knowledge and requisite skills for:

Eliciting and recording a health history;

Making physical and psychosocial assessments, recognizing the range of "normal" and the manifestations of common abnormalities;

Assessing family relationships and home, school, and work environments;

Interpreting selected laboratory findings;

Making diagnoses, choosing, initiating, and modifying selected therapies;

Assessing community resources and needs for health care;

Providing emergency treatment as appropriate, such as in cardiac arrest, shock, or hemorrhage; and

Providing appropriate information to the client and his family about a diagnosis or plan of therapy.

FIGURE 10-1 Some primary care functions of nurses

Adapted from Charlotte Cumbie, "The Shifting Emphasis in the Delivery of Health Care—Viewpoint of a Nurse," *Primary Health Care: Everybody's Business* (New York: National League of Nursing, 1973).

LEADERSHIP AND PROFESSIONAL NURSING

Terminology and Popular Theories

The term professional is constantly used to describe nursing. It is important to know what criteria determine a profession. Professions are characterized by:

> intellectual operations accompanied by large individual responsibility;
>
> continuous learning based on research and discussion;
>
> practical as well as theoretical goals;
>
> techniques that must be communicated through a specialized formal educational discipline;
>
> self-organization with activities and responsibilities that engage participants and develop group consciousness; and
>
> responsiveness to public interest and concern with the achievement of social ends. [35, Flexner as cited therein, p. 17]

The life processes suggested by these criteria are teaching/learning, self-responsibility, problem solving, communication, leadership, change, and caring.

Moloney has defined *leadership* as the interpersonal process of influencing the activities of an individual or group toward goal attainment in a given situation. [35, p. 11] Leadership, management, and administration are three terms that are often confused. They are distinctly different and the nurse will most probably find herself performing functions of each. Leadership is seen as a *function* of management, but concerns itself with achieving leadership goals which are not necessarily those of the organization.

The leader has the ability to see beyond immediate survival needs and fosters creative stimulation as well as guidance to followers. *Management* includes controlling, organizing, planning, and budgeting skills, but it should include leadership skills in order to be effective. A good leader should likewise be versed in management techniques in order to achieve institutional changes. *Administration* is concerned with the organizational structure and official channels of communication of an organization. It is possible to administer and manage and not lead, but innovation and change will not characterize this individual's tenure. There is no one best way to lead, although several definitive leadership theories have been researched and described.

Early theories of leadership focused on inherent traits that typified leaders. Leaders were born not made. This leadership belief persisted until the late 1950s when situational theories of leadership dominated the scene for the next decade. They remain a powerful force today. Situational theorists feel that leadership must be geared to the level of followers, the task, and the position power of the leader. Leadership style shifts to meet the needs of each, since leadership is of its very nature dynamic.

In 1970, psychological research was applied to leadership and suggested a leadership style based on supporting the follower's problem solving and goals, helping him identify alternatives, conflicts, and rewards associated with decision making. Other theorists took a human development approach based on the maturity of the worker. (For example, high task-low relationship style was considered best for an immature follower, and so on.) Most of these theories were used in the labor and management areas in which motivation and efficiency were valued in order to increase productivity.

In the 1930s, Kurt Lewin, the father of Gestalt psychology, expanded his revolutionary theory of change. In 1947 he presented his theory of leadership styles based on research conducted at the Group Dynamics Center in Massachusetts. Lewin's three styles were divided into (1) autocratic or authoritarian, (2) participative, supportive, or democratic, and (3) laissez-faire or free-rein leadership categories. [33] Characteristics of each type of leadership are listed below:

Autocratic Leader	Participative	Laissez-Faire Leader
Directive	Permissive	Leader serves only as a
Dogmatic	Follower participation	resource to the group
Demanding	Encourages self-direction	(similar to Rogerian
Scare tactics	Self-actualization and	approach)
Close supervision	Creative performance	
High tension level	Human relations	
Decreased freedom	approach	
Aloof from members	Worker as part of "team"	
	Employee morale	
	important	
	Workers seen as resource	

Based on these styles of leadership, Rensis Likert has developed four management systems which incorporate the following characteristics:

Likert's Four Management Systems [35]

Exploitative— Authoritative	Benevolent— Authoritative	Consultative	Participative
Little confidence expressed in subordinates. Does not seek input. Receives a very small amount of inaccurate communication. Policing and punishment used for control. Informal organization offers resistance.	Rewards and punishments used to control behavior. Little communication. No input into goal-setting by subordinates. An informal parallel organization often develops.	Confidence in subordinates expressed. Communications are open and flow from bottom to top. Superiors are knowledgeable about subordinates' problems. Rewards and self-guidance are used to control behavior.	Most effective system. Communications are open and flow in all directions. Problems are shared, superiors help problem solve. Informal and formal structure have the same goals.

The four systems are not unlike the self-care grid shown in Chapter 1. A participative management system and leadership style is consistent with a humanistic holistic philosophy, at the same time as it is still considered orthodox leadership and management. It is the responsibility of the nurse to choose a leadership style appropriate to her personality, philosophy, goals, clients, as well as to the situation.

The nurse should begin by acquiring a sound leadership and management theory base and by evaluating her own attitudes and experiences with different management sytems and leadership styles. The self-evaluation tool in Figure 10–2 may provide some data for the nurse to begin developing self-awareness regarding leadership and management.

Douglass and Bevis emphasize the importance of awareness of self or "the ability to be sensitive to one's own needs, motives and responses to stimuli," to nursing leadership. [16, p. 252] Self-awareness fosters self-acceptance in the nurse, which encourages her to accept clients as total persons capable of growth and change. Awareness and acceptance in a nurse-leader allow her to face challenge, conflict, and criticism without defensiveness. Understanding of her own feelings and the transactions of others enables the nurse to see the opportunity criticism brings for expressing views, feelings, and hostilities.

Human relations training as described in Chapter 9 is one way of helping the nurse-leader sensitize herself to her own needs and the needs of others. Self-acceptance helps the nurse to recognize realistic challenges and goals and to face failure and disappointment when a goal is not achieved.

Assertiveness is the term used to describe a person's/nurse's ability to:

express positive and negative feelings in a socially acceptable, respectful manner, recognizing others' rights and feelings;

make requests and have needs met;

refuse unrealistic demands or requests without feeling guilty; and

initiate and terminate interactions. [16, p. 256]

Assertiveness is a basic leadership quality in advocating the rights of self and others. The first part of Chapter 6 elaborated on assertiveness-training techniques that nurses can develop individually or in a group.

The qualification that a nurse-leader should possess (besides a working knowledge of the life processes) is a familiarity with initiating, maintaining, and terminating relationships with clients, colleagues, and groups. The nurse, after evaluating her own strengths and weaknesses, moves into nurse-client relationships. Asserting self and performing leadership functions does not negate encouragement of self-care in the client. The nurse-leader recognizes individual and group process theory and uses it to encourage achievement of individual and group health goals. A brief review of individual and group process theory follows.

Interpersonal Nurse-Client Relationships: Beginning Leadership in Action

A nurse-client relationship is an interaction process between two persons. The nurse offers self and a series of purposeful activities and practices that are useful to a client. It differs from the small group process and social relationships in which peo-

1. What value system operates in the work and/or educational setting in which you find yourself?
2. What rewards are offered for what behaviors?
3. What items appear on evaluation forms?
4. Are you being socialized into dependent, passive functioning, or functioning that encourages decision making, accountability, responsibility, independence?
5. Are you functioning passively and dependently or more actively and independently?
6. In which role are you the most comfortable and why?
7. List ten of your abilities and strengths:
    1.
    2.
    3.
    4.
    5.
    6.
    7.
    8.
    9.
    10.
8. Are you using your strengths?
9. Does your work or educational environment make use of those strengths and allow and encourage you to build on them?
10. Are other people in your setting aware of your strengths?
11. Have you told anyone about them?
12. Identify the last time you performed successfully.
13. Did you feel your success was due to your ability? Did you tell others about it?
14. What about the last time you failed at a task? Did you feel your failure was due to your inability?
15. Did you share your failure with others? Did they support you through it?
16. What is your salary? Do you feel it reflects your responsibilities, performance, and worth?
17. Is it comparable to other groups of workers within your salary system who have the same education, experiential qualifications, and similar levels of responsibility?
18. Identify the last time you felt powerless. Who or what was more powerful?
19. Why did you need the power?
20. What stood in your way?
21. Identify the last time someone working or studying with you was very successful at something. How did you feel?
22. What did you feel? Did you congratulate that person? What did you say?
23. How did you support that person?

FIGURE 10-2 Self-evaluation of leadership and management potential

Adapted from Dorothy A. Brooten and others, *Leadership for Change: A Guide for the Frustrated Nurse* (Philadelphia: J. B. Lippincott, 1978).

ple interact primarily to meet their own basic interpersonal needs, in that one person—the nurse—is primarily concerned with helping a person whose needs and problems require the help of a person with specific knowledge and skills.

There are, however, many similarities between interpersonal and small group interactions. The small group process can be compared to and analyzed in terms of the nurse-client relationship. Similar problems and phases occur in both. The development of the process in the nurse-client relationship is facilitated by the nurse in order to reach a collaborative working phase more quickly than is expected in small group work in which the interpersonal needs of all participants must be comfortably integrated.

The Orientation Phase

The orientation, initiating, or establishing phase centers upon mutual attempts to know each other. It serves as a testing phase for the client to determine how safe it is for him and how much he can trust and rely on the nurse. It also serves as a learning phase for the nurse to find out how the patient feels, responds, and reacts. Expectations can be clarified and contracts negotiated. Both can choose not to establish the relationship. Once the nurse commits herself to participation in the relationship, she is not free to drop the relationship and "contract."

The Working or Continuing Phase

Both nurse and client are active participants. Both have agreed to certain expectations, limitations, and commitments. The client is free to expose self and problems and to use the nurse and the relationship for his benefit. It is a time for learning about self and solving problems, a time for mutual planning and progression to interdependence or self-care. The client is allowed to meet needs for dependence, independence, and interdependence depending on the situation.

The Concluding or Termination Phase

Ideally, it is mutually agreed that the client no longer needs the help of the nurse. Reasons for concluding may vary. Knowledge of termination begins in the orientation-establishing phase and is continuous throughout the relationship. Many feelings are aroused: happiness, affection, love, sadness, and even depression, which take time to work through. The client becomes more aware of the nurse as a person distinct from the relationship. He may seek additional knowledge of the nurse as "person" and of her personal life. The nurse may begin to withdraw from the relationship. Client or nurse may wish to have the relationship become a social one. The client may have difficulty acknowledging and expressing the value of the relationship—and may withdraw; he may express gratitude verbally or with a gift. If the nurse has difficulty accepting gratitude or a gift it can be an awkward time for both. If handled openly, with feeling and honesty, termination can be a loving human experience. Both nurse and client will find it easier to establish meaningful relationships with another person after having experienced such a termination. No energy is tied up with an unresolved parting or with uncommunicated feelings or messages if termination is handled properly.

Group Dynamics: The Phases of Group Growth and Leadership Skill Development

Schutz (1961) sees groups on a continuum from those in which members are compatible according to their interpersonal needs to those who are extremely incompatible in regard to *inclusion, control,* and *affection.* According to Schutz, a group leader should be matched with the members in regard to inclusion and affection, but in regard to control, they should be different. That is, a person with a high need to control others needs to be matched with people who have high needs to be controlled. Compatible members learn to work together in a relatively short time; incompatible members may never learn to work together. Schutz sees group development centered around these three interpersonal needs. Every group, no matter what its function or composition, goes through the interpersonal phases of *inclusion, control* and *affection* (in that sequence). These are not distinct, clearly identified phases, but *problem areas* that are emphasized at certain points in a group's growth. All three problem areas are always present. Some members do not always go along with the central issue for the group. The area of concern for any individual will result from his own problem areas and continue with the work at hand. Later, they are worked over to a more satisfactory degree.

1. *Phase of Inclusion* (belonging in or out of the group). Problems of identity are: Will I belong? Will I be accepted? How much of myself will I devote to this group? How important will I be? Characteristically, members find problems with attendance: "I forgot we were meeting." Members attempt to find a common base of interaction for dealing with more important future issues. Discussion centers around rules of procedure and exchanging personal information not directly related to a task. It is a testing period. How safe will it be here for me? Some members commonly drop out at this time or talk about not coming, if it is a voluntary membership group, or discuss past experiences in groups.

2. *Phase of Control* (power, influence, and responsibility). Once members are fairly well-established as being together in a group, issues of decision making arise. Characteristically, leadership struggles occur. Competition, discussion of orientation to task, structure, rules of procedure, and sharing of work are worked out. Primary conflicts revolve around having too much or too little responsibility or influence. Each member is trying to establish himself in the group so that he has the most comfortable degree of initiation with other members with regard to control, influence, and responsibility.

Authority problems may occur fairly early in the group's development. Each member brings a "unique" orientation to authority, that is, to the official leader of the group. It is the nature of such relationships that members have ambivalent feelings toward the authority figure compared to ambivalence of adolescence regarding parental control. Dependence versus independence struggles occur.

3. *Phase of Affection* (closeness, liking, and warmth). After members have become differentiated with respect to influence, responsibility, and power, they must become emotionally integrated. In business settings and task groups, this need is seldom made overt. At one extreme, individuals like very close and personal relationships with each individual they meet. At the other extreme, individuals like their personal relationships in groups to be quite impersonal and distant—friendly perhaps, but not intimate. In seating arrangements, all members may sit close, or two members may always sit together. Some pairing and jealousy of members becomes evident. Characteristically, some positive feelings are expressed, either verbally, nonverbally, or by such behavior as bringing candy or coffee for the group. Members may plan a "social activity." *Termination* and problems with it become predominant when the group is near conclusion of its task. In groups in which members do not expect to be in contact, reunions or plans to exchange letters for time may be planned; generally, however, this effort at maintaining contact "dies out." Occasionally, members redefine another task to keep the group together. If communications were good all along, the members are apt to deal with termination honestly and openly with a review of the group's process and satisfactory termination.

THE CHANGE PROCESS AND THE CONTINUING NEED FOR PLANNED CHANGE IN THE HEALTH CARE SYSTEM

Change in self and self-awareness are inseparable from change in nursing, medicine, and society. The Taoist view of change is that differences and conflict do not breed separation, but rather, unity and wholeness. Orthodox medicine is not considered evil or in direct opposition to holistic approaches; in fact, they share more than they disagree on. Any change at the cellular, psychic, electromagnetic field level of the person affects the whole person, and any change affected by one person or family affects the neighborhood, community, and so on.

Massive changes in lifestyle are occurring in this country. No longer can one person, family, state, or nation act in isolation. What one person does affects the total environment. One person's political consciousness can swing a local election. Political apathy or passiveness has become a definite stance. No one can abrogate their rights and not have their actions affect the group of which they are a part. No one can give up responsibility and not stifle the rights of others. Decisions become complex matters when self-interest cannot be the sole motivator. Not being able to easily discriminate between issues and values also causes stress. In moderate amounts, stress motivates change. In order to mediate undue amounts of stress, however, certain lifestyle elements must be incorporated for the human organism and community to survive.

At such a crucial stage of professional development, it is necessary for every nurse to understand the nature of the change and the leadership processes. A leader is an advocate for change and facilitates it in self and others. Leadership, like caring, can be learned. The theories centering around "born leaders" have been superseded by other more exciting concepts of leadership. This chapter strives to describe a few of these theories in relation to holistic nursing. Examples of leadership and change in nursing, in the health care system, and in society as they shift toward a new paradigm of holistic consciousness will be emphasized.

Critics of the current state of health, nursing, and the health-care system will be cited, and suggestions for alternative solutions will be offered. Some realistic leadership and change strategies that have worked in the past or are being tested currently are suggested for practitioners.

Chapter 10 will bring together all the previously mentioned processes and put them to the test. Can they work? Can a graduate adapt to the "reality shock" of the health care marketplace? Can a practitioner reconcile her "ivory tower" holistic values with those of a system based on cost accountability? Examples of grass roots as well as hierarchical attempts at incorporating the holistic approach will be mentioned. There are still precedents to be set in applying holistic nursing to many areas of health care. A thorough understanding of evolution and revolution is a prerequisite for nurses who accept the charge.

Change can rightfully be associated with the learning process as product or effect. Learning has been defined as change in:

cognitive structure (knowledge)
motivation
group belongingness, ideology, or culture

Planned change is a rapidly growing area requiring knowledges and skills distinct from the teaching/learning process. It is best seen as a function of leadership. Since change is often seen as a natural outcome of so many other processes in nursing (for example, adaptation, stress or crisis, human development, teaching/learning, problem solving, communication), it is often assumed or even excluded from formal courses of study. As in the other life processes, planned change needs to be tested and applied in order for facility to develop.

Bevis has defined the process of change as one which deals with alterations by choice and deliberation as opposed to change by indoctrination, coercion, natural growth, and accident. In nursing, changing is a result of mutual, collective, and collaborative choice—that is, participatory changing. [16, p. 226] In this section we will focus on client, group, community, and specifically, institutional change.

Change process terminology usually includes the change agent or facilitator, the setting or organization, the institution in which change is to occur, and the target of the changing process—for example, a client or population to benefit from the change. Nursing as a profession should be a target of change on an individual and group level. Nursing has found itself in the midst of so many political, societal, and technological changes that it has difficulty adapting to changes in progress, much less planning for the future. The feeling expressed by many exhausted nurses is one of anger, frustration, and powerlessness in the face of changes "beyond their control."

Specific change techniques derived from theory will be advocated later in this section. The problems of change that nurses face among professionals are the focus for the following discussion. It is important for nurses to recognize that most nursing settings are authoritarian and pyramidal organizations. These hierarchical structures have chains of command and communication channels that make rapid change a discouraging task. Much valuable time is spent working through the bureaucracy instead of focusing on proposed pressing changes. Figure 10–3 depicts a typical organizational tree for the Department of Health and Human Services. (Since the department is undergoing reorganization, the chart is described as "hypothetical.") The purpose of such structures is to minimize disruption of services and maintain smooth functioning of the organization.

Although organizations appear to resist change, wise administrators acknowledge that institutions that don't respond to new input—technological advances, research findings, funding patterns, and changing client needs and social conditions, do not survive. [16, p. 93] If presented in a planned fashion, change can be a dynamic and creative experience. Stress is a normal byproduct of change, but it can be anticipated and reduced through the use of various group development and maintenance tactics. All the techniques mentioned in Chapter 6 can be adapted to help individuals and groups cope with rapid change.

Theories of Planned Change

Kurt Lewin

Most change theories are based on the work of Kurt Lewin who described his force field theory and defined three stages of change—unfreezing, moving, and refreezing [51, pp. 308–09]:

> Stage I (unfreezing) occurs when an individual or group recognizes a need to change. This is a cognitive state not accompanied by behavior. This can arise from lack of confirmation of another behavior (for example, a miracle diet does not produce desired results), a feeling of guilt or anxiety accompanies a certain behavior or lifestyle, or an obstacle to change is removed.
>
> Stage II (moving) includes redefining the problem and looking at it in a way that promotes change. This can occur through identification with an influential, admired, or powerful change agent or through "scanning"—obtaining various sources of information and choosing a solution. In either case the change is planned out and initiated.
>
> Stage III (refreezing) is the phase in which changes are integrated or stabilized as the person incorporates the new idea or behavior into his or her own value system. The forces at work in the energy field of change are called driving forces which facilitate change, or restraining forces which impede the changing process. Anticipation of these forces should be factored into any plan.

Agnes Reinkemeyer

Agnes Reinkemeyer has devised seven stages of planned change (based on Lewin's theory) which fit neatly with a systematic problem-solving approach. [51] Considerable fluctuation back and forth between stages is anticipated. The stages include:

1. development of a felt need and desire for change, which corresponds to "unfreezing";
2. development of a change relationship between the agent and the client system, which is an extremely important step and incorporates all the characteristics of a caring relationship;

UNITED STATES DEPARTMENT OF HEALTH AND HUMAN SERVICES

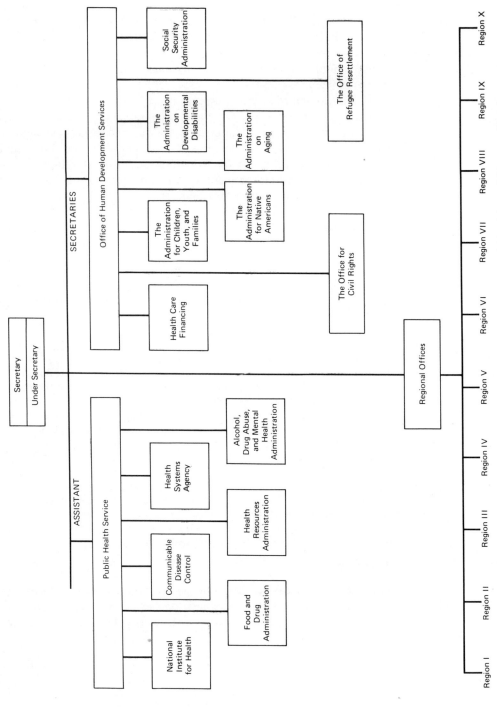

FIGURE 10-3 Hypothetical organizational chart for the U.S. Department of Health and Human Services

3. clarification or diagnosis of the client system's problem, need, or objective (as determined in Chapter 8);

4. determining alternate routes and tentative goals and intentions of actions, which is a generative nursing activity that requires brainstorming, intuitive insights, new research findings, etc.;

5. transformation of intentions into actual change behavior, which may take practice, backsliding, developing new alternatives, etc.;

6. stabilization, which occurs when the individual is achieving a change behavior goal an acceptable (predetermined) percent of the time; and

7. termination of the relationship between the change agent and the client system using all the knowledge, intuition, and experience the nurse possesses to smooth this transition. [51, p. 329]

Gordon L. Lippitt has also developed a problem-solving approach to change which includes initiating the nurse-client relationship *before* proceeding to change.

Another useful theory is Shirley Smoyak's confrontation model to implement change. This is a very direct approach and should be used to discuss a clearly defined issue. [37, pp. 330–31] It is not recommended for novice negotiators or for nurses with precarious senses of self-esteem. The client or institution being challenged should be capable of handling this technique.

Phase I calls for "planning the confrontation," by reading, researching, discussing, interviewing, and role playing the strategies to be used. Phase II, or "confronting the system," includes progress review, evaluation, and sharing of data with others in preplanned meetings in which the change agent maintains focus and composure. Phase III is composed of strengthening new images and relationships following the confrontation. [37, p. 331]

When Phase II is operating at a confrontation meeting, the participants should adhere to agreed upon mediation/arbitration procedures so that the problem is exposed, but no blame is placed. The purposes of a confrontation meeting can include such things as opening up communication, creating a dialogue, involving all members in "ownership" of the problem, and clarifying problems. Openness, interest, and readiness to listen are characteristics of change agents in such a situation. [37, p. 335]

One need not look far to find diatribes against the state of the nation's health-care delivery system both from those within and outside it. Ivan Illich, in his now classic book, *Medical Nemesis,* painted one of the most coherent (albeit grim) pictures of it, in which little hope for change without accompanying drastic change in group consciousness and responsibility was seen. [26]

Problems in health care delivery appear to center around five major issues—increasing accessibility to health care services for all, not just for the privileged few; improving the quality of health care; improving and increasing health care services; increasing consumer input and participation in planning and decision making; and lowering astronomical costs. Tentative solutions have included national health insurance proposals, governmental control of distribution of physicians to underserved areas, reducing specialization through institution of family practice residencies, improving access through Medicare and Medicaid community satellite clinics, and neighborhood health centers. Quality assurance has supposedly been legislated through peer standard review organizations (mentioned in Chapter 8) and increasing mandatory continuing education for relicensure of professionals.

Most of these solutions have been implemented to some degree, with the exception of National Health Insurance (NHI). The enthusiasm for NHI has diminished after observing England's experience with such a plan, and with the recognition that an affordable health insurance plan will probably only cover catastrophic illness at best and still leave the remaining health care financiers (third-party payment companies, private group financed, private insurance, and health maintenance organizations) untouched. Evaluating the other "solutions" does not bring much encouragement. For example, physicians can be forced to work to pay back government loans in underserved areas, but they invariably leave when their tour of duty is complete for urban, cultural, and educational centers. Thus, the distribution problem remains unresolved.

Regarding spiraling costs, Peer Standards Review Organization legislation is still being evaluated, but it may actually decrease "leave of stays" (and their costs) in the hospital even if it does not guarantee improvement of care. Although participation of consumers on federally financed Boards of Directors and Health Systems Agencies is mandated, such input into private corporations such as insurance companies, hospitals, and some government bureaucracies is limited.

Shifting the emphasis away from illness care and hospitalization in favor of outpatient and self-health maintenance services also has some disastrous political implications. Nursing alone contributes a large portion of its one million person labor force to institutions. Decreasing the number of hospital beds directly effects the employment of these and the other three and one-half million health care workers. Changing job descriptions from acute-care or custodial-type services to prevention and education requires a major planning and implementation effort at the intrapersonal, interpersonal, and community levels.

Planning for change in the future will involve heavy input from professional lobbying and pressure groups, in which nurses should play a big part. Consumers have been given access to areas in which they have never before had a voice. Unfortunately, the decision-making mechanisms have not been designed for their input; therefore, they often find themselves isolated, bored, and uninformed and underutilized. Consumer education must include an introduction to the decision-making structure and process of political and health organizations. It goes without saying that the nurse must have a working knowledge of this content as well.

Assessments

The following pages enumerate some self-assessment questions which can help nurses evaluate the leadership and change potential in themselves and the groups of which they are a part.

Intrapersonal: Are You a Community Activist?

1. Do you recognize the possibility of change?
2. Do you believe in a particular project or plan?

3. Are you willing to invest a few hours to gather some data and to do some critical thinking?
4. Are you willing to help bring a few other interested people together to formulate a plan or project?
5. Do you enjoy eliciting information, suggestions, and ideas from people?
6. Can you patiently allow others to arrive at decisions at their own pace?
7. Can you keep a sense of humor when under pressure?
8. Do you get defensive when attacked?
9. Can you educate poeple without preaching to them?
10. Can you avoid taking sides and remain impartial and objective in a situation that requires it?

Interpersonal: Assessing Motivation and Capacity for Change in a Group

1. What are the possible solutions to the problem?
2. What are the pros and cons of each possible solution?
3. How would each of these solutions be implemented?
4. What are the possible roadblocks to the completion of the change project lying within each possible solution?
5. What are the factors that are motivating people to participate in the change project?
6. How can these driving forces be capitalized on for each participant?
7. What are the limiting factors, that is, the restraining forces in the environment that will inhibit the implementation of the change project?
8. What are the factors or forces that would facilitate the implementation of each possible solution?
9. What are the costs, financial and otherwise? [51, p. 315]

Assess your motivation as the change agent. Are you up to it? Answer the following questions:

1. Does your motivation stem from a genuine desire to improve something?
2. Does your motivation stem from a personal desire for power or recognition?
3. Do you want to change simply for change's sake or to keep things from stagnating?
4. Does the situation call for interpersonal or highly developed organizational skills? Do you have them?
5. How much experience have you had with this particular type of problem?
6. What are your credentials? Are you regarded as an expert according to the key people in your situation?
7. Is your personality suited to the particular situation?

Nurses who have served as change agents have been described as socially aware, people-oriented, and competent in interpersonal relationships. [37, p. 323] The following three questions will bear this out:

1. Are you aware of your attitudes, approaches to other people, and feelings about the change to occur?

2. Are you persistent and flexible? Can you handle frustration and delay?

3. Can you help people involved in the change feel that the change is theirs rather than your personal coup?

Olson suggests some guidelines for change which will help people at the bottom of any organizational hierarchy to familiarize themselves with those at the top.

Guidelines for Change

For those working from below, rather than from positions of top power, the following guidelines may be of assistance:

1. Diagram the organization as a system. Ask the related questions: What are its goals, key subsystems, and key people? Knowledge of the organization's goals and norms will aid in ascertaining specifics about the orientation and philosophy of the system. Key people will be utilized to facilitate the change process.

2. Look for allies and potential allies either inside or outside the organization. It is generally more effective to initiate change by enlarging the group in favor of the change.

3. Know your change inside and out, including strengths and weaknesses. Also, know what evaluations have been conducted and what objections might be raised. Try diligently to have answers to these objections; resistance is decreased when people perceive that the change agent is aware of the ramifications of the proposed change.

4. If you have an adversary, analyze the situation from his or her point of view. This provides a better perspective and therefore should give greater insight into ways of coping.

5. Develop a sense of timing; act strategically and only when forces are in your favor. Remember that there is a limit to the extent of assimilation of change for an organization and/or a group. [37, p. 326]

Assessing Resistance to Change in Groups and Organizations

1. Is the nature of the change and its effect clear to those involved?

2. Has information been distorted in the past? Is there a feeling of distrust, discomfort, and threat stemming from past experience?

3. Is the change occurring because of personal preferences rather than in consideration of the needs and requirements of the group or organization?

4. Does the change ignore the established norms or customs of the group?

5. Is excessive work pressure involved in the change?

6. Has the planning of change failed to consider in detail how the change will be brought about?

7. Has consideration been given to problems that are likely to arise? Have specific strategies been developed for dealing with these problems?

8. Is there fear of failing in the group? Is there a feeling that the change is inadequate or being handled ineptly?

9. Has provision been made for two-way communication and feedback? [37, p. 332]

After resistance has been assessed, think of the possible reasons that may be causing it. If resistance is present, a step in the planning for change process has probably been overlooked. Some other common reasons for resistance that can be prepared for ahead of time are: clinging to existing structure and satisfactions, cost, threat, fear of failure, or disorganization.

Another element that can surface in any changing process is conflict, that is, a struggle due to the threat of harmony and balance among thoughts, feelings, and behaviors. Conflict can be either destructive or constructive. If it can be channeled into a constructive conflict, it will lead to growth and enhance the change. [37, p. 334] Creativity and increased communication can also result.

Four major factors need to be monitored in order to ensure a positive outcome of a conflict: (1) the issue should be kept in focus and not be turned into something it is not (for example, a power struggle); (2) power should not be allowed to enter the process; (3) a commitment by all parties to a solution that answers the majority's needs should be obtained beforehand; and (4) clear, effective communication should be used to keep everyone focused and informed. [37, p. 335]

Rules for Radicals

Douglass and Bevis have suggested ten guidelines for any group attempting to make changes:

1. Try to have no surprises. Let everyone know in advance about any plans that are underway.
2. Provide as much informational input as possible. Part of the backbone of any planned change is the collection of data phase. "Handouts," consultation with experts, training sessions, television, movies and other audiovisual materials, circulation of helpful articles, and data discussion sessions prior to the time the information must be used help to provide the data base necessary to planned changes.
3. Make conflicts explicit and legitimate. Bring out hidden agenda items so that real issues can be handled.
4. Identify areas of high feelings and elicit the help of a neutral facilitator either from within the group or from a source unrelated to the problem or issue itself.
5. Make risks legitimate and failure salvageable and acceptable. Operating in small task areas allows greater risks to be taken. If one small part fails, the whole system of changes is not likely to fall apart. Back-up systems are other options for handling the problem if an original plan fails.
6. Make change in the middle of a trial run acceptable. Then, if a plan being instituted is not working, alterations in the plan can be made.
7. Try to make it necessary to analyze failure or the reasons a part of a program is not working so that alterations and changes do not go without fair trial.
8. Agree to respond verbally or nonverbally to *each* member's contributions to the group—comments, needs, and behaviors. Acknowledgment reinforces and encourages continuing contributions and provides feedback.
9. When complete win-lose deadlocks occur, agree to some form of action that will allow unlocking and saving of pride. Delay the issue or shuttle it to another time.
10. Delay making "final" decisions. Make tentative decisions, take a consensus, decide on a "trial" basis, or accept something as a "provisional" or "working" copy. Voting and recording in the minutes create a feeling of finality that makes it more difficult for members of the change group to accept alterations. [16, pp. 228–29]

Douglass adds a few other helpful pointers:

Make sure that group members are acquainted with one another. Composition of nursing groups changes almost daily in some settings. Reflecting a warm, friendly, respectful attitude toward all group members encourages participation.

Plan each meeting in relation to predetermined goals. Knowledge of the purpose and expectations of a meeting gives the members opportunity to prepare for the meeting. Encourage group participation by keeping the group focused on the intent of the meeting, accepting member contributions, encouraging member-member discussion (perhaps member-leader discussion, if giving directions), and by helping the group to see their accomplishments and weaknesses, to plan for progress, and to know when errors in action or reasoning occur.

Utilize resources within the group as much as possible. Special knowledge and skills are useful in moving groups along. Develop the potential of all members. [16, p. 114]

Brooten and associates have formulated a problem-solving model for planning change. They suggest choosing a situation that should be changed and working through the steps of the change process:

1. *Situation.*
2. *Assessment:*
   Interest (extent and nature of)
   Motivation (depth and nature)
   Environment (in which change will occur)
3. *Planning:*
   Support Group
   Goals
   Sources of Power
   Resistance (blocking, power playing, uncooperativeness, disinterest, withdrawal, controlling, threatening with punishment, disapproval)
   Strategies
4. *Implementation.*
5. *Evaluation.* [7]

Change and the Health Care Delivery System

The so-called "crisis" in health care is primarily one of inadequate economic coping responses. It lacks what economists call effective market controls, that is, consumer choice and supplier competition to restrain demand, output, and prices. [31, p. 457] Health insurance has encouraged consumption and increased the cost of health care. The physician has been stimulated to request every possible diagnostic test because the insurance covers it. These luxuries can be afforded no longer. Health insurance companies are beginning to research the cost of health education and prevention maintenance programs as compared to crisis-oriented reactive health care in a hospital at $500+ per day.

The health-care industry in the United States is the nation's third largest, spending $139 billion in 1976 and with projections for 1981 of $264.3 billion or 10.2

percent of the Gross National Product. It maintains over 7,000 hospitals, 2,000 of them public (federal, state, or local), 1,000 privately owned, and the rest private, nonprofit, or voluntary institutions. In addition, there are 16,000 skilled nursing homes, all utilizing laboratories, equipment, drugs, and services. Administrating and financing these organizations is carried out by a combination of private and government representatives, boards, and committees. Coordinating the activities and spending of these organizations has been attempted in various ways through legislation (Hill-Burton Act, Regional Medical Programs, Comprehensive Health Planning) over the last twenty years. The most recent effort—the National Health Planning and Resources Development Act (PL 93–641)—was passed in 1975. The act makes use of the regionalization concept to develop resources, facilities, and programs in a unified fashion with the focus on ambulatory, intermediate, and home health care as opposed to inpatient services. This act also reinforces some of the Canadian Task Force ideas about actions of self-responsibility for health.

Consumer Activism

One of the ways individuals and groups are responding to their own health problems and access to a responsive health care system is to practice the "artful complaint," [2] in their relationships with health professionals. Self-help and consumer advocacy and education are encouraging assertive clients, who are aware of their rights and who do not blindly accept whatever the health care delivery system happens to give them.

Holistic nurses should be practicing, teaching, and supporting self-advocacy whenever possible. Clients should be encouraged to prepare for a visit to a health care delivery system by:

talking to others about recommended doctors and clinics;

calling consumer groups and women's groups to inquire about costs, attitudes, and competence of various doctors and clinics;

calling the doctor or clinic for a cost breakdown and the professional's expertise specialty and hospital affiliation;

if a contact or good rapport with a doctor, nurse, or health worker exists, getting information on various practitioners or clinics from them;

when possible, checking the health practitioner's credentials by calling local medical society and/or looking the practitioners up in The Directory of Medical Specialists in the library;

joining a consumer's group which exchanges the kind of information needed.

During a visit, clients should be prepared to:

fill out a family history and their own medical history, using some of the suggestions given in Chapter 8 as a guide;

write down any pertinent information, symptoms, etc., gathered, if there is a problem;

bring a friend for support and to act as another listener to give feedback later;

make sure the doctor explains everything that is done, such as any side effects of drugs (use generic name, not brand name) or remedies prescribed, and that all tests are explained in a language that is understandable;

ask the nurse or medical assistant to reiterate or explain in more detail anything that is unclear;

ask for a written summary of the results of the visit; and

obtain a second opinion, if desired; do not hesitate to get it. This is standard acceptable practice and is now covered by most insurance companies.

After a visit, clients should:

record what went on and their reaction to it;

shop drugstores for best prices, using generic names of drugs; ask for package inserts, if possible, or go to a medical library and look up the drug in a Physicians Desk Reference (PDR);

call the health practitioner and discuss them, if any side effects are experienced;

write down the details of any bad experience that should occur as soon as possible, including: the name of the clinic and practitioner, address, referring agent, the head of the clinic, hospital, etc., the public relations director or Director of Community Relations, the local medical society, the insurance carrier, the local health department, the neighborhood health council, local women's groups, women's health centers, magazines, and newspapers.

Any group wishing to organize around self-help and self-care issues can:

start a self-help, self-care course or group;

organize to change a health care facility;

get child-care centers into clinics and hospitals;

organize a local health project around a legitimate need;

create a women's counseling center and a hot-line or crisis intervention service;

start a childbirth educational group that offers holistic alternatives;

gather information, materials, and resources that consumers don't ordinarily have access to, for example, Physician Desk Reference, names of organizations which defend clients' rights and advocate for others, lists of names and addresses of appropriate consumer protection agencies and committees of local, state, and federal representatives in government; and

have a file on alternative health care resources, education, etc. [6, pp. 362–64]

Health Systems Agencies

One legislative attempt to solve some of the problems associated with the present health care system is Public Law 93–641 which set up regional Health Systems Agencies (HSAs). These may be private nonprofit corporations, public regional planning bodies, or units of local government. The agencies must be governed by a majority of consumers (50 percent to 60 percent) with the remainder comprised of physicians, dentists, nurses, health care institutions, professional and allied health schools. Since 1975 over 30,000 consumer members have been attracted to the nation's 200 HSAs and have volunteered their time and energy to them.

The purposes of the HSAs are to:

1. improve the health of residents of a health service area;
2. increase accessibility, continuity, and quality of health services provided;
3. restrain increases in the cost of providing health services; and
4. prevent unnecessary duplication of health resources. [10, p. 10]

Once the HSA is organized it must submit a Health Systems Plan or a statement of long-range goals for the community. An Annual Implementation Plan stating specific yearly objectives must be completed. Each area's health plan forms the basis for the State Health Plan which is administered by the State Health Planning and Development Agency (SHPDA). The consumer-dominated statewide health coordinating council reviews and coordinates the plans of the HSAs as well as other state health plans, grant applications, and so forth. It should be noted that the overall thrust of PL-93-641 is to decrease costs and duplication of services and equipment in an HSA area. Approval of funding for building new facilities is limited primarily to use for ambulatory and new client services, *not* for more hospital beds. Political parties and administrations may change, but the basic questions and positions remain:

1. How can we effectively evaluate cost control measures to arrest the astronomical spiraling?
2. How can we increase our knowledge base in regard to rational systematic health planning?
3. Can community-based health planning agencies make tough negative decisions in the face of the all-powerful health care industry?
4. Can consumers and providers work together to reach common goals?

In order to involve the community and consumer membership of HSAs, client/consumer education must occur. To actively bring members into the planning process the educational program must be designed based on articulated needs which may or may not pinpoint the basics of data gathering, analysis, and the health planning process. Building this awareness must be directly tied into the activities of the HSA. Change cannot occur on a large scale until people and communities change the ways they think and act in relation to health. An aware, motivated community can determine the pace, direction, and quality of change, at least on a local level. [11, p. 14]

Experience with the HSA health planning concept has yielded the following critique:

1. HSAs do not have enough real power, and although they promise to help reduce duplication and unnecessary expenditures, they have not—partially due to their own impotence at the state and federal levels which supersede them.

2. Regionalization, while seeming like a sound approach, can and has led to backroom deals and alliances between large hospitals and self-interested providers. [38, p. 3]

One way of using HSAs to change the illness focus of our health care delivery system is to develop sound "subarea" political bases dedicated to breaking up regional monopolies, exposing and protesting the imbalances of power, and promoting wellness and self-responsibility. HSA legislation allows for such small councils, although the exact communication channels need to be clarified. Such communication needs to be heard as acute-care, high-technology, high-overhead corporate medicine continues to divert "public hope and attention from the difficult task of prevention with its many ramifications for social and political change." [38, p. 14] Figure 10–4 summarizes the community health planning and problem-solving cycle.

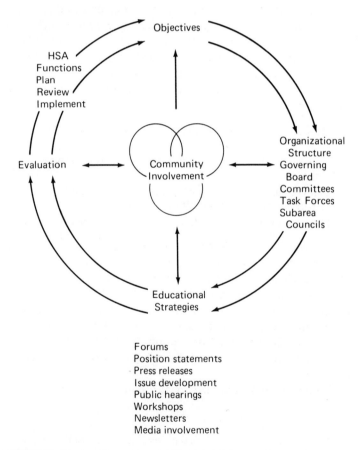

FIGURE 10-4 The community involvement circle of HSAs

Adapted from Jeanne A. Coombs and others, "A Systematic Approach to Community Education," *American Journal of Health Planning, 2,* no. 1 (July 1979), 14–18.

Health Planning and the Political Role of Nurses

How can nursing have more of a social and professional impact on the aforementioned issues? What is the role of nursing in the health-planning political process? As the largest professional group in the health field, nursing, if organized, can present a considerable power and lobbying force. Two hundred thousand nurses belong to nursing's professional organization, the American Nurses Association, which represents them in labor and management negotiations (collective bargaining) and provides benefits and guidance to its membership through state and local chapters. It also lobbies on a state and national level in support of the positions the organization takes on various pieces of legislation. Nurses collectively can work through this and other professional organizations of which they are a part.

A lobbyist is a person, usually paid, who represents a group's interests to government decision makers. For small organizations, hiring a lobbyist is unrealistic. For these groups, it is important to have staff who have the knowledge and experience to perform this function. An executive secretary of a state organization usually wields a considerable amount of power and influence. Issues need to be brought to her attention if they are to have statewide implications. Help can be solicited from such leaders in designing a package using appropriate terminology which will affect policymakers.

Nurses must begin to see themselves as political persons, despite one traditional image of nurses as apolitical, dedicated to service at all costs, ever-loyal, and submissive. Incorporating political consciousness into nursing theory and practice will not negate its humanistic goals, but will help make it more than a dream. Nursing *needs* to transform its image.

Nurses can begin the transformation by articulating their needs and wants to each other. If a group feels strongly about the changes they want, this becomes a demand when those in authority are asked to consider it. How can nurses get those in power to consider their demands? The answer is by converting a demand into an issue. [27, p. 165] An issue is defined as a conflict between two or more identifiable groups over procedural or substantive matters. Raising a demand to the level of an issue increases the visibility of the issue, mobilizes more persons and groups, and gives the demand more weight.

An issue will not get before a decision maker unless it commands attention. Issues that command attention are those that affect a significant portion of a constituency. Three prerequisites for a nursing or health issue to become part of a political agenda are:

1. widespread attention, or at least, awareness;
2. shared alarm of at least a sizable portion of the public that some action is required; and
3. a shared perception that the matter is the concern of a particular decision maker (or committee) or in that area of influence. [27, p. 166]

The major factor is that the issue be supported by a large and/or wide variety of groups. This support can be achieved through the petition process, sending letters or telegrams, phone calling campaigns, and other more dramatic methods involving the media. Helping elect a person to a position of power is another way to achieve a goal. The person must commit himself or herself to the cause and often these promises are not binding.

Another way of exerting pressure is to organize a group of interested people who are willing to contribute the necessary money, provide volunteer workers, and proceed without official sanction. An effective approach to getting an issue into the public eye is to organize an educational campaign which will stimulate strong public reaction and exert pressure on an existing official, agency, or committee. Identifying the appropriate focus of power or authority is an important prerequisite to this approach.

Conditions Paralyzing Nurses

Reality Shock

Several intrapersonal issues plague nurses attempting to apply the change process. The first is endemic to the new nurse who tries to apply an idealistic philosophy to a reality-based bureaucracy. This syndrome has been labeled "reality shock" by nurse researcher Marlene Kramer. It consists of feelings of shock, disappointment, and disillusionment when faced with staffing shortages, unsympathetic supervision, and inflexible administration. The eventual reaction of the neophyte nurse is to be "resocialized" into the pattern desired by the agency. Otherwise, a nurse may struggle to make changes and finally leave the institution—a 50 percent annual turnover rate for nurses is common—or even leave nursing altogether.

The costs of reality shock are staggering, with agencies constantly reorienting new staff, clients and staff experiencing lack of continuity and innovation, and change processes being hopelessly interrupted. Nurses who stay in the profession are said to have a high professional-low bureaucratic mentality. (This also keeps them in a position of performing high-level client care without making any broader system waves.) Some reality coping methods have been suggested:

1. orientation to "reality shock" in nursing education from the beginning of a program;
2. early clinical exposure and guided expression of feelings in conference;
3. careful selection of first employment based on mutual sharing of expectations on the part of both nurse and employer, coupled with a good orientation program;
4. recognition and joint efforts of education and service of transitional problems of new nurses. These "neophyte nurse" projects have been funded by the United States Department of Health and Human Services in various parts of the country;
5. setting up a method whereby the graduate can expect frequent feedback on performance;
6. coping workshops; and
7. choosing primary care, total-care situations in which holistic care can be performed.

Burn-Out

Another syndrome, peculiar not only to nursing, although very commonly experienced by nurses, is called "burn-out." As identified by Ayala Pines, "burn-out" occurs when a traumatic or stressful situation seems to become chronic and never ending—an indeterminate sentence. It involves a feeling of irritation and of being "out of control" in a situation. The helping professions, particularly nursing, are very prone to "burn-out." The ability to care for others appears to be lost. Some possible reasons for the syndrome include the lack of feedback, a job that is unclearly defined and in which there is role confusion, and a job in which the individual feels like another victim of the bureaucracy.

A cluster of physical, emotional, and attitudinal symptoms that nurses experience describe the seriousness of burn out:

1. Tired
2. Depressed
3. Powerless
4. Exhausted (physically, emotionally, and spiritually)
5. Unhappy
6. Run down
7. Trapped
8. Worthless
9. Weary
10. Troubled
11. Disillusioned
12. Resentful
13. Hyperirritable
14. Weak
15. Hopeless
16. Anxious
17. Pessimistic
18. Introverted and withdrawn
19. Cannot recall last good day

Some common responses of nurses to "burn-out" are:

1. to remain on the job but to do as little as possible;
2. to change jobs;
3. to leave the profession and retire to private life; or
4. to go through "burn-out," recognize it as a growth experience, and attempt to cope and revitalize self; [6] to identify the sources of stress, seek out a collegial social support system and use it. (The usual methods of stress reduction and management, mentioned in Chapter 6, can also assist the "burn-out" victim.)

What happens while the nurse struggles through reality shock and burn-out? The holistic aspects of nursing—the very qualities that differentiate it from other professions, technical specialties, and paraprofessions—are pushed aside as the nurse attempts to cope. If, however, the nurse is aware of herself, the potential problems, and effective methods of coping, she will be prepared to meet these challenges, to seek support, and to make the transition a period of growth.

LEADERSHIP, CHANGE, THE HOLISTIC HEALTH MOVEMENT, AND HOLISTIC NURSING

The holistic health movement exemplifies change in many of its innovative systems and approaches that have been incorporated in this text. What holistic health seems to lack is a working use of the leadership and change processes advocated in this chapter. It is correct to state that this is a grass roots movement and that leadership, organization, and process are difficult to isolate in such a diverse population. Although a considerable constituency is identifiable, very few attempts at politicization of this support group have occurred or been successful. If holistic health is to survive and become an acceptable part of this country's health consciousness, then some definite plans, strategies, and leaders must be developed.

This section will survey a few current opinions on the evolution of the holistic health movement, cite some examples of the state of leadership and change as it exists in the movement, and finally, make some suggestions for nursing leadership and its role in promoting the growth of holistic health and holistic nursing.

Self-Responsibility—Bane or Boon?

One of the basic tenets of holistic health—self-responsibility—has been criticized as part of the reason for its apolitical, highly individualistic tendencies. Current holistic practices center around the individual rather than on the larger social group or society as a whole. Berliner and Salmon point out, perhaps constructively, that such an orientation produces an individual who works on altering himself to deal with a pathological environment rather than on changing that environment. [3, p. 45] Disease, stress, and society are related in holistic health, but very little guidance is given on how to change that society. The environment is seen as an extension of self, but the primary means of bettering it are on a personal conservationist scale (a valid approach). Merely coping with a hostile environment and actually changing it are worlds apart. The same authors see this as a problem which can be resolved by viewing health in a collective context. Stresses are alleviated "as people form their own comradely support. Secondly, energy and support are generated and increase resistance to outside assault." [3, p. 48]

Conservative Milton Friedman is enthusiastically supportive of the holistic health movement's self-help aspects because they decrease reliance on the overinflated health care delivery system and take responsibility from government. He cites the summer 1978 Holistic Health Conference held in Washington, D.C.— "Holistic Health: A Public Policy"—as the first in a series of steps toward bringing holistic health into the political arena.

Policy resolutions made at that meeting advocated the governmental initiation of committees to study holistic health principles. Parallel informal structure had been doing just that at the National Institute of Health Hospital, but they have not been officially recognized. The Congressional Clearinghouse on the Future has been monitoring futurist periodicals which identify emergent concepts and facilitate the transformation of government. [22, p. 19] Currently, however, the feeling in Washington is that personal health and growth practices cannot be mandated by HHS guidelines.

Other socialistically-oriented writers see the self-responsibility ethic as a way for government and insurance companies to abrogate their own responsibilities by placing blame on the "self-destructive" client. Another potential problem centers around legislating the protection of individuals from themselves by outlawing cigarettes, intoxicants, and so on. This seems a highly unlikely prospect, given the strength of those respective lobbies.

What is happening in occupational settings and in insurance policies is that individuals with negative lifestyle habits are being penalized either through increased premiums or decreased eligibility or in some cases discrimination in hiring, especially in job situations in which certain risk factors might have an effect on job performance or an increased risk of disability payments on the part of the employer.

On the positive side, privately initiated offshoots of the holistic health movement continue to appear. Some physicians formed the American Holistic Medical Association in 1978. The Holistic Health Association has been convening national conferences since 1976 with its first international symposium taking place in 1979. Governmental, quasi-governmental, and professional associations have been including holistic health speakers on their meeting schedules. Professional continuing education in nursing, medicine, dentistry, and so on, are continually sponsoring weekend symposia on various holistic practices.

The East West Academy of Healing Arts

One of the earliest attempts to bring holistic health to the attention of the medical and lay communities was the East West Academy of Healing Arts. The Academy was founded in 1973 by nurse/acupuncturist Dr. Effie Poy Yew Chow to promote education and research in holistic health and cultural practices. Among its many activities the East West Academy sponsors professional and lay conferences and symposia in various parts of the United States several times a year with continuing support and success.

Also co-founded by Dr. Effie Chow in 1977 was the Council of Nurse Healers. This support group of nurses is dedicated to the use of self to promote health and "mobilize the client's recuperative powers through the intentional, therapeutic transmission of energy within a nurse-client interaction, integrating body/mind/ spirit in a unitive effort." (Taken from page 2 of the brochure from the First Congress of Nurse-Healers, June 11–12, 1977.)

Concepts incorporated in the holistic philosophy serve as the basis for countless continuing education courses for professionals, with titles such as: "The Healing Brain," "The Search for Health," "Holistic Health: The Renaissance Nurse," "The Nurse-Healer of Tomorrow." All of these programs indicate the need nurses and other professionals have to learn more about holistic health and how to incorporate it into their practices and their own lives.

"Self-Determination": Holistic Politics

Assemblyman John Vasconcellos of San Jose, California helped to found Self-Determination, a personal/political network designed to broaden the humanistic holistic vision of humanity, and through politics, to find better ways of living in the world.

The group claims a membership of over two thousand, and it also carries on the following activities:

1. Publication of the *Self-Determination Quarterly Journal* which acts as a forum for activists and writers to explore personal experience and social theories, to describe

creative community projects and institutional alternatives, and to promote community-based alternatives. [19, p. 9]

2. The Network Exchange, a statewide program to locate, disseminate information about, and facilitate use of resources which assign persons and groups in becoming more active and effective in personal and/or community exchange.

3. A skills workshop program, which brings to local communities workshops which fuse personal growth and interaction with political skills and processes.

The Committee for Integrated Health

Another California group, The Committee for Integrated Health Policy (CIH), formed in 1976, is working toward the following goals:

Integration of mental, physical, emotional, spiritual, and environmental components of health;

Reform of medical care delivery systems;

Enlightenment of the public to the opportunities for transforming our caring and curing systems;

Pilot projects to demonstrate integrated, multidisciplinary, and holistic health concepts in practice;

Research on quality, cost effectiveness, and accessibility of new integrated delivery systems and treatment programs;

Recognition of alternative healing arts and affirmative health strategies;

Legitimation of "nonprofessional" specialists and educators in healing and health;

Absorption of alternative modalities into traditional practice;

Realization that health is an ever-increasing state of well-being and a continuing growth process, not merely the absence of clinical disease;

Pursuit of recommendations for legislative action;

Dedication to the educational process for community involvement, action, and volunteer work;

Training of health practitioners in new integrated, multidisciplinary, and holistic concepts and skills; and

Initiation of policy-planning processes: to assess public needs and expectations in utilization of alternative healing and health practicies, programs, and systems.

Major project areas include reshaping local, state, and national health policy and supporting innovative community action programs including:

1. a healing center project involving the development of a detailed plan for model healing centers utilizing integrated multidisciplinary and holistic approaches and practices; procurement of funds and creation of facilities to provide clinical, education, research, and training services; and

2. an education project including development of conferences, seminars, and programs for in-service and continuing education of health professionals; agencies and the public create educational materials for schools, government agencies, professions, business, industry, and the general public; provide speakers, papers, literature, and audiovisual media as a public course service for organizations, planning conferences, seminars, and educational programs.

Models for alternative healing centers are being suggested and implemented, for example, The Holistic Health Centers in Chicago, a joint project of the University of Illinois Medical Center and the W. K. Kellogg Foundation. In it, a health team approach is utilized. [47]

California established its first Council on Wellness and Physical Fitness in 1980. Wellness was defined by Governor Brown as a "state of well-being through responsibility, nutritional awareness, stress management, environmental sensitivity and physical fitness . . .an optimal state of being." The Council's job is to focus government programs and assist schools and private enterprise in "promoting" the "wellness" of the California population.

Well-Being Centers: An Idea Whose Time Has Come

Henrik Blum has suggested that a Well-Being Center (WBC) be integrated into a medical care delivery system that is a subscription-supported total health maintenance program (HMO). Positive aspects include primary care screening for immediate problems and access, no financial barriers, multiple small competitive WBCs to allow diversity in philosophy and community outreach services, a single convener or advocate to facilitate entry and progress through the system, caregivers who have a humanistic philosophy, and secondary- and tertiary-level services that are available when needed.

All WBCs and health-care delivery systems (HCDSs) do the following:

1. involve clients in accepting the possibility of prospective, personally-oriented new health behaviors which strengthen health and decrease risks;
2. provide practice for the same behaviors they preach;
3. make nutrition services available with economic and cultural ramifications;
4. make physical fitness and meditation guidance services available;
5. provide for broad involvement and responsibility of subscribers in:
   a. evaluating utilization, quality, and outcomes of service on both health and costs in well-being centers and health-care delivery systems;
   b. policy setting for WBCs and HCDSs regarding services, access, cost utility, controls of various sorts, etc.;
   c. consumer product safety, utility, and cost;
   d. consumer-dominated planning and governing entities of WBCs and HCDSs;
   e. regional and statewide health planning efforts;
   f. ecologic, zoning, environmental, nursing, employment, etc., activities of their communities and states; and
   g. public resource allocation politics between sectors such as housing, transit, education, and health. [5, p. 15]

Legal Considerations

The self-responsibility issue has other ramifications, one of the most important being the legal considerations of practicing holistic health. Like any new area, holistic health suffers from the absence of objective standards and guidelines by which

9. The exact text of Business and Professions Code Section 2903 reads as follows:

No person may engage in the practice of psychology, or represent himself to be a psychologist, without a license granted under this chapter, except as otherwise provided in this chapter. The practice of psychology is defined as rendering or offering to render for a fee to individuals, groups, organizations or the public any psychological service involving the application of psychological principles, methods and procedures of understanding, predicting and influencing behavior, such as the principles pertaining to learning, perception, motivation, emotions, and interpersonal relationships; and the methods and procedures of interviewing, counseling, psychotherapy, behavior modification and hypnosis; and of construction, administering and interpreting tests of mental abilities, aptitudes, interests, attitudes, personality characteristics, emotions and motivations.

The application of such principles and methods includes, but is not restricted to: diagnosis, prevention, treatment, and amelioration of psychological problems and emotional and mental disorders of individuals and groups. Psychotherapy within the meaning of this chapter means the use of psychological methods in a professional relationship to assist a person or person to acquire greater human effectiveness or to modify feelings, conditions, attitudes and behavior which are emotionally, intellectually or socially ineffectual or maladjustive. As used in this chapter, "fee" means any money or other valuable consideration paid or permitted to be paid for services rendered.

8. The exact text of Business and Professions Code Section 2141 reads as follows:

Any person who practices or attempts to practice, or who advertises or holds himself out as practicing, any system or mode of treating the sick or afflicted in this state, or who diagnoses, treats, operates for, or prescribes for any ailment, blemish, deformity, disease, disfigurement, disorder, injury or other mental or physical condition of any person, without having at the time of so doing a valid, unrevoked certificate as provided in this chapter, or without being authorized to perform such act pursuant to a certificate obtained in accordance with some other provision of law, is guilty of a misdemeanor.

FIGURE 10-5 Excerpts from the California Business and Professions Code

clients can judge competence. A review of the various definitions of holistic health alone reveals the confusion that abounds. The California Business and Professions Code includes two sections which speak specifically to the unlicensed practitioner. Figure 10-5 contains excerpts from this law.

The debate on this issue is only beginning and will become more and more intense as the holistic health movement expands and the inevitable fraud, malpractice, and neglect suits increase. The coming years will be a crucial time for holistic practitioners to influence policy and make law regarding their futures.

In the meantime, *no* group is free from a fringe of quackery, and holistic health is no exception. The aforementioned debate on licensure offers no guarantees or protection of the consumer from unsound practice in the near future. Marilyn Ferguson has formulated ten rules for helping the client differentiate the "Healers from the Wheeler Dealers": [20]

1. Beware of outrageous claims.
2. Beware the practitioner who relies on a single technique.
3. Ask for references.
4. Don't accept mystification.
5. Look for the practitioner who looks at the whole person, not just a collection of symptoms.
6. Beware of outrageous fees.
7. Beware the fanatic who advocates throwing away Western medicine.
8. Beware of combined affects of various treatments, especially if you are seeing several different practitioners.
9. Be willing to accept responsibility for participating in the healing process; do not just be a passive recipient.
10. Educate yourself as much as you can rather than taking everything a practitioner offers you without question or background information.

Toward a Holistic Paradigm

In summary, holistic nursing faces a major challenge—like and unlike every revolutionary change nursing has weathered in the past. Like their ancestors, holistic nurses are primarily concerned with prevention of illness, nurturance, and generation of optimal health in all their clients. Like their heroic forebears, holistic nurses are willing to work and prepare to assume more responsibility for total health care delivery by mastering an enormously sophisticated body of knowledges and skills organized around the basic life processes of self-responsibility, caring, human development, stress, lifestyling, communication, problem solving, teaching/learning, and leadership and change. Figure 10-6 depicts the changes our concepts of health and health status assessment have undergone since 1900.

Holistic nurses are looking at their own life processes, evaluating them, and recognizing their special abilities and weaknesses. Holistic nurses are taking responsibility as well as nurturing the same in their clients and colleagues. The knowledge and use of caring-assertiveness with self, clients, and colleagues makes the dialogue between orthodox medical values and holistic ones open and honest, with each side

Time	Epidemiologic Methods	Concepts of Health	Health Measurement
1900	Single-Cause Model (Infectious Diseases)	Ecology Model (Agent-Host-Environment)	Mortality from Infectious Diseases (Death Rates: Crude, Specific, Adjusted)
1920	Multiple-Cause Model (Infectious/Chronic Diseases, Transition Cycle)	Social Ecological Model (Host, Environment, Personal Factors)	Morbidity Measurement (Incidence, Prevalence) Disability Measurement (Work Loss, Disability Days)
1940		W.H.O. Model (Physical, Mental, Social)	
1970	Multiple Cause/ Multiple Effect Model (Chronic Disease Cycle)	Holistic Model (Life Style, Environment, Biology, Health Care System) High-Level Wellness Model (Physical Exercise, Stress Management, Nutrition, Self-Responsibility)	Holistic and Wellness Measurement (Prospective Measures, Health Risk Assessments, Self-Inventories)
1980	Psychosomatic or Stress Disorders	Content/Context Model (What's in Health/ How to Hold on to Health) Holistic Nursing Model (Basic Life Processes underlying all of the above concepts and content)	Measurement of the Content and Context of Health (Mind/Body Relationships) Holistic *and* Allopathic Assessment; discrete and qualitative, individual and community health status indicators

FIGURE 10-6 Changing concepts of health and health measurement

Adapted with permission from G. E. Alan Dever, *Community Health Analysis: A Holistic Approach* (Germantown, Md.: Aspen Systems, Inc., 1980).

recognizing the contributions of the other and incorporating aspects of each that are comfortable at that particular point in time.

With a coherent philosophy and cohesive spirit of dedication, holistic nursing, echoing the words of Carl Rogers, is moving toward the following:

Life Processes Implied	Goals of Holistic Paradigm
Caring/Leadership Communication	Toward a nondefensive openness in all interpersonal relationships—within the family, the working task force, the system of leadership.
Lifestyling Teaching/Learning	Toward the exploration of self, and the development of the richness of the total, individual, responsible human soma-mind and body.
Caring	Toward the prizing of individuals for what they are, regardless of sex, race, status, or material possessions.
Lifestyling	Toward human-sized groupings in our communities, our educational facilities, our productive units.
Lifestyling	Toward a close, respectful, balanced, reciprocal relationship to the natural world.
Lifestyling	Toward the perception of material goods as rewarding only when they enhance the quality of personal living.
Lifestyling/Change	Toward a more even distribution of material goods.
Change/ Self-Responsibility/ Human Development	Toward a society with minimal structure; human needs taking priority over any tentative structure that develops.
Leadership	Toward leadership as a temporary, shifting function, based on competence for meeting a specific social need.
Caring/Stress/ Lifestyling	Toward a more genuine and caring concern for those who need help.
Problem solving/ Caring	Toward a human conception of science—in its creating phase, the testing of hypotheses, the valuing of the humanness of its applications.
Problem solving/ Change	Toward creativity of all sorts—in thinking and exploring—in the areas of social relationships, the arts, social design, architecture, urban and regional planning, science, and the study of psychic phenomena. [40, p. 282]

A partial listing of some organizations involved in the politics of the New Age and Holistic Health appears in the appendices. Certainly, change begins, as Lewin theorized, with unfreezing and gathering information. This text is a start in that direction. Exploring some of the references here presented, critiquing and conducting research, and finally, making contact with some of the groups that are attempting to promote holistic health are further steps toward change for holistic nursing.

REFERENCES FOR CHAPTER 10

[1] George J. Annas, *The Rights of Hospital Patients* (New York: Avon Books, 1975).

[2] Donald B. Ardell, *High-Level Wellness* (Emmaus, Pa.: Rodale Press, 1977).

[3] Howard S. Berliner and J. Warren Salmon, "The Holistic Health Movement and Scientific Medicine: The Naked and the Dead," *Socialist Review*, no. 43, vol. 9, no. 1 (January-February 1979), 31–52.

[4] William W. Biddle, *The Cultivation of Community Leaders* (New York: Harper & Row, 1953).

[5] Henrick Blum, "National Health Policy," *AJHP*, 1, no. 1 (July 1976), 4–21.

[6] The Boston Women's Health Book Collective, *Our Bodies, Ourselves* (New York: Simon and Schuster, 1976).

[7] Dorothy A. Brooten, Laura Hay, and Mary Naylor, *Leadership for Change: A Guide for the Frustrated Nurse* (Philadelphia: J.B. Lippincott, 1978).

[8] California Office of Statewide Health Planning and Development, "California State Health Plan, 1980–1985," (Sacramento, Ca.: Office of State Health Planning and Development, 1979).

[9] Mary Helen Castillo and Dorothy F. Corona, "Coping with Reality," in Ann Marriner, ed., *Current Perspectives in Nursing Management*, vol. 1 (St. Louis: C. V. Mosby Co., 1979), pp. 184–202.

[10] Harry P. Coin and Helen N. Darling, "Health Planning in the United States; Where We Stand Today," *Health Policy and Education* (1979), 5–25.

[11] Jeanne A. Coombs and others, "A Systematic Approach to Community Education," *AJHP*, 2, no. 1 (July 1977), 14–18.

[12] Norman Cousins, "The Holistic Health Explosion," *Saturday Review*, March 31, 1979, pp. 17–20.

[13] Rob Crawford, "Sickness as Sin," *Health-Pac Bulletin*, no. 80 (January-February 1978), 10–16.

[14] G. E. Alan Dever, *Community Health Analysis: A Holistic Approach* (Germantown, Md.: Aspen Systems, Inc., 1980).

[15] Laura Mae Douglass, *Review of Leadership in Nursing* (St. Louis: C. V. Mosby Co., 1977).

[16] Laura Mae Douglass and Em Olivia Bevis, *Nursing Management and Leadership in Action* (St. Louis: C. V. Mosby Co., 1979).

[17] Peter F. Drucker, *Management, Tasks, Responsibilities, Practices* (New York: Harper & Row, 1973).

[18] Barbara Ehrenreich and Deirdre English, *For Her Own Good* (Garden City, N.Y.: Anchor Press, 1978).

[19] "The Esalen Catalogue," April-July 1979, p. 9.

[20] Marilyn Ferguson, "How to Tell the Healers from the Wheeler-Dealers," *New West*, January 3, 1977, p. 68.

[21] Ellen Frankfurt, *Vaginal Politics* (New York: Bantam Books, 1973).

[22] Milton Friedman, "Holistic Health: Is Washington Listening?" *New Realities*, II, no. 1 (1978), 17–20.

[23] Sarah Fuller, "Humanistic Leadership in a Pragmatic Age," *Nursing Outlook*, 27, no. 12 (December 1979), 770–73.

[24] Vivian Gornick and Barbara K. Moran, eds., *Women in Sexist Society* (New York: New American Library, 1971), pp. 555–75.

[25] John Huensfeld, *The Community Activist's Handbook* (Boston: Beacon Press, 1970), pp. 4–10.

[26] Ivan Illich, *Medical Nemesis* (New York: Bantam Books, 1977).

[27] Philip A. Kalisch and Beatrice J. Kalisch, "The What, Why, and How of the Political Dynamics of Nursing," in Ann Marriner, ed., *Current Perspectives in Nursing Management*, vol. 1 (St. Louis: C. V. Mosby Co., 1979), pp. 156–74.

[28] Spencer Klaw, *The Great American Medicine Show* (New York: Penguin Books, 1976).

[29] John H. Knowles, ed., *Doing Better and Feeling Worse* (New York: W. W. Norton & Co., 1977).

[30] Marlene Kramer, *Reality Shock* (St. Louis: C. V. Mosby Co., 1974).

[31] Marvin M. Kristein, "Health Economics and Preventive Care," 195, no. 4277 (February 4, 1977), 457–62.

[32] Thomas S. Kuhn, *The Structure of Scientific Revolutions,* vols. I and II, Foundations of the Unity of Science, vol. II, no. 2 (The University of Chicago Press, 1958).

[33] Kurt Lewin, *Field Theory and Social Science* (New York: Harper & Row, 1951), pp. 30–80.

[34] C. Maslack and A. Pines, "Burn Out, The Loss of Human Caring," in *Experiencing Social Psychology* (New York: Random House, 1978).

[35] Margaret M. Moloney, *Leadership in Nursing, Theory, Strategies, Action* (St. Louis: C. V. Mosby Co., 1979).

[36] National League for Nursing, *Primary Health Care . . .Everybody's Business* (New York: National League for Nursing, 1973).

[37] Elizabeth Mosdiez Olson, "Strategies and Techniques for the Nurse Change Agent," *Nursing Clinics of North America,* 14, no. 2 (June 1979), 323–36.

[38] "Part of the Way with HSAs," *Health-Pac Bulletin,* II, no. 1 (September 1979), 1, 2, 14.

[39] Kay B. Partridge, "Nursing Values in a Changing Society," *Nursing Outlook,* 26, no. 6 (July 1978), 356–60.

[40] Carl Rogers, *On Personal Power* (New York: Delacorte Press, 1977).

[41] Michael Rossman, "Notes on the Tao of the Body Politic," *The Self-Determination Quarterly Journal,* 2, no. 2 (1978), 33–38.

[42] Mark Satin, *New Age Politics* (Vancouver, B.C.: White Cap Books, 1978).

[43] Barbara J. Stevens, "Improving Nurses' Managerial Skills," *Nursing Outlook,* 27, no. 12 (December 1979), 774–77.

[44] Source Collective, *Organizing for Health Care* (Boston: Beacon Press, 1974).

[45] Alvin Toffler, *Future Shock* (New York: Bantam Books, 1972).

[46] Alvin Toffler, *The Third Wave* (New York: William Morrow & Co., 1980).

[47] Donald A. Tubesing, "A Practical Approach to Creating Holistic Health Centers," *Journal of Holistic Health,* III (1978), 66–74.

[48] United States Department of Health and Human Services, "This is HHS," (Washington, D.C.: U.S. Government Printing Office, 1980).

[49] United States Public Health Service, *Forward Plan for Health* (Washington, D.C.: United States Government Printing Office, 1976).

[50] Dennis M. Warren, "Legal Consideration in the Search for Holistic Health," *Journal of Holistic Health,* III (1978), 102–08.

[51] Lynne Brodie Welsh, "Planned Change in Nursing: The Theory," *Nursing Clinics of North America,* 14, no. 2 (June 1979), 307–21.

[52] John D. Williamson and Kate Danaher, *Self-Care in Health* (London: Croom-Helm, 1978).

appendices

APPENDIX A: THE ROTTER INTERNAL-EXTERNAL CONTROL SCALE

*1. a. Children get into trouble because their parents punish them too much.
   b. The trouble with most children nowadays is that their parents are too easy with them.
2. *a.* Many of the unhappy things in people's lives are partly due to bad luck.
   b. People's misfortunes result from the mistakes they make.
3. a. One of the major reasons why we have wars is because people don't take enough interest in politics.
   b. There will always be wars, no matter how hard people try to prevent them.
4. a. In the long run people get the respect they deserve in this world.
   b. Unfortunately, an individual's worth often passes unrecognized no matter how hard he tries.
5. a. The idea that teachers are unfair to students is nonsense.
   b. Most students don't realize the extent to which their grades are influenced by accidental happenings.
6. *a.* Without the right breaks one cannot be an effective leader.
   b. Capable people who fail to become leaders have not taken advantage of their opportunities.
7. *a.* No matter how hard you try some people just don't like you.
   b. People who can't get others to like them don't understand how to get along with others.
*8. a. Heredity plays the major role in determining one's personality.
   b. It is one's experiences in life which determine what they're like.
9. *a.* I have often found that what is going to happen will happen.
   b. Trusting to fate has never turned out as well for me as making a decision to take a definite course of action.
10. a. In the case of the well prepared student there is rarely if ever such a thing as an unfair test.
   b. Many times exam questions tend to be so unrelated to course work that studying is really useless.
11. a. Becoming a success is a matter of hard work, luck has little or nothing to do with it.
   b. Getting a good job depends mainly on being in the right place at the right time.
12. a. The average citizen can have an influence in government decisions.
   b. This world is run by the few people in power, and there is not much the little guy can do about it.
13. a. When I make plans, I am almost certain that I can make them work.
   b. It is not always wise to plan too far ahead because many things turn out to be a matter of good or bad fortune anyway.

* Items with an asterisk preceding them are filler items. Score is the number of italicized alternatives chosen.

From J. B. Rotter, Generalized expectancies for internal versus external control of reinforcement. *Psychological Monographs,* 1966, *80,* No. 1 (Whole No. 609). Copyright 1966 by the American Psychological Association. Reprinted by permission.

*14. a. There are certain people who are just no good.
  b. There is some good in everybody.
 15. a. In my case getting what I want has little or nothing to do with luck.
  b. Many times we might just as well decide what to do by flipping a coin.
 16. a. Who gets to be the boss often depends on who was lucky enough to be in the right place first.
  b. Getting people to do the right thing depends upon ability; luck has little to do with it.
 17. a. As far as world affairs are concerned, most of us are the victims of forces we can neither understand nor control.
  b. By taking an active part in political and social affairs the people can control world events.
 18. a. Most people don't realize the extent to which their lives are controlled by accidental happenings.
  b. There really is no such thing as "luck."
*19. a. One should always be willing to admit mistakes.
  b. It is usually best to cover up one's mistakes.
 20. a. It is hard to know whether or not a person really likes you.
  b. How many friends you have depends upon how nice a person you are.
 21. a. In the long run the bad things that happen to us are balanced by the good ones.
  b. Most misfortunes are the result of lack of ability, ignorance, laziness, or all three.
 22. a. With enough effort we can wipe out political corruption.
  b. It is difficult for people to have much control over the things politicians do in office.
 23. a. Sometimes I can't understand how teachers arrive at the grades they give.
  b. There is a direct connection between how hard I study and the grades I get.
*24. a. A good leader expects people to decide for themselves what they should do.
  b. A good leader makes it clear to everybody what their jobs are.
 25. a. Many times I feel that I have little influence over the things that happen to me.
  b. It is impossible for me to believe that chance or luck plays an important role in my life.
 26. a. People are lonely because they don't try to be friendly.
  b. There's not much use in trying too hard to please people, if they like you, they like you.
*27. a. There is too much emphasis on athletics in high school.
  b. Team sports are an excellent way to build character.
 28. a. What happens to me is my own doing.
  b. Sometimes I feel that I don't have enough control over the direction my life is taking.
 29. a. Most of the time I can't understand why politicians behave the way they do.
  b. In the long run the people are responsible for bad government on a national as well as on a local level.

APPENDIX B: A CASE STUDY OF CARING THROUGH TOUCH

"Think how good it will feel to have your tired feet anointed in oil—soothed, stroked, rubbed and kneaded. Imagine the delightful sensations that will be yours if you win this massage," hawked the auctioneer.

The bidding was slow. After a few half-hearted offers, Stefan bought that foot massage—a four dollar bargain at the local cooperative nursery school auction.

Since I had donated the massage, for the next few days, I waited for Stefan to call. But the phone never rang. Perhaps he sensed my discomfort or felt some of his own. We don't exactly live in a society that encourages people to touch.

Months—even years went by without a request for the massage. Most of the time, I'd forget about it. But every once in a while, it would pop into my head like an unpaid bill. Occasionally, I'd see Stefan at a school party or baseball game.

"When are you going to collect your massage?" I'd ask. "You know I still owe it to you."

He'd laugh. "Gee, I sure could have used one the other night. My feet were just aching."

"You paid for it. Just call when you want it," I'd say.

He was a captain in the fire district. He always looked immaculate in his navy blue uniform. He was a handsome guy—tall and muscular, with dark brown hair that was always neatly groomed.

He worked at the parent co-op nursery school on my day, Thursdays. He loved the kids at school with a passion and they loved him.

But life is not always a series of smooth steps forward. There are jolts that seem to come from nowhere. The school grapevine was bristling with bad news. Stefan had cancer and was expected to live for only a few more weeks.

My mind flashed on the debt I owed him. There is not much you can do or say to a person who is dying. But I wondered if a massage wouldn't be among the few things that could still be appreciated. When you are born and when you die, soothing touches are the only things that matter.

When Stefan first heard about my offer, he just laughed. His closest friends told me he didn't want to see or talk to anyone. They doubted he was even strong enough to have a massage anymore.

But late one afternoon, he said, "You know, I want that massage. It just might feel good."

As I got into bed that night, I could only think about giving that massage. It's not going to be easy, my husband warned. Like a fortune-teller, he predicted, "Once you give that massage, you are going to be different."

"What do you mean?" I asked.

"I just can't tell you how. I can only feel it. When you touch a person who's dying, you touch your own mortality. It's frightening. Our society does as much as it can to separate the living from the dying."

Enid Rubin, "Touching and Saying Goodbye," *San Francisco Sunday Examiner and Chronicle,* May 8, 1977. Reprinted with permission from California Living Magazine of the *San Francisco Examiner and Chronicle,* Copyright © 1977, San Francisco Examiner.

I couldn't fall asleep for what seemed like hours. I was practicing dialogues inside my head.

"Stefan, I'm so sorry you are dying. There are so many things I enjoyed sharing with you. I liked the way you treated the kids when they came to the fire station. I'm really glad you could let me give you this massage. I'm sorry it has to be in these circumstances."

Tears slipped down my cheeks as I rehearsed the melodramatic scenario. Finally, my fear melted into exhaustion, and I fell asleep.

In the morning, I knew I would have to call Stefan. The anticipation of making that call was like a weight that hung over me. I don't know what to say or how to say it. I sat down on the kitchen floor and leaned on the cabinets. I wanted all the support I could get.

Stefan's friend answered the phone. I was relieved that I didn't have to talk to him yet. We made an appointment for the following day.

Friday morning I got up and ready. I packed the soaking tub, the massage oil, and the cream into my trunk. The directions were already tucked into my purse. I was shaky when I got into the car. This was going to be my moment to understand something terribly important about the world I lived in.

I looked at the road and the landscape for some kind of clue about the experience. The boats bobbed silently in the bay and the restful green hills made no sign that I could fathom. I followed the signs to Sausalito. "Keep Right," they said, and "Food Ahead."

I climbed up a big hill and found the house. The number 108 was clearly marked. Stefan's friend Sandy came out and said hello. I smiled back, glad to have her there.

I unlocked the trunk and took out my equipment. How I needed something to hold onto. My plastic basin and my bottles of cream and oil felt so solid, so tangible, I could hide my discomfort behind them.

Sandy opened the door and we walked in. The first thing I saw was the motorized hospital bed facing the window. "Stefan is dozing, but I'll wake him now that you're here," she said.

Visually, there were so many things I understood in that split second of entering. Myriads of information were communicated with one step inside. Stef was lying in bed asleep. I saw his face. It was jaundiced, not a yellow but an orange color. His cheeks were sunken and most of his hair had fallen out from the chemotherapy.

"You know Stef," said Sandy.

Stef and I both laughed. But my insides were saying I don't know this Stef, not the one lying there so weak and sick.

"Hi, Stefan, how are you?" I asked in my everyday pattern of conversation. There was no answer to that question. Well, that's not the best beginning, I thought to myself.

Stef was a lot weaker than I could have imagined. Next to his bed was a small table filled with bottles of medicine, get-well cards, a bouquet of roses, and assortment of iced drinks—tea, water, soda—all with that familiar hospital trademark, the bendable straw.

"Sandy, water," Stefan called. He could not even lean over to pick up a glass.

When Sandy brought the glass to his mouth, he reached for the straw with a trembling hand. Beneath layers of blankets and white sheets, Stefan was tucked tightly into the hospital bed.

"Well I'm really glad I'm able to give you this massage," I said. "You've waited three years to collect it."

"You should be an expert by now," he joked.

I was relieved to be able to get busy. Busy never felt better or safer. I knew just what I was supposed to do and began doing it. There were so many things to get ready. I had to take the tops off all the bottles, roll up my sleeves and take off my rings, run the water until it was warm, then fill the basin. I had to lay the towels on the bed, and finally adjust the bed so Stefan could be comfortable. It's nice to be here now, I thought, going through the preparations.

As I stood at the foot of the bed and looked into Stefan's face, I could see vague traces of the person that I knew. The distance between us felt like the gulf of eternity.

I began to pull the covers away from his feet. They were tucked in tightly. Underneath the covers, his body seemed locked up full of mysterious secrets. I thought when the covers were ruffled and his body exposed, the truth would be exposed as well.

I began working on his right foot first. His foot was sheathed in a woolen sock. I took his sock off as gently as I could and slid a towel underneath to keep the bed dry. There were bruises all over his foot and leg. I bathed his foot and smoothed on the oil and cream. I soothed and rubbed the entire area. I ran my fingers through his toes. I worked on his heel, his sole, his tendons. Occasionally I was interrupted from my own world of physical sensations by the sound of a heavy sigh. I looked up into his face. It seemed so faraway, yet there was such a sense of peace and calm.

His feet were on an escalator moving swiftly and unswervingly toward death. There was no stopping to explain, there was just movement forward. Looking into his face, I could only see sickness and pain and suffering. There was the discomfort that came from his physical body no longer functioning at optimum conditions. I heard effort and strain in his voice. But when I felt his foot, I was able to enjoy his serenity. Could that be the secret that lurked underneath those covers?

My other senses would have misled me, making me fearful in the face of my friend's dying. I know the body does not lie. It cannot pretend. A tense person feels tense. A calm person feels calm. Muscles open and close, relax and flex in perfect harmony with our mental state.

As I worked loving circular strokes around his ankles, tarsals, metatarsals, fleshy parts and bony parts, a surge of feeling welled up inside me. I knew that I was transmitting the message which said, "Stefan, this is my good-bye. This is my way of loving you and letting you know how I feel about you as another human being. I just want to surround you with my love which I am transmitting through your feet. I know you can feel it by the open way you are receiving the strokes. You are not pulling away or making any attempt to be in control of your feet. For the time being, you have given me complete charge."

I wanted to give everything. Everything that was possible in the whole world to a thirty-one year old friend, dying of cancer who merely had the strength to lie in a hospital bed and look out at the San Francisco skyline and the hills of Sausalito.

How much can you feel through your feet? I looked up at Stef's face and wondered if I should stop, if this was too exhausting. I wanted to go on. He's only partly here, I thought. He comes and he goes, back and forth from this world to the next. I don't like letting go of him but there's no choice. This is the only way that he can experience this massage—on his terms, not on mine.

I stayed with his feet as he dozed. In a short while, he came back and opened his eyes again. I was relieved to see him and know that he was still here. I kept going until I felt finished. I capped his foot with my hands and wrapped it back up beneath the blankets.

I felt complete and full and satisfied. But I was surprised that instead of feeling like falling apart, I felt calm and peaceful.

There was no fear—there was simply being. Stefan was being exactly where he was—partly here and partly there. And he let me into the space beneath the covers.

APPENDIX C: TYPE A BEHAVIOR PATTERN QUESTIONNAIRE

Directions: Please place a check mark to the left of the question if your answer is affirmative.

1. Do you have (a) a habit of explosively accentuating various key words in your ordinary speech even when there is no real need for such accentuation, and (b) a tendency to utter the last few words of your sentences far more rapidly than the opening words?

2. Do you always move, walk, and eat rapidly?

3. Do you feel (particularly if you openly exhibit to others) an impatience with the rate at which most events take place?

4. Do you find it difficult to restrain yourself from hurrying the speech of others and resort to the device of saying very quickly over and over again, "Uh huh, uh huh," or, "Yes yes, yes yes," to someone who is talking, unconsciously urging him to "get on with" or hasten his rate of speaking?

5. Do you attempt to finish the sentences of persons speaking to you before they can?

6. Do you become unduly irritated or even enraged when a car ahead of you in your lane runs at a pace you consider too slow?

7. Do you find it anguishing to wait in a line or to wait your turn to be seated at a restaurant?

8. Do you become impatient with yourself as you are obliged to perform repetitious duties (making out bank deposit slips, writing checks, washing and cleaning dishes, and so on), which are necessary but take you away from doing things you really have an interest in doing?

9. Do you find yourself hurrying your own reading or always attempting to obtain condensations or summaries of truly interesting and worthwhile literature?

10. Do you indulge in polyphasic thought or performance, frequently striving to think of or do two or more things simultaneously?

11. Do you always find it difficult to refrain from talking about or bringing the theme of any conversation around to those subjects which especially interest and intrigue you, and when unable to accomplish this maneuver, you pretend to listen but really remain preoccupied with your own thoughts?

12. Do you almost always feel vaguely guilty when you relax and do absolutely nothing for several hours to several days?

13. Do you no longer observe the more important or interesting or lovely objects that you encounter in your milieu? For example, if you enter a strange office, store, or home, and after leaving any of these places you cannot recall what

Adapted from Mayer Friedman and Ray H. Rosenman, *Type A Behavior and Your Heart* (New York: Fawcett Crest, 1974), pp. 100–03.

was in them, you no longer are observing well—or for that matter enjoying life very much.

14. Do you not have any time to spare to become the things worth being because you are so preoccupied with getting the things worth having?

15. Do you attempt to schedule more and more in less and less time, and in doing so make fewer and fewer allowances for unforeseen contingencies?

16. If, on meeting another severely afflicted Type A person, instead of feeling compassion for his affliction do you find yourself compelled to "challenge" him? This is a telltale trait because no one arouses the aggressive and/or hostile feelings of one Type A subject more quickly than another Type A subject.

17. Do you resort to certain characteristic gestures or nervous tics? For example, if in conversation you frequently clench your fist, or bang your hand upon a table or pound one fist into the palm of your other hand in order to emphasize a conversational point, you are exhibiting Type A gestures.

18. Do you believe that whatever success you have enjoyed has been due in good part to your ability to get things done faster than your fellow men?

19. Do you find yourself increasingly and ineluctably committed to translating and evaluating not only your own but also the activities of others in terms of "numbers"?

The characteristics above mark the fully developed hard-core Type A. Many people properly classified as Type A exhibit these characteristics to a lesser degree, however. If you exhibit *none* of the traits or habits mentioned above, you probably possess a Type B behavior pattern.

APPENDIX D: HEALTH RISK INDEX

Your Health Risk Index Questionnaire

A questionnaire designed to provide an analysis of your medical history, current habits, and other factors that influence your life expectancy.

NOTE: *Read instructions provided and follow directions carefully. If you consider a question too personal, you may skip it. Medical Datamation warrants that it will provide medical reports resulting from this questionnaire to you and / or your designated medical facility, if applicable, and it will not otherwise release your reports without your written consent.*

1-203

IDENTIFICATION

10 **Name** |_|_|_|_|_|_|_|_|_|_|_|_|_|_|_|_|_|_|_|_|_|_|_|_|_|_|_|_|_|
Last Name, First Name, Middle Name

11 **Today's Date** |__|__| - |__|__| - |__|__| 12 **Date of Birth** |__|__| - |__|__| - |__|__|
     Mo.   Da.   Yr.   Mo.   Da.   Yr.

15 __ **Female**   16 __ **Male**

17 **Height** __ ft. __ in.   18 **Weight** _____ lbs.

PERMANENT HOME ADDRESS

19 **Street** |_|_|_|_|_|_|_|_|_|_|_|_|_|_|_|_|_|_|_|_|_|_|_|_|_|_|_|_|_|

20 **City** |_|_|_|_|_|_|_|_|_|_|_|_|_|_|_|_|_|_|_|_|_|_|_|_|_|_|_|_|_|

21 **State or Province** |_|_|_|_|_|_|_|_|_|_|_|_|_|_|_|_|_|_|_|_|_|_|_|_|

22 **Zip** |_|_|_|_|_|_|

23 **Country** |_|_|_|_|_|_|_|_|_|_|_|_|_|_|_|_|_|_|_|_|_|_|_|_|_|_|_|

1-602

DEMOGRAPHIC Background

Race
10 ____ American Indian
11 ____ Black
12 ____ Caucasian
13 ____ Oriental
14 ____ Spanish American
15 ____ Other

Family income level
16 ____ Low
17 ____ Middle
18 ____ High

Marital Status
19 ____ Single
20 ____ Married
21 ____ Widowed
22 ____ Separated
23 ____ Divorced

2-104

ILLNESSES and MEDICAL PROBLEMS

Check the problems you have or have had that have been diagnosed or treated by a physician or other health professional.

Yes	No	Problem	Yes	No	Problem
10 __	__	Alcoholism			High blood fats, specify.
11 __	__	Anemia-sickle cell	50 __	__	*Cholesterol*
12 __	__	Bleeding trait	51 __	__	*Triglycerides*
13 __	__	Bronchitis, chronic	52 __	__	High blood pressure
		Cancer	53 __	__	High blood pressure, uncontrolled
14 __	__	*Breast*			
15 __	__	*Cervix*	54 __	__	Obesity - more than 20 lbs overweight
16 __	__	*Colon*			
17 __	__	*Lung*	55 __	__	Pneumonia
18 __	__	*Uterus*	56 __	__	Polyps in colon
19 __	__	*Other cancer*	57 __	__	Rheumatic fever
20 __	__	Cirrhosis - liver	58 __	__	Rheumatic fever, with resultant heart murmur
21 __	__	Colitis - ulcerative			
22 __	__	Depression	59 __	__	Stroke
23 __	__	Diabetes	60 __	__	Suicide attempt
24 __	__	Diabetes, uncontrolled	61 __	__	Tuberculosis
25 __	__	Emphysema	**Yes**	**No**	**In the past year, have you had -**
26 __	__	Fibrocystic breasts	62 __	__	Chest pain on exertion, relieved by rest?
		Heart problem			
27 __	__	*Heart attack*	63 __	__	Shortness of breath lying down, relieved by sitting up?
28 __	__	*Coronary disease*			
29 __	__	*Rheumatic heart*			
30 __	__	*Heart valve prob*	64 __	__	Unexplained weight loss, more than 10 lbs?
31 __	__	*Heart murmur*			
32 __	__	*Enlarged heart*	65 __	__	Unexplained rectal bleeding?
33 __	__	*Heart rhythm prob*			
34 __	__	*Other heart prob*	66 __	__	Unexplained vaginal bleeding?

2-105

FEELINGS

Mark the frequency with which you have the feelings listed by placing a checkmark in the appropriate column.

M-Most of time   S-Some of time   R-Rarely or none

M	S	R	
10 __	__	__	Feel sad, depressed?
11 __	__	__	Wish to end it all?
12 __	__	__	Feel tense and anxious?
13 __	__	__	Worry about things generally?
14 __	__	__	More aggressive, hard-driving than friends?
15 __	__	__	Have an intense desire to achieve?
16 __	__	__	Feel optimistic about the future?

FAMILY MEDICAL HISTORY (Blood Relatives)

Check items that apply for your blood relatives. Your blood relatives include your children, brothers, sisters, parents, and grandparents.

30 ____ **Do not know my family medical history.**
(Go to question 50)

Yes	No	Illness	Yes	No	Illness
31 __	__	Anemia-sickle cell	36 __	__	High blood press
32 __	__	Bleeding trait	37 __	__	Mental illness
33 __	__	Cancer	38 __	__	Stroke
34 __	__	Diabetes (sugar)	39 __	__	Suicide
35 __	__	Heart disease	40 __	__	Tuberculosis

Yes	No	Check the items that apply.
50 __	__	Father died of a heart attack before age 60?
51 __	__	Mother died of a heart attack before age 60?
52 __	__	Mother or sister had cancer of the breast?
53 __	__	Did your mother take DES (diethylstilbestrol) when she was pregnant with you?

HABITS and RISK FACTORS

Your habits influence your ability to achieve and maintain good health and long life. The questions on this page concern factors that are known to influence your health.

4-201

EXERCISE

Specify the amount of exercise you get each day.

10 ___ None or very little

The equivalent of-

11 ___ 10 flights of stairs, or 1 mile walking
12 ___ 20 flights of stairs, or 2 miles walking
13 ___ Over 20 flights of stairs, or over 2 miles walking

SMOKING

Yes	No	Do you-
14 ___	___	Smoke a pipe and inhale 5 or more times/day?
15 ___	___	Smoke cigars and inhale 5 or more times/day?
16 ___	___	Currently smoke cigarettes?
17 ___	___	Have a history of cigarette smoking, but stopped?

If no longer smoking, specify number of years since you stopped.

18 ___ 1 yr.		21 ___ 4 yrs.		24 ___ 7 yrs.	
19 ___ 2 yrs.		22 ___ 5 yrs.		25 ___ 8 yrs.	
20 ___ 3 yrs.		23 ___ 6 yrs.		26 ___ 9 yrs.	

If you have ever smoked cigarettes, specify amount and duration.

Daily amount	Number of years
27 ___ 1/2 pack/day or less	31 ___ Less than 1 year
28 ___ 1/2 to 1 pack/day	32 ___ 1 to 5 years
29 ___ 1 to 2 packs/day	33 ___ 5 to 10 years
30 ___ Over 2 packs/day	34 ___ Over 10 years

ALCOHOL

Yes	No	
35 ___	___	Do you currently drink alcohol?
36 ___	___	Did you formerly drink alcohol but stopped?

If you have ever drunk alcohol, specify details

Amount per week	Number of years
37 ___ Less than 2 drinks/wk.	42 ___ Less than one year
38 ___ 2 to 10 drinks/wk.	43 ___ 1 to 5 years
39 ___ 10 to 25 drinks/wk.	44 ___ 5 to 10 years
40 ___ 25 to 40 drinks/wk.	45 ___ 10 to 20 years
41 ___ Over 40 drinks/wk.	46 ___ Over 20 years

TRAUMA, ACCIDENTS and OTHER HAZARDS

Yes	No	Do you-
47 ___	___	Often carry a weapon at work or otherwise?
48 ___	___	Have an arrest record for a violent crime?
49 ___	___	Drive after drinking or taking drugs?

How many miles do you travel in a car or other motor vehicle each year (average is 12,000 miles)?

50 ___ Up to 10,000	52 ___ 15,000 to 20,000
51 ___ 10,000 to 15,000	53 ___ Over 20,000

What percent of the time do you wear a seat belt?

54 ___ 0 to 25%	56 ___ 50% to 75%
55 ___ 25% to 50%	57 ___ 75% to 100%

What percent of the time do you wear a shoulder strap?

58 ___ 0 to 25%	60 ___ 50% to 75%
59 ___ 25% to 50%	61 ___ 75% to 100%

9-102

SELF-CARE

The early evaluation of symptoms, self-exams, and various professional health exams are important in detecting diseases. Regular medical follow-up is important in keeping problems under control and avoiding complications.

Yes	No	Have you-
10 ___	___	Ever had a chest x-ray?
11 ___	___	Had an abnormal chest x-ray?
12 ___	___	Ever had an EKG (Electrocardiogram)?
13 ___	___	Had an abnormal EKG?
14 ___	___	Had a TB skin test?
15 ___	___	Had a positive TB skin test?
16 ___	___	Had eyes checked in past two years?
17 ___	___	Had hearing tested (audiometry) in past 2 years?
18 ___	___	Had dental exam in the past year?
		Do you-
19 ___	___	Regularly follow your physician's advice?
20 ___	___	Plan annual medical symptom review with your physician or health service?
21 ___	___	Plan annual rectal exam after age 30?

WOMEN (Men go to "Tests")

Yes	No	Do you or have you-
30 ___	___	Had a PAP test within past year?
31 ___	___	Had at least three PAP tests in past 5 years?
32 ___	___	Had an abnormal PAP test in past?
33 ___	___	Plan annual PAP tests in the future?
34 ___	___	Check your breasts once a month for lumps?
35 ___	___	Have a breast exam by a doctor once yearly?

TESTS For these tests, if ever done, find out results from your physician. Check values shown that are closest to your own results. If measured more than once, use most recent value.

Blood Pressure				Cholesterol	
Systolic		Diastolic			
40 ___ 120 or less	45 ___	82 or less	50 ___	180 or less	
41 ___ 140	46 ___	88	51 ___	210	
42 ___ 160	47 ___	94	52 ___	240	
43 ___ 180	48 ___	100	53 ___	270	
44 ___ 200 or more	49 ___	106 or more	54 ___	300 or more	

INFORMATION

Check items for which you would like educational information

60 ___	Alcohol	68 ___	Legal problems
61 ___	Birth Control	69 ___	Loneliness
62 ___	Diet	70 ___	Marital problems
63 ___	Drug abuse	71 ___	Medical emergencies
64 ___	Emotional problems	72 ___	Self-breast exam
65 ___	Exercise	73 ___	Sexual problems
66 ___	Financial problems	74 ___	Smoking
67 ___	Health hazards	75 ___	Venereal disease

CONCLUSION

Yes	No	
80 ___	___	Do you have any other problem not covered by this questionnaire?

Please give us your opinion of this system.

81 ___	Great	83 ___	Generally good, criticism minor
82 ___	Good	84 ___	Don't like it

Thanks for completing this questionnaire. Please review for accuracy, then mail in postpaid envelope.

January 23, 1980

CHARLES A. TAYLOR
2571 HILLCREST AVE
WOODLAND, MI 54321

Dear Mr. Taylor:

Enclosed is your personal HEALTH RISK INDEX. This analysis of
your health risks is based on information supplied in your
health questionnaire. It projects likely causes of your death,
points out contributing factors, and suggests specific risk
reduction actions to improve your life expectancy.

Based on this analysis, your life expectancy is less than
that of an average person of your age and sex. If you take all
indicated risk reduction actions now, and follow through on
them during the rest of your life, you can add 14.1 years to
your life expectancy.

The major factors that increase your risk of dying, and which
you can reduce through your own efforts, are:
  Exercise habits
  Smoking habits
  High cholesterol level

You are already doing well in some areas of risk reduction:
  Limiting alcohol to less than 2 drinks/week
  Using seatbelt regularly

The reverse side of your HEALTH RISK INDEX gives a detailed
explanation of the report. Also enclosed is a personal
booklet that describes in depth various health hazards and how to
reduce them. We hope that the information provided will help
you to make decisions and take actions that will lead to a longer,
healthier life.

Sincerely,

Medical Datamation, Inc.

Enclosures

Your Health Risk Index

SOUTHWEST AND HARRISON   BELLEVUE, OHIO 44811

TAYLOR, CHARLFS A.
2571 HILLCRFST AVE
WOODLAND, MI . 54321

Date: 1/ 9/80
Number: 200- 2508465
Birthdate: 5/19/61
Ht: 5'10"   Wt: 205 lbs.
BP: 160/94   Chol: 270 mg%

Your HEALTH RISKS and CONTRIBUTING FACTORS

FOR THE NFXT 20 YEARS — RISK CF DYING

Potential Causes of Death	Yours	Average	Reduced	Contributing Factors
1 Suicice	0.5%	0.5%	0.5%	none identified.
2 Coronary heart disease	0.4	0.1	<0.1	Blood pressure, cholesterol, exercise habits, family history, smoking habits, weight.
3 Motor vehicle accicent	0.3	1.1	0.3	none identified,
4 Homicice	0.3	0.3	0.3	none identified,
5 Drowning accicent	0.1	0.1	0.1	none identified.
Other causes	1.3	1.4	1.2	
TOTAL RISK NEXT 20 YEARS	2.9%	3.5%	2.4%	

FOR THE NEXT 40 YEARS — RISK CF DYING

Potential Causes of Death	Yours	Average	Reduced	Contributing Factors
1 Coronary heart disease	20.2%	4.3%	2.0%	Blood pressure, cholesterol, exercise habits, family history, smoking habits, weight.
2 Cancer of lungs	1.1	1.0	0.2	Smoking habits.,
3 Suicice	1.1	1.1	1.1	none identified.
4 Stroke	1.1	0.5	0.2	Blood pressure, cholesterol, smoking habits.
Other causes	7.8	9.6	7.4	
TOTAL RISK NEXT 40 YEARS	31.3%	16.5%	10.9%	

Your LIFE EXPECTANCY PREDICTIONS

Comparative Ages			Life Expectations	Life Remaining		Total Lifespan	
Actual Age	18.6	yrs.	For an *average* person of your age, race, sex	53.0	yrs.	71.6	yrs.
Health Age	28.0	yrs.	For *you* based on your current analysis	44.5	yrs.	63.1	yrs.
Achievable Age	12.7	yrs.	For *you* based on maximum risk reduction	58.6	yrs.	77.2	yrs.
			Potential gain in *your* life expectancy	+14.1	yrs.	+14.1	yrs.

HOW *You* CAN LIVE LONGER

Rank	Actions You Can Take	Gain in Life Expectancy
1	Follow a program of regular vigorous exercise	2.5 yrs.
2	Stop smoking	2.2 yrs.
3	Reduce, control cholesterol level	1.9 yrs.
4	Reduce, control high blood pressure	1.2 yrs.
5	Reduce weight to 151, maintain	0.9 yrs.
6	Get annual rectal exam after age 30	0.1 yrs.
7	Added benefit from doing ALL of the above	5.3 yrs.

TOTAL GAIN IN LIFE EXPECTANCY   +14.1 yrs.

HEALTH RISK INDEX

Background

During the last 20 years, medical and actuarial experts developed a health education tool known as "health hazard appraisal" to help people identify and reduce their health risks. This technique forms the basis of your Health Risk Index. Causes of death by age, sex, and race are analyzed in terms of contributing causes. Group statistics are applied to individuals so that a person can identify his risk of dying by various causes, take note of contributing factors, and follow through on improving his chances of staying alive and healthy by taking risk reduction actions.

Your Health Risks and Contributing Factors

Health risks are problems or conditions that can kill you. This section lists possible causes of your death in order of decreasing frequency for the time period shown. Risk of dying during that period of time is expressed on a percentage basis. Your risk is based on your current analysis and is derived from information you supplied in your health questionnaire. The risk of an average person of your age, sex and race is shown for comparison. Your achievable risk indicates a favorable change in your chances of living based on risk reduction actions you can take.

Contributing factors to your possible causes of death stem from a variety of sources, including your habits, family medical history, and existing conditions such as high blood pressure. Some factors cannot be altered, such as having a family history of heart attack. However, many factors can be altered favorably and your risk of dying reduced by actions that you take.

Your risk of dying is determined for a specific period of time. This period of time is dependent on your age. Generally, young people are interested in both their chances of reaching middle age and in how long they will live. For young people, the Health Risk Index projects risks for two time periods, one for reaching middle age and one for a "lifetime." For people who are already nearing middle age or beyond, risks are projected for only one time period. In any case, the goal is to present you with information which will be useful to you in reducing your risks.

Your Life Expectancy Predictions

How old are you in terms of your health risks, and how long are you likely to live? This section answers these questions and suggests how much your "age" and life expectancy might be improved. Your actual age is your real or chronologic age. The years of life remaining and total lifespan for an average person of this age are shown. Your health age is based on your current risk level; it was determined through calculating your years of life remaining and total lifespan. For instance, if you are 25 years old and have a health age of 30, you might expect to live the same number of years as the average 30-year-old person (instead of the average 25-year-old). If you are 25 and have a health age of 20, you are better off than the average person your age and can expect to live as long as the average 20-year-old.

Your achievable age was determined by considering your life expectancy in terms of what it would be like should you now reduce all risks possible and continue to follow through on these risk reduction actions in the future. If you are 25 years old, have a health age of 30, and an achievable age of 20, it means you can have the life expectancy of an average 20-year-old rather than a 30-year-old. Your potential gain in life expectancy is shown on the bottom line of this section. NOTE: Your actual age should be added to your life remaining in any category to obtain your total lifespan in that category.

How To Live Longer

Specific actions for you to take to reduce your risks and improve your life expectancy are listed here. Actions are listed in order of decreasing importance with regard to impact on your life expectancy. Please note that the gain shown is entirely dependent on you and what actions you take now and continue to follow through on. These actions generally take one of three forms: 1) eliminating a dangerous habit, such as smoking; 2) starting a healthy habit, like getting regular exercise; or 3) keeping a condition under control, such as high blood pressure or obesity. Most of these actions will not only improve your life expectancy, but allow you to feel better during the rest of your life.

Conclusion

The Health Risk Index does not show all health hazards. It deals only with those that have been studied enough to use in making reasonable predictions regarding their effect on health. Many other hazards are known, but they have not been sufficiently studied to permit reasonable predictive analysis. There are many other hazards that are suspected, and probably many more that are yet unknown. However, health care professionals must use information and tools that are available now in an effort to prevent problems from arising, or keeping problems under control if they are already present. The Health Risk Index is an information tool that you can use to begin taking actions that will reduce your health risks. Health care professionals may assist you in understanding risk reduction techniques, but the motivation to take appropriate action rests with you.

Warranty

Medical Datamation warrants that this report is based on existing techniques for analyzing and applying national mortality statistics in conjunction with hazards contributing to the causes of death. It further warrants that such techniques are generally meaningful in regard to the health risks of individuals. However, Medical Datamation asserts that these techniques are subject to statistical variation, and that particular individuals may experience events differing from those specified in this report. Consequently, Medical Datamation makes no warranties regarding the application of this report to particular individuals or its use for specific purposes.

APPENDIX E: NUTRITION, HEALTH, AND ACTIVITY PROFILE*

Nutrition, Health, and Activity Profile

Introduction

Over the past ten years, researchers in the health field have discovered and re-discovered numerous factors which relate to physical and mental performance, sexual functioning, and aging.

The importance of nutrition has been emphasized. At the same time, however, it has been shown that nutrition alone is just not enough to attain the best possible health. To keep the body functioning at peak performance and to increase resistance to diseases like heart attack and possibly cancer, several other aspects of life-style must be considered as well. Exercise, financial security, general health habits, exposure to pollution, stress, etc., are among these other important factors.

Even if you had all this information for yourself, it would be extremely difficult to evaluate and determine where to start a personal program for better health. As an aid to you and your doctor in overcoming these difficulties, this computerized Nutrition, Health, and Activity Profile was developed. Experts in nutrition, biochemistry, statistics, and exercise collaborated in the design and development of this test to bring you the very latest findings in these areas as they apply to you personally. Your doctor can review the results together with your case history to develop a comprehensive personal health program for you.

This computerized profile will determine your dietary intake of proteins, carbohydrates, fats, vitamins, minerals, fibers, calories, etc., compare them to established requirements, and discuss their meaning and interpretation for your particular case. In fact, each major area of life-style critical to health and longevity will be contrasted with essential requirements for a healthier and longer life. Suggestions will be made for supplemental reading, where necessary, to further clarify important points. For those concerned with losing weight, a safe and sane approach will be discussed for losing extra pounds sensibly and keeping them off permanently. These recommendations can be carefully reviewed by your doctor and modified, as necessary, to suit your life-style.

The knowledge you will gain about your life and your health from the results of this test can play a significant role in your future health and longevity. So please be sure to answer all the questions to the best of your ability.

---

*Both lay people and doctors can take advantage of the Nutrition, Health, and Activity Profile which follows. Lay people are advised to take the analysis to their doctor for best results. Doctors should write for the special Doctor packet on their letterheads.

This is only a sample profile. It cannot be analyzed in its present form. Those desiring a personal analysis may write to Pacific Research Systems, P.O. Box 64218, Los Angeles, CA 90064. The computerized form will be mailed to the student and analyzed for a student rate of $10.00.

Doctor's
Name: _____

Phone
Number: ( ) _____

Doctor's
Address: _____

Number　　　　　Street　　　　　City　　　　　State　　　　　Zip

Name of
Patient: _____

Date of Birth: _____　Sex: _____

Month　　Day　　Year

Pregnant? _____　　　　　Lactating? _____

Occupation: _____

Height: _____ft._____ins.　Weight: _____　Ideal Weight: _____

Number of pounds
you want to lose: _____

Frame
Size: small ( ) medium ( ) large ( )

Are you currently
losing weight ( ), gaining weight, ( )
or staying about the same ( )?

```
For Doctor's
Use Only
[ ] [ ] [ ]
```

There are five sections to complete, each provided with instructions and examples where necessary.

　　—Nutrition I: Important Nutritional Factors
　　—Nutrition II: Food Consumption
　　—Vitamin and Mineral Supplementation
　　—Health Factors
　　—Physical Activities

Be certain to answer the questions as they appear—please do not change any questions and then answer. You may find that this questionnaire does not cover some food or activity that is an important part of your everyday living. You will find spaces provided in each section to write in your additions.

NUTRITION I: IMPORTANT NUTRITIONAL FACTORS

Please answer the questions below as follows:

　A) Complete each square with a numerical response. If you do not know the answer or the question does not apply to you, leave it blank.

　B) Complete each parenthesis with a check ( ) for a "Yes" response. If the answer is "No" or if you do not know the answer, leave it blank.

1. How many cups of the following beverages do you drink per week?

Regular
Coffee ☐   Decaf ☐   Regular
Tea ☐   Low
Calorie ☐
Soft Drinks   Regular
Soft ☐
Drinks

2. Do you use cream with your . . .

Coffee? (   )   Decaf? (   )   Tea? (   )

3. Fill in the number of teaspoons of sugar used with each cup of . . .

Coffee ☐   Decaf ☐   Tea ☐

4. How many teaspoons of sugar do you use with each serving of cereal? ☐

5. Beyond beverages or cereal, how many teaspoons ☐
of sugar do you add to your food per week?

6. Do you use any artificial sweeteners? (i.e., saccharine, sucaryl, etc.)   (   )

7. How many times per week do you eat:

convenience
foods like TV ☐
dinners?   fried
foods? ☐   at hamburger
or taco ☐
stands?   in
restau- ☐
rants?

8. Are you a regular meat eater? (   )   If yes, how is it prepared?

medium to
well done   (   )   rare (   )   very lean (   )   with gravy (   )

9. Do you eat:

less than
average?   (   )   more than
average?   (   )   foods with
extra salt?   (   )   breakfast
5 or more
days per week?   (   )

10. Do you drink tap water? (   )

11. Do you use iodized salt? (   )

In percentage (%) terms, what form of the following two food groups do you consume? The percentage must total 100%.

Example:
If one quarter of your vegetables are frozen, just under three quarters are fresh-cooked, very little are fresh-raw, and none are canned, your numerical response should be:

What percentage of the vegetables that you consume are . . .

Fresh-raw   Fresh-cooked   Frozen   Canned

☐ %   +   ☐ %   +   ☐ %   +   ☐ %   = 100%

---

12. What percentage of the vegetables that you consume are . . .

Fresh-raw		Fresh-cooked		Frozen		Canned		
☐ %	+	☐ %	+	☐ %	+	☐ %	=	100%

13. What percentage of the fruits that you consume are . . .

Fresh-raw		Fresh-cooked		Frozen		Canned		
☐ %	+	☐ %	+	☐ %	+	☐ %	=	100%

NUTRITION II: FOOD CONSUMPTION

Nutrition II lists foods or groups of foods together with serving sizes in parentheses:

Please: 1) For each food you consume, fill in how often you eat the specified serving size under one of the columns: "daily," "weekly," or "monthly." Do not change the specified serving sizes. Fill in only one box under "daily," "weekly," or "monthly" for each food.

2) Leave the line entirely blank if you do not consume the food or foods listed (do not use zeros). Remember, your answers are to represent your nutrition as of now. Do not include any foods which have not been consumed over the past month.

3) If you are certain about how often you eat a given food, just ask yourself how frequently you have eaten it over the last week to two weeks, to a month at most, and answer accordingly. It may be helpful to discuss your answers with someone familiar with your eating habits.

4) Be sure to enter all your snacks as well as regular meals.

To make sure that you don't forget any foods, it may be helpful to write down your intake of food and drink for a week and then check the list again.

Example 1: If you drink 2 cups of whole milk per day, the correct response is:

	Daily	Weekly	Monthly
Whole milk (1 cup)	☐	☐	☐

IMPORTANT: Do not fill in unused boxes with zeros.

Example 2: If you have 3 waffles (3 servings) and six pancakes (2 servings) per week, your answer will be:

	Daily	Weekly	Monthly
Waffle (3), pancakes (2)	☐	☐	☐

IMPORTANT: Fill in one box only - leave the other two blank.

	Daily	Weekly	Monthly
1) Whole milk (1 cup, 8 oz.)	☐	☐	☐
2) Skim/nonfat milk (1 cup, 8 oz.)	☐	☐	☐
3) Low-fat milk (1 cup, 8 oz.)	☐	☐	☐
4) Yogurt (1 cup, 8 oz.)	☐	☐	☐
5) Yogurt, low-fat (1 cup, 8 oz.)	☐	☐	☐
6) Regular cottage cheese (½ cup, 4 oz.)	☐	☐	☐
7) Low-fat cottage cheese (½ cup, 4 oz.)	☐	☐	☐
8) Cream cheese (1 oz.)	☐	☐	☐
9) Sour cream (1 Tbsp., ½ oz.)	☐	☐	☐
10) Other cheeses (1 oz.)	☐	☐	☐
11) Milk shake (16 oz.)	☐	☐	☐
12) Egg (one)	☐	☐	☐
13) Protein powder (1 Tbsp.)	☐	☐	☐
14) White bread (1 slice)	☐	☐	☐
15) Whole wheat bread (1 slice)	☐	☐	☐
16) Corn bread (1 square, 2 oz.)	☐	☐	☐
17) Oatmeal (1 cup)	☐	☐	☐
18) Cereal, wheat germ (½ cup), whole grain (1 cup)	☐	☐	☐
19) Bran (2 Tbsp.)	☐	☐	☐
20) Cereal, hi vitamin (1 cup)	☐	☐	☐
21) Cereals without sugar (1 cup)	☐	☐	☐
22) Cereals, sugared or frosted (1 cup)	☐	☐	☐
23) Waffle (1), pancakes (3, 2½ oz.)	☐	☐	☐

	Daily	Weekly	Monthly
24) French toast (2 slices, 1½ oz.)	☐	☐	☐
25) Sweet roll (one, 1¾ oz.)	☐	☐	☐
26) Muffin or roll (one, 1¾ oz.)	☐	☐	☐
27) Bagel (3" diam., 2 oz.)	☐	☐	☐
28) Spaghetti with meat sauce (1 cup)	☐	☐	☐
29) Spaghetti or macaroni with cheese (1 cup)	☐	☐	☐
30) Macaroni, plain (1 cup)	☐	☐	☐
31) Noodles, egg enriched (1 cup)	☐	☐	☐
32) Pizza (1 slice, 2½ oz.)	☐	☐	☐
33) Brown rice (1 cup)	☐	☐	☐
34) White rice (1 cup)	☐	☐	☐
35) Doughnut, or cupcake (one, 1 oz.)	☐	☐	☐
36) Cake with icing (1 slice, 4 oz.)	☐	☐	☐
37) Cake without icing (1 slice, 4 oz.)	☐	☐	☐
38) Fudge (1 square, 3 oz.)	☐	☐	☐
39) Brownies (1 square, 2 oz.)	☐	☐	☐
40) Pumpkin or custard pie (1 slice, 4 oz.)	☐	☐	☐
41) Any other pie (1 slice, 4 oz.)	☐	☐	☐
42) Ice cream (1½ cup)	☐	☐	☐
43) Cookie (one, 3" diam., ½ oz.)	☐	☐	☐
44) Butter (1 Tbsp., ½ oz.)	☐	☐	☐
45) Margarine (1 Tbsp., ½ oz.)	☐	☐	☐
46) Vegetable oil (1 Tbsp., ½ oz.)	☐	☐	☐

	Daily	Weekly	Monthly		Daily	Weekly	Monthly
47) Salad dressing Thousand/French (2 Tbsp., 1 oz.)	☐	☐	☐	70) Sardines (3 oz.)	☐	☐	☐
48) Italian dressing (2 Tbsp., 1 oz.)	☐	☐	☐	71) Tuna, swordfish (3 oz.)	☐	☐	☐
49) Roquefort/Blue cheese (2 Tbsp., 1 oz.)	☐	☐	☐	72) Other fish (3 oz.)	☐	☐	☐
50) Steak (6 oz.)	☐	☐	☐	73) Soybeans (½ cup)	☐	☐	☐
51) Hamburger (one, 3 oz.)	☐	☐	☐	74) Tofu (½ cup)	☐	☐	☐
52) Hot dog (one regular size)	☐	☐	☐	75) Lima, Kidney, navy beans (½ cup)	☐	☐	☐
53) Taco, tamale, tostada (one)	☐	☐	☐	76) Green beans (½ cup)	☐	☐	☐
54) Chicken, duck, fowl (6 oz.)	☐	☐	☐	77) Bean sprouts (1 cup)	☐	☐	☐
55) Lamb, beef (6 oz.)	☐	☐	☐	78) Avocado (½ large, 4 oz.)	☐	☐	☐
56) Pork, ham (5 oz.)	☐	☐	☐	79) Olives, ripe (10, 2 oz.)	☐	☐	☐
57) Pork sausage (3 oz.)	☐	☐	☐	80) Asparagus (6 spears, 3½ oz.)	☐	☐	☐
58) Bacon (2 slices, ½ oz.)	☐	☐	☐	81) Broccoli (½ cup)	☐	☐	☐
59) Veal (4 oz.)	☐	☐	☐	82) Beets (½ cup)	☐	☐	☐
60) Corned beef (4 oz.)	☐	☐	☐	83) Cabbage (½ cup)	☐	☐	☐
61) Beef liver (3½ oz.)	☐	☐	☐	84) Peas, brussels sprouts, rutabagas (½ cup)	☐	☐	☐
62) Chicken liver (3½ oz.)	☐	☐	☐	85) Sauerkraut, eggplant (½ cup)	☐	☐	☐
63) Organ meat, kidney, heart etc. (3½ oz.)	☐	☐	☐	86) Spinach, chard, mustard greens (½ cup)	☐	☐	☐
64) Liverwurst, liver pate (2 oz.)	☐	☐	☐	87) Cucumbers radishes (½ cup)	☐	☐	☐
65) Other luncheon meats or sausages (2 oz.)	☐	☐	☐	88) Kale, carrot-pea mix (½ cup)	☐	☐	☐
66) Chicken, beef pot pie (1, 8 oz.)	☐	☐	☐	89) Turnips, kohlrabi (½ cup)	☐	☐	☐
67) Oysters, clams (6 oz.)	☐	☐	☐	90) Carrots (½ cup)	☐	☐	☐
68) Shrimp, crab, lobster (3 oz.)	☐	☐	☐	91) Celery (1 stalk)	☐	☐	☐
69) Salmon (3 oz.)	☐	☐	☐	92) Corn (1 ear or ½ cup)	☐	☐	☐
				93) Mushrooms (¼ cup)	☐	☐	☐

	Daily	Weekly	Monthly			Daily	Weekly	Monthly
94) Tomatoes (½ cup)	☐	☐	☐	119) Almonds, other nuts (½ cup)		☐	☐	☐
95) Tomato juice (1 cup)	☐	☐	☐	120) Milk chocolate, candy bar (2 oz.)		☐	☐	☐
96) V-8 juice (1 cup)	☐	☐	☐	121) Jam, jelly, honey, syrup (2 Tbsp.)		☐	☐	☐
97) Squash (½ cup)	☐	☐	☐	122) Potato chips (10 2" Diam.)		☐	☐	☐
98) Artichoke (1 large)	☐	☐	☐	123) Wine (1 glass, 4 oz.)		☐	☐	☐
99) Cauliflower (½ cup)	☐	☐	☐	124) Scotch, whiskey, gin, etc. (1 oz.)		☐	☐	☐
100) Green pepper (½ large)	☐	☐	☐	125) Drink mixer, sweet (1 glass, 8 oz.)		☐	☐	☐
101) Onions, raw (¼ cup, 2 oz.)	☐	☐	☐	126) Cola drink (12 oz.) Not low calorie		☐	☐	☐
102) Lettuce (⅛ head)	☐	☐	☐	127) Other soft drink (12 oz.) Not low calorie		☐	☐	☐
103) Potato (1 med.) mashed (½ cup)	☐	☐	☐	128) Beer (12 oz.)		☐	☐	☐
104) French fries (10 pieces, 2 oz.)	☐	☐	☐	129) Orange or grapefruit juice (½ cup, 4 oz.)		☐	☐	☐
105) Coleslaw (½ cup)	☐	☐	☐	130) Orange (1 med.) grapefruit (½ med.)		☐	☐	☐
106) Bean soup (1 cup)	☐	☐	☐	131) Peaches, canned (½ cup)		☐	☐	☐
107) Chicken soup (1 cup)	☐	☐	☐	132) Peach, fresh (1 mcd.)		☐	☐	☐
108) Vegetable soup (1 cup)	☐	☐	☐	133) Apricot, canned (½ cup)		☐	☐	☐
109) Beef & vegetable soup (1 cup)	☐	☐	☐	134) Apricot, fresh (3 med.)		☐	☐	☐
110) Clam chowder (1 cup)	☐	☐	☐	135) Applesauce (½ cup)		☐	☐	☐
111) Tomato soup (1 cup)	☐	☐	☐	136) Apple juice (½ cup, 4 oz.)		☐	☐	☐
112) Split pea soup (1 cup)	☐	☐	☐	137) Apple, pear canned (½ cup)		☐	☐	☐
113) Other creamed soup (1 cup)	☐	☐	☐	138) Apple, pear, fresh (1 med.)		☐	☐	☐
114) Crackers (2 med.)	☐	☐	☐	139) Pineapple (½ cup)		☐	☐	☐
115) Popcorn, popped (1 cup)	☐	☐	☐	140) Strawberries, fresh (½ cup)		☐	☐	☐
116) Peanuts (⅓ cup), peanut butter (5 Tbsp.)	☐	☐	☐	141) Other berries, fresh (½ cup)		☐	☐	☐
117) Sunflower seeds (½ cup)	☐	☐	☐					
118) Pecans, walnuts (½ cup)	☐	☐	☐					

	Daily	Weekly	Monthly			Daily	Weekly	Monthly
142) Berries, canned (½ cup)	☐	☐	☐	147) Raisins (¼ cup)	☐	☐	☐
143) Banana (1 med.)	☐	☐	☐	148) Grapes (½ cup)	☐	☐	☐
144) Cantaloupe (½ med.)	☐	☐	☐	149) Lecithin granules (1 Tbsp.)	☐	☐	☐
145) Dates, dried (½ cup)	☐	☐	☐	150) Brewers yeast (1 Tbsp.)	☐	☐	☐
146) Papaya, fresh (½ med.)	☐	☐	☐	151) Bone meal (½ Tsp.)	☐	☐	☐

Additional Foods

Please write in the names and serving sizes of any additional foods that you eat at least twice monthly

Food	Serving size	Daily	Weekly	Monthly
152) _____ _____		☐	☐	☐
153) _____ _____		☐	☐	☐
154) _____ _____		☐	☐	☐
155) _____ _____		☐	☐	☐
156) _____ _____		☐	☐	☐
157) _____ _____		☐	☐	☐
158) _____ _____		☐	☐	☐
159) _____ _____		☐	☐	☐
160) _____ _____		☐	☐	☐

Vitamin and Mineral Supplementation

Check (✔) the supplements that you presently use.

Blank spaces are provided for your additions.

(1)	Multivitamin with minerals	( )
(2)	Multivitamin (only)	( )
(3)	Multimineral (only)	( )
(4)	Vitamin B-complex	( )
(5)	Vitamin A	( )
(6)	Vitamin C	( )
(7)	Vitamin E	( )
(8)	Calcium	( )
(9)	Magnesium	( )
_____		_____
_____		_____

(10) How long have you been taking the supplements checked above?

more than 1 year ( )
more than 3 mos. ( )
less than 3 mos. ( )

HEALTH FACTORS

Please answer the questions below with the usual check (✔) for a "Yes" response. If the answer is "No" or you do not know the answer, leave it blank.

1) Have you had a medical examination in the past 6 months? ( )

2) Do you have high blood pressure? ( )

3) Do you know your blood triglyceride level? ( )

4) Do you know your blood cholesterol level? ( )

5) Do you have a tendency to get ulcers? ( )

6) Is there a history of diabetes in your family? ( )

7) Is there a history of cancer in your family? ( )

8) Is there a history of heart disease in your family? ( )

9) Is there a history of respiratory ailments in your family? ( )

10) In your personal life, are you often under stress? ( )

11) At work, are you often under stress? ( )

12) Do you take a drink before you do something important? ( )

13) Do you often go 3 or more days without alcohol? ( )

14) Do you take any form of tranquilizers? ( )

15) Have you had a dental check-up in the past year? ( )

16) Do you drink diet beverages regularly? ( )

17) Will you or do you have a monthly income for retirement other than social security? ( )

18) Physically, are you often tired, sluggish? ( )

19) Physically, do you feel average, could be better? ( )

20) Physically, do you feel full of energy? ( )

21) Is your stamina poor? ( )

22) Is your stamina average? ( )

23) Is your stamina excellent? ( )

24) Do you get enough sleep (7–8 hours)? ( )

25) Are you most often in a good mood and at ease with the world? ( )

26) Are you often depressed and moody? ( )

27) Is your mood mostly average? ( )

28) Do you smoke cigarettes? ( )

29) Do you often spend time in closed rooms with cigarette smokers? ( )

30) Do you live in highly polluted air? ( )

31) Do you work in highly polluted air? ( )

32) Do you use air purifiers where needed? ( )

33) Do you take any drugs on a regular basis? ( )

PHYSICAL ACTIVITIES
PART A

The profile is designed to provide information on the calories burned during physical activity. Those activities you are now doing are to be entered in part A below. Part B provides spaces for activities you are not doing but would like to do. If you indicated a desire to lose weight on page one of this questionnaire, the calories burned from the activities of both parts A and B will be properly combined to help meet your goal. But you must specify at least two physical activities.

From the Activity Table below, please select physical activities in which you are now (this season) participating. Select only those which you are doing at least twice a month and place their numbers in the squares provided after the example. Be sure to complete each line for the selected activity indicating, in the appropriate square provided, how many minutes you spend each day, week, or month at that activity. Please do not include any activities which are part of your daily work routine. A few spaces are provided for you to add more entries in the Activity Table, if necessary.

For example, if you jog for 15 minutes a week and practice yoga 15 minutes each morning, your response should be:

Activity Number	Daily	Weekly In Minutes	Monthly
☐	☐	☐	☐
☐	☐	☐	☐

IMPORTANT: On each line, fill in an activity number plus the time spent. Use only one box from the "daily", "weekly" or "monthly" columns.

	Activity Number		Daily	Weekly in Minutes	Monthly		Activity Number		Daily	Weekly in Minutes	Monthly
1.	☐		☐	☐	☐	6.	☐		☐	☐	☐
2.	☐		☐	☐	☐	7.	☐		☐	☐	☐
3.	☐		☐	☐	☐	8.	☐		☐	☐	☐
4.	☐		☐	☐	☐	9.	☐		☐	☐	☐
5.	☐		☐	☐	☐	10.	☐		☐	☐	☐

ACTIVITY TABLE

1. Back packing with heavy pack
2. Baseball
3. Basketball
4. Bicycling, slow
5. Bicycling, fast
6. Bowling
7. Boxing
8. Boxing (punching bag)
9. Calisthenics/Tai Chi
10. Canoeing, slow
11. Canoeing, fast
12. Climbing stairs
13. Dancing, slow
14. Dancing, vigorous
15. Fencing
16. Football, tackle
17. Football, touch
18. Gardening
19. Golf
20. Handball
21. Hockey, ice
22. Hockey, field
23. Horseback riding
24. Horse vaulting
25. Horseshoes
26. Housework
27. Hunting
28. Isometrics
29. Jai Alai
30. Jogging (over eight minutes per mile)
31. Karate
32. Motorcycling
33. Mountain climbing
34. Parallel bars

35. Polo
36. Racquetball
37. Rugby
38. Running (under eight minutes per mile)
39. Shuffleboard
40. Skating, ice
41. Skating, roller
42. Skiing, snow
43. Skiing, cross country
44. Skiing, water
45. Skin diving
46. Soccer
47. Softball
48. Squash
49. Surfing
50. Swimming, competitive

51. Swimming, recreational
52. Tennis, singles
53. Tennis, doubles
54. Volleyball
55. Walking, slow
56. Walking, moderate
57. Walking, fast
58. Water polo
59. Weight lifting
60. Yoga/Akido
61. Working out in a gym or spa with varied equipment
62. _____
63. _____
64. _____

PART B

Referring again to the Activity Table, please select physical activities that meet all of the following requirements:

—you are not now doing them
—the activities are currently in season
—you would enjoy doing these activities and could do them in your present state of health
—the activities are both practical and convenient for your personal circumstances and environment.

Place the numbers which correspond to the selected activities in the squares provided below. Do not include any activities listed above in Section A.

1. ☐   2. ☐   3. ☐   4. ☐

5. ☐   6. ☐   7. ☐   8. ☐

NUTRITION HEALTH AND ACTIVITY PROFILE
OF MR AMERICAN ANY STREET

This profile is designed for you personally and is meant to be your guide to much improved health. Thousands of error free calculations have been made to determine the average daily level of key nutrients in your diet. These results along with your health habits have been compared with standards adjusted for your own personal characteristics. Wherever appropriate, easy to understand explanations and suggestions are offered to help you make the changes necessary to avoid disease and to attain your best possible health.

THE CONTENTS OF YOUR PROFILE

   I. Your intake of protein, fat, fiber and carbohydrate
  II. Understanding your need for vitamins, minerals, and other nutrients
 III. Your food vitamin/mineral content vs the RDA (Recommended Daily Allowance)
 IV. Your vitamins and minerals below RDA and corresponding good food sources
  V. Further nutritional considerations
 VI. Other critical health factors *Stress, smoking, dental care, air polution, lack money –*
VII. The importance of exercise and an analysis of your current program
VIII. Suggested weight loss program
 IX. Conclusions
  X. Doctor's summary page

I. PROTEIN

There are two standards against which your intake of protein can be compared. The first standard, the RDA (Recommended Daily Allowance), suggests 109.1 grams per day for you. It is based solely on your weight and does not take into account whether you are over or under weight, very active or sedentary. The second standard, a more precise method of estimating your protein requirement, is based on caloric expenditure and recommends that your intake be between 68.6 and 87.0 grams per day.* (Scrimshaw—*The New England Jl. of Medicine,* Jan. 22, 1976)

Even slightly more protein may be needed if you are very active or have low absorption or when disorders like hypoglycemia exist. Just be sure your intake of complex carbohydrates are not sacrificed for increased protein. (For a detailed discussion of the relative importance of all the nutrients and health factors read Dr. Kugler's *Seven Keys to a Longer Life*—H. Kugler, Ph.D.)

Your total protein from all food sources averages 95.6 grams per day.

Protein is one of the most important nutrients the body requires for maintaining good health. Protein from different sources is comprised of varying amounts of different amino acids. There are about 22 different amino acids which can form a protein. They have been classified as essential and non-essential.

Foods rich in all the essential amino acids are eggs, cheese, meat, poultry and fish. When one or more of these foods are present at each meal and comprise more than 50 percent of your protein intake, specific amino acid deficiencies are much less likely. Each meal should be comprised of foods that individually or taken together are rich in all the essential amino acids to assure good nutrition. This task is particularly difficult if your diet is restricted to vegetables and grains only.

FATS

The average American diet derives about 40% of its calories or energy from fat. Experts in heart disease and diseases of the arteries agree that an across the board recommendation to lower fat intake would benefit the majority of people. Some experts feel fat should be about 34% while others feel it should be as low as 10%. A range of 20 to 34% seems reasonable (atherosclerosis, Medcom).

53.5% of the calories in your diet come from fats.

---

* Calculations include a 20% excess.

Reduced consumption of animal source fats such as gravies, fatty sauces, fried foods, whole milk, butter, oils and fats is advisable when your overall fat intake is high.

Fat intake can influence serum cholesterol and triglycerides, the fat in the blood. Studies have shown a high correlation between coronary heart disease and increased triglyceride levels. This is one important reason for seeing your doctor regularly and having these factors checked. Your doctor can interpret the results and/or you can read Richard Passwater's book, *Supernutrition for Healthy Hearts,* for a detailed explanation.

With respect to heart disease, there are two important fractions of cholesterol in the blood, HDL and LDL. The HDL fraction should be high and the LDL fraction should be low. Good exercise, especially of the endurance type, like running, can change these values for the better.

Learn your present cholesterol and triglyceride levels, check them on a regular basis, keep a running written record and watch for any changes.

Serum cholesterol levels of about 170 to 190 or lower and triglyceride levels of about 100 or lower are desirable. Some experts accept values slightly higher; others feel even lower levels are desirable. Often if one is high, so is the other. Should these values be high, achieving normal values is very important. Some of the factors that can greatly help to normalize these important indicators of heart disease risk are: achieving normal weight, carefully increased exercise, lowering fat intake, and being sure you have no vitamin/mineral deficiencies. Fiber (discussed later on) also helps in lowering cholesterol levels (Trowell, H. C., *Amer. Journal of Clinical Nutrition,* 25:464, 1972).

It is possible for a person with a high fat intake to have normal triglycerides. In most cases this will not be so. In any event do not go to extremes, you may have a disorder requiring medical treatment.

There is, of course, a need for some essential fatty acids. The most important of these is linoleic acid. It plays a very important role in maintaining proper cholesterol metabolism, hormonal control, the development of new cells and the maintenance of healthy body tissues, particularly of the skin, liver and kidneys. Your average daily linoleic acid intake is 9.5 grams.

According to the latest studies, a daily intake of 3 to 5 grams is desirable. You may fulfill this need by taking only 1 teaspoon to 1 tablespoon daily of a rich source of unsaturated fatty acids such as sunflower seed oil, safflower oil or corn oil. Sunflower seed oil is also richer in vitamin E than safflower oil or corn oil, which gives it an added plus. Such oils should be refrigerated and sealed tightly, when not in use, to protect from rancidity.

Note: Increased exercise, especially endurance type exercises, increases the need for polyunsaturates.

FIBER

Fibers are recognized as important substances in the daily diet. Researchers have shown that a diet high in fiber helps prevent cancer of the colon and disorders of the digestive tract (Burkitt). No minimum daily requirements have been established. Experts consulted on the issue have indicated that 6 grams per day is a minimal amount for your weight range. Your average daily fiber intake was 2.5 grams which is too low. Consider dietary changes geared to increasing your fiber intake.

Foods rich in natural fibers are bran, whole wheat, other whole grain products, fruits and vegetables, especially in the raw state.

CARBOHYDRATES

Nutritionists often refer to carbohydrates as refined (sugar, white flour, etc.) and complex (carbohydrates in the natural state as found in vegetables, whole grain products, etc.). Foods which are usually high in refined carbohydrates are ice cream, candy, white flour, cakes, soft drinks, etc. The ratio of refined carbohydrates to total carbohydrates should be kept as low as possible.

Refined carbohydrates, in excessive quantities, may have drug-like activity, cause tooth decay, lower blood sugar, cause overweight and take the place of important nutrients. They are also suspect in a host of other disorders. However, these foods in very small quantities are not considered to be harmful as long as all other nutritional requirements are fulfilled.

Even though experts have not yet established guidelines for refined carbohydrates, an intake greater than 30% such as your intake of 80% seems too high. In fact your daily intake is equal to the calories from 43 teaspoons of sugar. Including alcohol, it is 54 teaspoons of sugar daily on average.

Experts recommend moderation in carbohydrate consumption for people, such as yourself, who show a history of diabetes in their family. Be sure and follow the doctor's advice on this topic.

	Refined carbohydrates you eat at least once per week (servings/week)
Scotch, Gin, Vodka, etc. (1 oz.)	12
Drink mixers, sweet (8 oz.)	12
White Bread (1 slice)	14
Ice cream (½ cup)	2
Potato chips (10)	1
Cola drink (12 oz.)	14
Beer (12 oz.)	3
Doughnut, cupcake (one, 1 oz.)	1
Cookie (one, 3 ins., diam.)	4
Pizza (1 slice, 2.5 oz.)	2

II. UNDERSTANDING YOUR NEEDS FOR VITAMINS, MINERALS AND OTHER NUTRIENTS

Listed in the table below are the latest Recommended Daily Allowances (RDA) set forth on certain nutrients by the United States Food and Drug Administration (FDA) in 1976. Asterisks, appearing in the RDA column above, mean that no RDA has yet been established for that nutrient. The RDA represents what the FDA considers to be an estimated approximate need for a healthy population.

The RDA values have been revised over the years to try to keep abreast of the latest nutritional knowledge. Many nutritionists recommend higher daily intake for many of these nutrients when a person has not been getting complete nutrition on a regular basis. Differences in metabolism, weight, lifestyle and other factors also have an effect on vitamin and mineral requirements. Therefore you might require more of some of these nutrients. The RDA should only serve as a yardstick against which your daily nutrition may be contrasted for about one half of the known essential nutrients. Remember, a very large excess of fat soluble vitamins, like vitamin A, may cause toxicity effects.

There are several circumstances which may greatly elevate the need for one or more of these or other essential nutrients. Some of these circumstances are:

1. Environmental factors—air pollution, alcohol intake, cigarette smoking, stress, polluted water, food contaminants, taking birth control pills, etc., are but a few environmental factors that can greatly change and/or elevate many of your nutritional requirements.

2. Decline in food quality—the nutritional quality of food has declined substantially in this century, with the advent of white flour, refined sugar and extracted oils, according to Dr. H. Rosenberg M.D., and A. N. Feldzamen, Ph. D., writing in their text, *The Doctor's Book of Vitamin Therapy.*

White flour was first produced to prevent spoilage and increase shelf life without realizing the nutritional ramifications. Years later, alarmed by the sad state of our national health, the government instituted a mandatory enrichment program for the flour used in bread.

Refining flour removes at least 22 known nutrients including vitamin E and most of the B complex vitamins as well as important oils and minerals. Enrichment, on the other hand, replaces only four nutrients: vitamin B1 (thiamine), vitamin B2 (riboflavin), vitamin B3 (niacin) and iron.

Consumption of large quantities of refined foods can substantially increase the need for many essential nutrients to maintain health. Obviously, whole grain products should be eaten in preference to ones made of refined flour and fresh vegetables should be used instead of canned ones. Note that whole grain products have a shorter shelf life and can be more harmful when stale or rancid than products made from refined flour, so be sure they are fresh before you eat them.

3. Attainment of your best state of health. To attain your best possible state of health frequently requires higher levels than the RDA values for several nutrients, especially after an illness, an extended period of stress or for physically very active people.

The vitamin question is far from being completely resolved. While some nutritionists feel a balanced diet will supply all the vitamins and minerals needed, others like Prof. Cheraskin, Chairman of the Department of Oral Medicine at Alabama School of Medicine, tell us our needs might be much higher. Prof. Cheraskin recently conducted a study on humans and concluded that the amounts of vitamin A, C and niacin needed by the average person for best health may be 4 to 6 times the RDA (Meeting of the International Academy of Preventive Medicine, Los Angeles, September 1975).

III. YOUR FOOD VITAMIN AND MINERAL CONTENT VERSUS RDA

(Daily intake below does not include Vitamin/Mineral supplements)

Vitamins	Daily intake	U.S. RDA	PCT of RDA	Currently takes this Vitamin
Vitamin A (int units)	11407.0	5000.0	228.1	Yes
Vitamin C (mgs)	34.0	60.0	56.7	Yes
Vitamin E (int units)	4.7	30.0	15.6	No
Vitamin B1 (mgs) Thiamine	0.4	1.5	29.0	No
Vitamin B2 (mgs) Riboflavin	1.2	1.7	72.1	No
Vitamin B3 (mgs) Niacin	21.1	20.0	105.6	No
Vitamin B6 (mgs) Pyridoxine	1.0	2.0	49.5	No
Folacin (mcgs) Folic acid	91.0	400.0	23.0	No
Vitamin B12 (mcg)	9.0	6.0	150.8	No
Pantothenic Acid (mgs)	4.5	10.0	45.2	No
Biotin (mcgs)	38.7	300.0	12.9	No
Choline (mgs)	388.0	* * * * *	* * * * *	—
Inositol (mgs)	149.0	* * * * *	* * * * *	—

Minerals	Daily intake	U.S. RDA	PCT of RDA	Currently takes this Mineral
Calcium (mgs)	629.0	1000.0	62.9	No
Phosphorus (mgs)	1848.0	1000.0	184.9	No
* * Calcium and phosphorus are out of balance.				
Magnesium (mgs)	98.0	400.0	24.7	No
Iron (mgs)	12.4	18.0	68.9	No
Copper (mgs)	0.3	2.0	13.3	No
Zinc (mgs)	8.4	15.0	55.7	No
Iodine (mcgs) in food only	11.0	150.0	7.9	No
Manganese (mgs)	0.3	* * * * *		
Potassium (mgs)	1879	* * * * *	* * * * * *	
Sodium (mgs) in food only	3434	* * * * *	* * * * * *	
Fluorine (mcg)	520	* * * * *	* * * * * *	

Iodine concentration in foods varies widely depending on their origin. We have been conservative in establishing your intake from foods. It is important to provide some dietary insurance against a possible deficiency by using kelp or by using iodized salt sparingly.

* * Your dietary intake of phosphorus is more than twice that of calcium which can lead to mineral loss, muscle spasms, and even hyperparathyroidism.

Since your calcium intake is below the recommended daily allowance, consider increasing your intake of foods richer in calcium than phosphorus such as swiss cheese, cheddar cheese, american cheese, milk (preferably non-fat milk), kale, mustard or dandelion greens and watercress.

Phosphorus intake should be reduced. The foods containing large amounts of phosphorus and little or no calcium are grains and meats.

Note: increased physical activity also slightly increases your vitamin and mineral needs.

IV. YOUR VITAMINS/MINERALS BELOW THE RDA

Your dietary intake of the following nutrients is below the RDA, however, you are supplementing these nutrients. Supplements can be a form of dietary insurance but you should fix your diet so it provides adequate amounts of these essential nutrients from foods. To help you bolster those nutrients in your diet that are below the RDA, rich food sources have been listed below.

If you have any food allergies or other nutrition-related disorders, you might want to check with your doctor before using any new foods in your diet.

Vitamins	Daily intake	U.S. RDA	PCT of RDA	Currently takes this Vitamin
Vitamin A (int units)	11407.0	5000.0	228.1	Yes
Vitamin C (mgs)	34.0	60.0	56.7	Yes
Vitamin E (int units)	4.7	30.0	15.6	No
Vitamin B1 (mgs) Thiamine	0.4	1.5	29.0	No

Vitamins	Daily intake	U.S. RDA	PCT of RDA	Currently takes this Vitamin
Vitamin B2 (mgs)				
Riboflavin	1.2	1.7	72.1	No
Vitamin B3 (mgs)				
Niacin	21.1	20.0	105.6	No
Vitamin B6 (mgs)				
Pyridoxine	1.0	2.0	49.5	No
Folacin (mcgs)				
Folic acid	91.0	400.0	23.0	No
Vitamin B12 (mcgs)	9.0	6.0	150.8	No
Pantothenic				
Acid (mgs)	4.5	10.0	45.2	No
Biotin (mcgs)	38.7	300.0	12.9	No
Choline (mgs)	388.0	* * * * *	* * * * *	
Inositol (mgs)	149.0	* * * * *	* * * * *	

Minerals	Daily intake	U.S. RDA	PCT of RDA	Currently takes this Mineral
Calcium (mgs)	629.0	1000.0	62.9	No
Phosphorus (mgs)	1848.0	1000.0	184.9	No
* * Calcium and Phosphorus are out of balance.				
Magnesium (mgs)	98.0	400.0	24.7	No
Iron (mgs)	12.4	18.0	68.9	No
Copper (mgs)	0.3	2.0	13.3	No
Zinc (mgs)	8.4	15.0	55.7	No
Iodine (mcgs)				
in food only	11.0	150.0	7.9	No
Manganese (mgs)	0.3	* * * * *	* * * * * *	
Potassium (mgs)	1879.0	* * * * *	* * * * * *	
Sodium (mgs)				
in food only	3434.0	* * * * *	* * * * * *	
Fluorine (mcgs)	520.0	* * * * *	* * * * * *	

Has taken supplements above more than 1 year.

Health factors:

1 Diabetes in family	2 Heart disease in family	3 Lives/works in pollution
4 Under stress	5 Physically sluggish	6 Stamina poor
7 Smokes cigarettes	8 No retirement security	9 Drinks tap water

Good Food Sources

Nutrient below RDA: Vitamin C (brussel sprouts, broccoli, cantaloupe, strawberries, green vegetables, and citrus fruit or juice).

Adding iodized salt to food, as you do, provides insurance against a deficiency of iodine.

Your dietary intake of the following nutrients is below the RDA and you have not indicated you are taking food supplements which could compensate for these needs. Continued long term intake below the RDA may lead to illnesses. Be sure to work at bolstering your intake of these nutrients. Study the table below and the corresponding list of foods rich in that nutrient.

Remember, if you have any food allergies or other nutrition-related disorders, you might want to check with your doctor before using any new foods in your diet.

Good Food Sources

Nutrient
below RDA

Vitamin E	sunflower seed oil, wheat germ oil, wheat germ
Vitamin B1	brewers yeast, split peas, sunflower seeds
Vitamin B2	liver, organ meats, mushrooms, milk (preferably non-homogenized), brewers yeast
Vitamin B6	brewers yeast, molasses, salmon, liver, wheat bran
Folic acid	liver, lima beans, cantaloupe, chicken, beef, whole wheat bread, asparagus, brewers yeast
Pantothenic acid	organ meats, eggs, peanuts, wheat bran, wheat germ, mushrooms, broccoli, beef and brewers yeast
Biotin	organ meats, peanuts, eggs, cauliflower, mushrooms, and molasses
Calcium and phosphorus	are plentiful and in good balance in milk (preferably non-homogenized), cheese, dark green leafy vegetables
Magnesium	wheat germ, almonds, peanuts, green vegetables, eggs, bran (in small amts, large amts can increase calcium reqd)
Iron	liver, meats, eggs, lentils, mushrooms, sunflower seeds
Copper	oysters, liver, whole wheat, oats, dry beans, avocado, molasses and apricots
Zinc	oysters, herring, oatmeal, sunflower and pumpkin seeds, brewers yeast, liver, eggs

While there are many other foods which may be good or even better dietary sources of one or more isolated nutrients, we have attempted to select foods which are readily available, balanced with respect to other nutrients, free from special preparation requirements and have a reasonable storage life.

You may also wish to take a good vitamin and mineral supplement to bolster these nutrients. If so, be sure to discuss the quantities with your doctor.

V. FURTHER NUTRITIONAL CONSIDERATIONS

An intake of 1 or 2 cups of coffee and/or tea per day or even less is advised by experts. Tentative research findings have linked caffeine to several disorders. Consider reducing your intake of 70 cups per week (Professor Jean Mayer, Harvard, *Los Angeles Times,* June 10, 1976).

One third or more of your meals are eaten away from home or are convenience foods. The freshness and nutritional quality of these foods is not comparable to that of a freshly prepared meal at home. If you must eat out frequently, or really hate to cook, try to find restaurants that serve fresh raw vegetables and/or begin to fix them yourself. It takes less time than cooking and provides many nutrients vital to your health and well being.

0 percent of your vegetables are consumed in the fresh, raw state. Using fresh raw vegetables increases roughage and promotes healthy elimination of waste products (see discussion of fibers above).

95 percent of the fruit you consume is fresh which is important since large amounts of sugar have been added to canned and frozen fruit. Keep it up.

Drinking tap water, as you do, may be a health hazard. Impurities in tap water are under investigation as possible contributing factors toward cancer and heart disease. Even though this is not 100% established, some caution seems advisable. Consider purchasing good well water or attaching a filter to your water faucet.

It is important to be sure you get an adequate supply of iodine daily. This can easily be accomplished through sparing use of iodized salt. Be sure to use salt in moderation since too much can cause high blood pressure and other problems.

VI. OTHER CRITICAL HEALTH FACTORS

Nutrition is important but it alone is not enough to achieve a healthier and longer life; several good health habits must be considered. At the UCLA School of Public Health seven good health habits were studied with respect to average life spans and it was found that there could be a difference of at least 12.5 years between doing things right or wrong.

When approximately the same 7 major good health habits were investigated in another study, it was found that only about 3 to 5% of all people came reasonably close to doing things right in all these major health habits (H. Kugler, Ph. D., meeting of the International Academy of Preventive Medicine, Denver, March 1976).

To protect your health, a check up at least once a year is advisable. Be sure to have your blood serum cholesterol and triglycerides tested, as discussed above in the section on fats. Record these values together with your blood pressure each time you have them measured. Watch for any changes that may occur. Should there be a change, be sure to discuss it with your doctor.

It is also important to have regular dental checkups every six months or at least once per year.

Stress can adversely affect your health and your daily life. However, you can learn to deal with it more effectively through consultation and improved nutrition.

Discuss your work stress situation with your fellow workers. Analyze the situation carefully and try to resolve it.

It is very important to be aware of the adverse effects of stress on your health and life. If you can not resolve your stress situation or would like to know more about this subject, there is an excellent paperback book by the authority on stress, Dr. Hans Selye, called *Stress Without Distress.*

Since there is a history of heart disease in your family, it is very important to correct faulty health habits, including environmental factors. These aspects of life are believed to be major contributors to cancer and heart disease.

Smoking cigarettes, as you do, is considered, by most experts, to have a very high risk of triggering cancer or heart disease. Further, it has been associated with premature aging, i. e., increased wrinkle formation and, in some cases, impotence in men due to the potential hormone lowering effect. For your long term health and well being, it is of great importance to stop smoking. If you try or have tried and have difficulty stopping, seek out one of the several organizations that help people break the habit.

The effect of air pollution is well established. It contributes to cancer, heart disease and emphysema. Consider installing air purifiers where the pollution is very high to protect yourself.

Lack of money has proven to be a major obstacle in the successful aging of the average American. Look into setting up an independent retirement account to be sure you do not face your advanced years with financial pressure.

Improved health habits of nutrition and exercise may significantly improve your physical well being and your mood too.

The role of food, exercise and other key health factors is explained in more detail by Dr. Kugler in his new book, *Dr. Kugler's Seven Keys to a Longer Life.*

VII. THE IMPORTANCE OF EXERCISE

You consume 3230 calories daily, on average. Calories, as you may know, are a measure of energy. Foods provide this energy which the body burns through performance of routine tasks and especially through vigorous exercise. By decreasing caloric intake and also increasing physical activities, the body can shed unwanted extra pounds. In fact, if sugar or refined carbohydrate intake were reduced 1 tablespoonful per day and fat intake also reduced 1 tablespoonful, you could lose approximately a half pound per week.

Experts have shown regular exercise to be a key link to longevity and essential to the attainment of your best possible state of health. So, it makes sense, in planning any weight reduction program to couple a regular exercise regimen with caloric food restrictions.

No recommended level of caloric intake is provided since your individual requirements depend on factors such as stress, environment, unique biochemical needs, etc. Further, it is not usually advisable that anyone try to lose more than 2 pounds per week or lower their caloric intake below 1200 calories per day without first consulting a doctor.

Your current exercises plus the exercises you want to add, if any, are listed below together with their corresponding caloric expenditure information.

Physical Activities

Exercise	Current weekly activity in min.	Calories burned in 10 min. exercise	Caloric expenditure per week
1 Jogging (over 8 min./mile)	60	113	680
2 Tennis, singles	60	71	425
3 Handball	0	129	0
4 Working out w. varied eqpt	0	50	0

Weekly total: 1105

VIII. SUGGESTED WEIGHT LOSS PROGRAM

A weight loss goal of 1.4 pounds per week is suggested. At this rate, you should lose your unwanted 45 pound(s) in 32 week(s), provided you are a normally healthy person. Remember that 3500 calories less per week coming from restricted food intake and/or increased physical activity will result in losing one more pound each week.

Your goal can be achieved through caloric restriction and increased physical activity equal to a total of 4886 calories per week.

Eating half as much of the refined carbohydrate foods listed in the table below will contribute 3263 calories to your total weekly goal. The balance of 1623 calories must be burned up by your exercise program. One such program is presented in the suggested physical activities table displayed following the foods table.

Foods for you to avoid	No. of servings you now eat per week	Calories saved if you eat half as much
1 Scotch, gin, vodka, etc. (1 oz.)	12	420
2 Cola drinks (12 oz.)	14	959
3 Drink mixers, sweet (8 oz.)	12	420
4 Beer (12 oz.)	3	257
5 White bread (1 slice)	14	427
6 Doughnut, cupcake (one, 1 oz.)	1	68
7 Ice cream (½ cup)	2	150
8 Cookie (one, 3 ins., diam.)	4	288
9 Potato chips (10)	1	64
10 Pizza (1 slice, 2.5 oz.)	2	210

Weekly total: 3263

Suggested Physical Activities Program

Exercise	Increase in weekly activity (min.)	Increase in caloric expenditure (calories)
1 Jogging (over 8 min./mile)	30	339
2 Tennis, singles	30	210
3 Handball	60	774
4 Working out w. varied eqpt	60	300
Weekly totals:	180	1623

This program may not be practical. Instead you may prefer to do more of some exercises and less of others. Be sure the total calories burned from increased exercise is at least 1623 or more so you can achieve your weight loss goal of 1.4 pounds per week. The caloric expenditure information, provided in the physical activities table above, has been prepared to serve as an aid in computing the needed additional minutes if you choose to build a plan of your own design.

You can aid your caloric restriction by consuming negative calorie foods instead of refined carbohydrate and animal fat. In the process of digesting the negative calorie vegetables and fruits listed below, the body uses an equal or greater amount of calories than they contain. The vegetables (steamed or eaten raw) are: broccoli, bean sprouts, beets, celery, carrots, asparagus, cucumbers, eggplant, lettuce, mushrooms, green pepper, summer squash and tomatoes. The fruits are: grapefruit, strawberries, honeydew, cantaloupe and watermelon.

Weight control and/or maintaining cardiovascular fitness should be everyone's goal. A good paperback book on the subject is *The New Aerobics* by Kenneth Cooper, M.D. Another good text is *Actevitics* by Charles T. Kuntzleman. Remember that any exercise program should be started slowly and carefully. Often, people over-do the first few days of exercise which can be harmful.

If you are a member of a health club, be sure to follow the instructor's advice. After you have built up to a certain level of exercise, your exercise should be vigorous. It should be done at least 3 times per week and for a minimum of 30 minutes at a stretch.

IX. CONCLUSIONS

Of all the factors considered in your profile, the most critical problem areas are summarized below in order of importance:

1. Stop smoking.
2. Reduce your percent calories from fat to help protect you from cancer and possible heart disease.
3. Increase your intake of all vitamins and minerals below the RDA.
4. Correct your calcium/phosphorous imbalance.
5. Eating less refined carbohydrates and more vegetables and whole grains is especially important due to your family history of diabetes.
6. Correct your stress situations.
7. Reduce your intake of regular coffee and/or tea.

This concludes your nutrition, health and activity profile. We enjoyed having the opportunity of bringing you the latest dietary and lifestyle findings that pertain to you. It would be a good idea for you to retake this test again in 3 to 6 months so we can appraise the changes you may make between now and then. Keep in mind that this test will be revised to incorporate new information and will remain an up to the minute medium of lifestyle evaluation.

In parting, we have three final notes of caution:

1. This program is designed to be educational, to point out risk factors, to teach good health habits and nutrition and is not meant to detect medical disorders or diseases.

2. Remember your analysis was based on standards for normal healthy people of your age and may not apply in some instances, especially when a medical condition such as heart disease, ulcers, etc., is present. See your doctor to determine if you may have a medical condition differentiating you from the normal healthy individual.

3. Throughout this evaluation of your lifestyle, suggestions for supplemental reading have been made. We feel, overall, that each of the recommendations are very worthwhile. However, we do not necessarily endorse all their contents.

Food intake amino acid composition is listed below for reference only, since some doctors require this information.

Amino Acid Composition
(in Milligrams, MGS Approximate)

Amino acid	Your intake	Amino acid	Your intake
Arginine	5968	Histidine	2459
Threonine	4467	Valine	5544
Leucine	8374	Isoleucine	5241
Lysine	6917	Methionine	2718
Phenylalanine	4688	Tryptophan	1156

Nutrition, Health, and Activity Profile
of Mr. American Any Street

X. Doctors
  Summary of 7/16/78

Age 38; Wt 240; Sex M

(See text for explanation)	Daily Intake	Recommended Intake	24740
weekly exercise calories 1105			
Total calories	3230		
Protein (grams)	95.6	109.1; 68.6 to 87.0	
Fat (grams)	191.9		
Calories from fat	1727		
PCT calories from fat	53.5	20% to 34%	
Linoleic acid (grams)	9.5	3 to 5	
Fiber (grams)	2.5	6	
Carbohydrates (grams)	198.4	(calories 896; PCT calories 28)	
Refined (grams)	159.0	(equals 43 tsps sugar)	
PCT refined	80	(including alcohol 83 PCT)	
Regular coffee/Tea 70 cups/wk			

APPENDIX F: THE WELLNESS INVENTORY[1]

Instructions

Please put a mark in the box before each statement which is true *for you*. Total each section, then copy the subtotals to the back page. Average total scores range from 65 to 75.

What is Meant by Wellness?

The ideas of measuring wellness and helping people attain high levels of wellness are relatively new. Most of us think in terms of illness and assume that the absence of illness indicates wellness. This is not true. There are many degrees of wellness as there are many degrees of illness. The diagram below is a model used by well medicine.

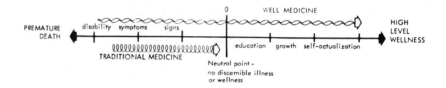

Moving from the center to the left shows a progressively worsening state of health. Moving to the right of center shows increasing levels of health and well-being. Traditional medicine is oriented towards curing evidence of disease, but usually stops at the midpoint. Well medicine begins at any point on the scale with the goal of helping a person to move as far to the right as possible.

Many people lack physical symptoms but are bored, depressed, tense, anxious or generally unhappy with their lives. These emotional states often lead to physical disease through the lowering of the body's resistance. The same feelings can also lead to abuse of the body through smoking, drinking and overeating. These behaviors are usually substitutes for other more basic human needs such as recognition from others, a stimulating environment, caring and affection from friends, and growth towards higher levels of self-awareness.

Wellness is not a static state. It results when a person begins to see himself as a growing, changing person. High level wellness means giving good care to your physical self, using your mind constructively, expressing your emotions effectively, being creatively involved with those around you, being concerned about your physical and psychological environment and becoming aware of other levels of consciousness.

This questionnaire will help to give you an idea about where you presently are on the wellness scale.

[1]Reprinted with permission from *Wellness Workbook for Health Professionals,* copyright 1977, John W. Travis, M.D., published by The Wellness Associates, 42 Miller Ave., Mill Valley, CA 94941.

*An asterisk at the end of a statement indicates that there is a footnote for that statement on p. 477 or p. 478.

1. Productivity, Relaxation, Sleep

00 ☐ I usually enjoy my work.
01 ☐ I seldom feel tired and rundown (except after strenuous work).*
02 ☐ I fall asleep easily at bedtime.
03 ☐ I usually get a full night's sleep.
04 ☐ If awakened, it is usually easy for me to go to sleep again.
05 ☐ I rarely bite or pick at my nails.
06 ☐ Rather than worrying, I can temporarily shelve my problems and enjoy myself at times when I can do nothing about solving them immediately.
07 ☐ I feel financially secure.
08 ☐ I am content with my sexual life.
09 ☐ I meditate or center myself for 15 to 20 minutes at least once a day.*

☐
Total
Checked

2. Personal Care and Home Safety

10 ☐ I take measures to protect my living space from fire and safety hazards (such as improper sized fuses and storage of volatile chemicals).
11 ☐ I have a dry chemical fire extinguisher in my kitchen and at least one other extinguisher elsewhere in my living quarters. (If very small apartment, kitchen extinguisher alone is adequate).*
12 ☐ I regularly use dental floss and a soft toothbrush.*
13 ☐ I smoke less than one pack of cigarettes or equivalent cigars or pipes *per week*.
14 ☐ I don't smoke at all (if this statement is true, mark item above true as well).
15 ☐ I keep an up-to-date record of my immunizations.
16 ☐ I have fewer than three colds per year.*
17 ☐ I minimize my exposure to sprays, chemical fumes or exhaust gases.*
18 ☐ I avoid extremely noisy areas (or wear protective ear plugs).*
19 ☐ I am aware of changes in my physical or mental state and seek professional advice about any which seem unusual.

WOMEN
100 ☐ I check my breasts for unusual lumps once a month.
101 ☐ I have a pap test annually.

MEN
102 ☐ If uncircumcised, I am aware of the special need for regular cleansing under my foreskin.
103 ☐ If over 45, I have my prostate checked annually.

☐
Total
Checked

3. Nutritional Awareness

20 ☐ I eat at least one uncooked fruit or vegetable each day.*
21 ☐ I have fewer than three alcoholic drinks (including beer) per week.
22 ☐ I rarely take medications, including prescription drugs.
23 ☐ I drink fewer than five soft drinks per week.*
24 ☐ I avoid eating refined foods or foods with sugar added.
25 ☐ I add little salt to my food.*
26 ☐ I read the labels for the ingredients of the foods I buy.
27 ☐ I add unprocessed bran to my diet to provide roughage.*

Total
Checked

28 ☐ I drink fewer than three cups of coffee or tea (with the exception of herbal teas) a day.*

29 ☐ I have a good appetite and maintain a weight within 15% of my ideal
weight.

4. Environmental Awareness*

30 ☐ I use public transportation or car pools when possible.

31 ☐ I turn off unneeded lights or appliances.

32 ☐ I recycle papers, cans, glass, clothing, books and organic waste (mark
true if you do at least three of these).

33 ☐ I set my thermostat at 68° or lower in winter.

34 ☐ I use air conditioning only when necessary and keep the thermostat
at 76° or higher.

35 ☐ I am conscientious about wasted energy and materials both at home
and at work.

36 ☐ I use nonpolluting cleaning agents.

37 ☐ My car gets at least 18 miles per gallon. (If you don't own a car, check
this statement as true).

38 ☐ I have storm windows and adequate insulation in attic and walls. (If you
don't own your home or live in a mild climate, check this statement
as true).

Total
Checked

39 ☐ I have a humidifier for use in winter. (If you don't have central heating
check this statement as true).*

5. Physical Activity

40 ☐ I climb stairs rather than ride elevators.

41 ☐ My daily activities include moderate physical effort (such as rearing
young children, gardening, scrubbing floors, or work which involves
being on my feet, etc.).

42 ☐ My daily activities include vigorous physical effort (such as heavy construction work, farming, moving heavy objects by hand, etc.).

43 ☐ I run at least one mile twice a week (or equivalent aerobic exercise).*

44 ☐ I run at least one mile four times a week or equivalent (if this statement
is true, mark the item above true as well).*

45 ☐ I regularly walk or ride a bike for exercise.

46 ☐ I participate in a strenuous sport at least once a week.

47 ☐ I participate in a strenuous sport more than once a week (if this statement is true, mark the item above true as well).

48 ☐ I do yoga or some form of stretching-limbering exercise for 15 to 20
minutes at least twice per week.*

Total
Checked

49 ☐ I do yoga or some form of stretching exercise for 15 to 20 minutes at
least four times per week (if this statement is true, mark the item above
true as well).

6. Expression of Emotions and Feelings

50 ☐ I am frequently happy.
51 ☐ I think it is OK to feel angry, afraid, joyful or sad.*
52 ☐ I do not deny my anger, fear, joy or sadness, but instead find constructive ways to express these feelings most of the time.*
53 ☐ I am able to say "no" to people without feeling guilty.
54 ☐ It is easy for me to laugh.
55 ☐ I like getting compliments and recognition from other people.
56 ☐ I feel OK about crying, and allow myself to do so.*
57 ☐ I listen to and think about constructive criticism rather than react defensively.

☐

Total
Checked

58 ☐ I would seek help from friends or professional counselors if needed.
59 ☐ It is easy for me to give other people sincere compliments and recognition.

7. Community Involvement

60 ☐ I keep informed of local, national and world events.
61 ☐ I vote regularly.
62 ☐ I take interest in community, national and world events and work to support issues and people of my choice. (If this statement is true, mark both items above true as well.)
63 ☐ When I am able, I contribute time or money to worthy causes.
64 ☐ I make an attempt to know my neighbors and be on good terms with them.
65 ☐ If I saw a crime being committed, I would call the police.
66 ☐ If I saw a broken bottle lying in the road or on the sidewalk, I would remove it.
67 ☐ When driving, I am considerate of pedestrians and other drivers.
68 ☐ If I saw a car with faulty lights, leaking gasoline or another dangerous condition, I would attempt to inform the driver.

☐

Total
Checked

69 ☐ I am a member of one or more community organizations (social change group, singing group, club, church or political group).

8. Creativity, Self Expression

70 ☐ I enjoy expressing myself through art, dance, music, drama, sports, etc.
71 ☐ I enjoy spending some time without planned or structured activities.*
72 ☐ I usually meet several people a month who I would like to get to know better.
73 ☐ I enjoy touching other people.*
74 ☐ I enjoy being touched by other people.*
75 ☐ I have at least five close friends.
76 ☐ At times I like to be alone.

☐

Total
Checked

77 ☐ I like myself and look forward to the future.
78 ☐ I look forward to living to be at least 75.*
79 ☐ I find it easy to express concern, love and warmth to those I care about.

9. Automobile Safety

If you don't own an automobile and ride less than 1,000 miles per year in one, enter 7 points in the box at left and skip the next 10 questions. (If you ride more than 1,000 miles per year but don't own a car, answer as many statements as you can and show this copy to the car's owner.)

80 ☐ I never drink when driving.
81 ☐ I wear a lap safety belt at least 90% of the time that I ride in a car.*
81a ☐ I wear a shoulder-lap belt at least 90% of the time that I ride in a car. (If this statement is true, mark the item above true as well.)*
82 ☐ I stay within 5 mph of the speed limit.
83 ☐ My car has head restraints on the front seats and I keep them adjusted high enough to protect myself and passengers from whiplash injuries.*
84 ☐ I frequently inspect my automobile tires, lights, etc. and have my car serviced regularly.
85 ☐ I have disc brakes on my car.*
86 ☐ I drive on belted radial tires.*
87 ☐ I carry emergency flares or reflectors and a fire extinguisher in my car.
88 ☐ I stop on yellow when a traffic light is changing.
89 ☐ For every 10 mph of speed, I maintain a car length's distance from the car ahead of me.

☐
Total
Checked

10. Parenting

If you don't have any responsibility for young children, enter 7 in the box at left and skip the next 10 questions. (If some of the questions are not applicable because your children are no longer young, answer them as you would if they were youngsters again.)

90 ☐ When riding in a car, I make certain that any child weighing under 50 pounds is secured in an approved child's safety seat or safety harness similar to those sold by the major auto manufacturers.*
91 ☐ When riding in a car, I make certain that any child weighing over 50 pounds is wearing an adult seat belt/shoulder harness.*
92 ☐ When leaving my child(ren), I make certain that the person in charge has the telephone numbers of my pediatrician or a hospital for emergency use.
93 ☐ I don't let my children ride escalators in bare feet or tennis shoes.*
94 ☐ I do not store cleaning products under the sink or in unlocked cabinets where a child could reach them.
95 ☐ I have a lock on the medicine cabinet or other places where medicines are stored.
96 ☐ I prepare my own baby food with a baby food grinder—thus avoiding commercial foods.*
97 ☐ I have sought information on parenting and raising children.
98 ☐ I frequently touch or hold my children.
99 ☐ I respect my child as an evolving, growing being.

☐
Total
Checked

Enter Subtotals on Last Page

Footnotes

Numbers before each statement refer to a statement above. Numbers following statements indicate references (see p. 479).

01. Fatigue without apparent cause is not a normal condition and usually indicates illness, stress or denial of emotional expression. (14)

09. Meditation or centering greatly enhances one's sense of well being. (1, 2, 12, 13)

11. Many injuries and much damage can be prevented by putting out fires when they first start. Dry chemical or CO_2 fire extinguishers are necessary for oil, grease and electrical fires.

12. Regular flossing and using a good soft toothbrush with rounded tip bristles prevent the premature loss of teeth in one's 40s and 50s. Be sure to learn the proper techniques of use from a dental hygienist or dentist. (3)

16. If you have more than three colds a year, you may not be getting enough rest, eating a good diet or meeting other energy needs properly. (4)

17. All such toxins have a harmful effect on the liver and other tissues over long periods of time.

18. Very loud noises which leave your ears ringing can cause permanent hearing loss which accumulates and is usually not noticeable until one reaches 40 or 50. Small cushioned ear plugs (not the type designed for swimmers), wax ear plugs and acoustic ear muffs (which look like stereo headphones without wires) can often be purchased in sporting goods stores.

20. Fresh fruits and vegetables provide vitamins, minerals, trace nutrients and roughage which are often lacking in modern diets. (5, 11)

23. Soft drinks are high in refined sugar which provides only "empty" calories and usually replace foods which have more nutritional value. Artificially sweetened soft drinks consumed in excess may have long-range consequences as yet not known. (Both types of soft drinks contain caffeine or other stimulants.)

25. Salting foods during cooking draws many vitamins out of the food and into the water which is usually discarded. Heavy salting of foods at the table may cause a strain on the kidneys and result in high blood pressure. (4)

27. Wheat bran, usually removed in the commercial milling of wheat, is the single best source of dietary fiber available. The use of approximately two tablespoons per day (individual needs vary) can substantially reduce colon cancer, diverticulosis, heart disease and other conditions related to refined food diets.

28. Coffee and tea (other than herbal teas) contain stimulants which, if abused, do not allow one's body to function normally. (4)
ENVIRONMENTAL AWARENESS. Taking care of your environment affects your own wellness as well as everyone else's.

39. Humidified heated air allows one to set the thermostat several degrees lower and still feel as warm as without humidification. It also helps prevent many respiratory ailments. House plants will require less watering and will be happier too.

43, 44. Vigorous aerobic exercise (such as running) must keep the heart rate at 150 beats per minute for 12 to 20 minutes to produce the "training effect." Less vigorous aerobic exercise (lower heart rate) must be maintained for much longer periods to produce the same benefit. The "training effect" is necessary to prepare the heart for meeting extra strain. (6)

48. Such exercise prevents stiffness of joints and musculo-skeletal degeneration. It also promotes a greater feeling of well-being. (7)

51. Basic emotions, if repressed, often cause anxiety, depression, irrational

behavior or physical disease. People can relearn to feel and express their emotions with a resulting improvement in their well-being. Some people, however, exaggerate emotions to control and manipulate others; this can be detrimental to their well-being. (8, 9)

52. Learning ways to constructively express these emotions (so that all parties concerned feel better) leads to more satisfying relationships and problem solving. (8, 9)

56. Crying over a loss or sad event is an important discharge of emotional energy. It is, however, sometimes used as a manipulative tool, or as a substitute expression of anger. Many males in particular have been erroneously taught that it is not OK to cry. (8)

71. Spending time spontaneously without relying on an external structure can be self-renewing. (8)

73, 74. Physical touch is important for the maintenance of life for young children and remains important throughout adult life. (10)

78. With proper self care, most individuals can easily reach this age in good health.

81. Shoulder/lap belts are much safer than lap belts alone. (Shoulder belts should never be worn without a lap belt.)

83. Whiplash injuries can be prevented by properly adjusted head restraints. These are required, in the U.S., on the front seats of all autos made since 1968 but are often not raised high enough to protect passengers and driver.

85. Disc brakes provide considerably better braking power than conventional drum brakes.

86. For most cars, radial tires maintain firmer contact with the road and improve braking and handling better than bias ply tires. They also have less rolling friction and give better gas mileage.

90, 91. Over 1,000 young children a year are killed in motor vehicle accidents in the U.S. Many deaths can be prevented by keeping the child from flying about in a car crash. Most car seats do not provide enough protection—as government standards are very low. Check consumer magazines for up-to-date information. Never use an adult seat belt for a child weighing less than 50 pounds.

93. The bare feet of young children are often injured at the end of escalators. Wearing tennis shoes is equally dangerous because their sturdy long laces get pulled into the mechanism and their thin canvas walls offer little protection.

96. Commercial baby foods contain high amounts of sugar, salt, modified starches and preservatives which may adversely affect a baby's future eating habits and health. Federal legislation has been introduced to help correct this problem. Portable baby food grinders and blenders can be used to prepare for an infant the same food as eaten by the rest of the family. Individual servings can be packaged and frozen for future meals.

Scoring

Enter subtotals from each section below and compute your total score.

1 ☐ Productivity

2 ☐ Care & Safety

3 ☐ Nutrition

4 ☐ Environment

5 ☐ Physical

6 ☐ Emotions

7 ☐ Community

8 ☐ Creativity

9 ☐ Auto

10 ☐ Parenting

Total _____

References

1. *Human Life Styling* - McCamy.
2. *Be Here Now* - Ram Dass.
3. *The Tooth Trip* - McGuire.
4. *Well Body Book* - Samuels and Bennett.
5. *Nutrition Against Disease* - Williams.
6. *The New Aerobics* and *Aerobics for Women* - Cooper.
7. *Fundamentals of Yoga* - Mishra.
8. *Born to Win* - James and Jongeward.
9. *The Angry Book* - Rubin.
10. *Touching* - Montague.
11. *Diet for a Small Planet* - Lappe.
12. *Center of the Cyclone* - Lilly.
13. *The Crack in the Cosmic Egg* - Pearce.
14. *Stress* - McQuade & Aiken

APPENDIX G: BILLS OF RIGHTS

Nurses' Rights*

1. The right to find dignity in self-expression and self-enhancement through the use of our special abilities and educational background.
2. The right to recognition for our contribution through the provision of an environment for its practice, and proper, professional economic rewards.
3. The right to a work environment which will minimize physical and emotional stress and health risks.
4. The right to control what is professional practice within the limits of the law.
5. The right to set standards for excellence in nursing.
6. The right to participate in policy making affecting nursing.
7. The right to social and political action in behalf of nursing and health care.

Patients' Rights

The American Hospital Association has adopted a "Patients' Bill of Rights" as a national policy statement and distributed it to its member hospitals throughout the country. The 12 rights, in summary, are:

1. The patient has the right to considerate and respectful care.
2. The patient has the right to obtain from his physician complete current information concerning his diagnosis, treatment, and prognosis in terms the patient can be reasonably expected to understand.
3. The patient has the right to receive from his physician information necessary to give informed consent prior to the start of any procedure and/or treatment.
4. The patient has the right to refuse treatment to the extent permitted by law, and to be informed of the medical consequences of his action.
5. The patient has the right to every consideration of his privacy concerning his own medical care program.
6. The patient has the right to expect that all communications and records pertaining to his care should be treated as confidential.
7. The patient has the right to expect that within its capacity a hospital must make reasonable response to the request of a patient for services.
8. The patient has the right to obtain information as to any relationship of his hospital to other health care and educational institutions insofar as his care is concerned.
9. The patient has the right to be advised if the hospital proposes to engage in or perform human experimentation affecting his care or treatment.
10. The patient has the right to expect reasonable continuity of care.
11. The patient has the right to examine and receive an explanation of his bill regardless of source of payment.
12. The patient has the right to know what hospital rules and regulations apply to his conduct as a patient.

* Excerpted from Claire M. Fagin, "Nurses' Rights," *AJN,* 75, no. 1 (January 1975), pp. 82–85.

Student Nurses' Rights and Responsibilities*

1. Students should be encouraged to develop the capacity for critical judgment and engage in a sustained and independent search for truth.

2. The freedom to teach and the freedom to learn are inseparable facts of academic freedom: students should exercise their freedom with responsibility.

3. Each institution has a duty to develop policies and procedures which provide and safeguard the students' freedom to learn.

4. Under no circumstances should a student be barred from admission to an institution or judged in grievance proceedings on the basis of race, creed, sex, marital status, weight, or height.

5. Students should be free to take reasoned exception to the data or views offered in any course of study and to reserve judgment on matters of opinion, but they are responsible for learning the content of any course of study for which they have enrolled.

6. Any student or group of students has the right to grieve any problems in the following areas: grading policies, validity of clinical evaluations, student-instruction or class-instructor conflicts, and school policies regarding curriculum, testing, and admissions or dismissals.

7. Students should have protection through orderly procedures against prejudiced or capricious academic evaluation, but they are responsible for maintaining standards of academic performance established for each course in which they are enrolled. Uniform evaluation forms reflecting course objectives should be used and shown to students at the beginning of each course. Students should have the right to comment in writing on the evaluation form, and have the right to grieve evaluations with which they disagree.

8. Information about student views, beliefs, and political associations which instructors acquire in the course of their work should be considered confidential and not released without the knowledge and consent of the student.

9. The student should have the right to a responsible voice in the determination of his/her curriculum. Students have the right to challenge the accuracy or the relevancy of material presented to them. They have the right to insist upon unbiased teaching or transcultural nursing, the right to insist that lecture and lab courses be correlated, and that they be taught the material.

10. Students should be tested only on material emphasized during a particular semester and from the resources used in the presentation of that material. Tests should be gone over in a reasonable amount of time during class sessions.

11. The grading policies of each instructor should be included in the introductory material for each course. Purpose, objectives, class content, and assignments will be presented in writing during the first week of instruction. The student has the right to know how the tests are to be graded and the type of grading curve to be used. Students should receive mid-term evaluations of class and clinical performance, which allow the student to improve as necessary before the end of the term.

12. Students have a right to know what information is to be kept as part of permanent records, and the conditions under which this information is disclosed.

13. Students have the right to belong or refuse to belong to any organization of their choice. Students and student organizations should have the right to examine and discuss all questions of interest to them, and to express opinions publicly or privately.

14. Students should be allowed to invite and hear anyone of their own choosing thereby taking the responsibility of furthering their own education.

15. The student body should have clearly defined means to participate in the formulation and application of departmental policy affecting academic and student affairs.

16. As citizens and members of an academic community, students are subject to the obligations which accrue them by virtue of this membership and should enjoy the same freedom of citizenship.

* Reprinted with permission from © National Student Nurse's Association, Inc.

APPENDIX H: A GENERAL GUIDE TO HOLISTIC ORGANIZATIONS

Groups and Associations

1. HOLISTIC HEALTH ORGANIZING COMMITTEE
P.O. Box 166
Berkeley, CA 94701

(415) 841-6500 Ext. 142

Stresses preventive medicine and health education as well as full recognition and legal protection for all forms of alternative healing and their qualified practitioners.

2. QUEST OF CARMEL
P.O. Box 6301
Carmel, CA 93921

(408) 624-8722

Florence Zellhoefer, MD, Director

Dedicated to helping individuals become self-healers of the body, mind, and spirit.

3. THE COMMITTEE FOR FREEDOM OF CHOICE IN CANCER THERAPY
146 Main Street, Suite 408
Los Altos, CA 94022

(415) 948-9475

Information available on alternative cancer therapies.

4. CENTER FOR INTEGRAL MEDICINE
P.O. Box 955
Pacific Palisades, CA 90272

(213) 459-3373

David Bresler, PhD, Executive Director

Founded by a group of physicians and psychologists dedicated to the maintenance of life and health through innovative approaches to healing and a realization of a benevolent universal life force.

5. ASSOCIATION FOR HOLISTIC HEALTH
P.O. Box 33202
San Diego, CA 92103

(714) 298-5965

David Harris, President

A nonprofit educational corporation dedicated to promoting and supporting holistic health, and to ensuring its continued development in professional methods, standards, and ethics.

6. THE EAST-WEST ACADEMY OF HEALING ARTS COUNCIL OF NURSE-HEALERS
117 Topaz
San Francisco, CA 94131

(415) 285-9400

Essie Poy Yew Chow, PhD, RN, Co-chairperson

Dedicated to expanding the existing body of knowledge relevant to healing modalities in nursing through theory development, research, and practice.

7. INSTITUTE FOR THE STUDY OF HUMANISTIC MEDICINE
Synthesis Graduate School
3352 Sacramento Street
San Francisco, CA 94118

(415) 826-7171

Naomi Remen, MD, Director

Believes that effective medicine mobilizes the multiple dimensions of the person who is the patient.

8. HAWAII HEALTH NET
2535 South King Street
Honolulu, HI 96814

(808) 955-1555

W. Stroude, MD, Director

A communications network to assist individuals in finding viable alternatives to personal health care.

9. THE FOUNDATION OF TRUTH, INC.
3941 Gateway Court
Indianapolis, IN 46254

Ikot Alfred Ekanem, Chief Executive Director

Dedicated to uplifting mankind both spiritually and physically, through Positive Health Community Centers.

10. CHILDREN IN HOSPITALS
31 Wilshire Park
Needham, MA 02192

(617) 878-7000

Barbara Popper, Chairperson

Reprinted by permission of Doubleday and Company, Inc., from *Holistic Dimensions in Healing* by Leslie Kaslof. Copyright © 1978 by Leslie Kaslof.

A nonprofit organization of parents and health care professionals seeking to support and educate parents wishing to remain in close contact with their children during a hospital experience. Personal counseling, a newsletter, information sheets and meetings are available. Also available is a 1972 survey of Boston area hospitals' pediatric and maternity departments' policies toward visiting and rooming in (50¢, or free with a $2.00 membership). Founded 1972.

11. AMERICAN MEDICAL-PSYCHIC RESEARCH ASSOCIATION
135 Madison Avenue N.E.
Albuquerque, NM 87123

(505) 265-0221

Aims to unite individuals in the fields of osteopathy, homeopathy, naturopathy, and other therapeutic fields who share common orientations toward healing.

12. THE EAST/WEST CENTER FOR HOLISTIC HEALTH
275 Madison Avenue, Suite 500
New York, NY 10016

(212) 689-1321

Marie Valenta, Director

Dedicated to promoting effective approaches to total health and wholeness with the recognition of mind-body-spirit unity.

13. FOUNDATION FOR ALTERNATIVE CANCER THERAPY, LTD.
P.O. Box HH
Old Chelsea Station
New York, NY 10011

(212) 741-2790

Information and resources on alternative cancer therapies.

Schools, Centers, and Clinics

1. HEALTH AWARENESS INSTITUTE
1224 East Northern
Phoenix, AZ 85020

(602) 943-8182

Stephen H. Grunfeld, DC, Director

Provides natural health care through chiropractic, nutritional guidance, massage therapy, psychological counseling, and clinical hypnosis.

2. BERKELEY COMMUNITY HEALTH PROJECT
(Free Clinic)
2339 Durant Avenue
Berkeley, CA 94704

(415) 548-2570

Harvey Smith, Coordinator of Outreach

Preventive and self-help approaches to health are emphasized in all four areas of the clinic: medical, dental, rap center, and switchboard/crisis intervention.

3. BERKELEY HOLISTIC HEALTH CENTER
2640 College Avenue
Berkeley, CA 94704

(415) 845-4430

Offers classes and workshops in many areas of holistic healing, stressing unity of mind, body, and spirit.

4. BERKELEY WOMEN'S HEALTH COLLECTIVE
2908 Ellsworth Street
Berkeley, CA 94705

(415) 843-1437

Provides extensive informational, educational, medical, and referral services for women in the Bay Area. Mental health counseling, pregnancy counseling, self-help groups are available.

5. THE PSYCHOSOMATIC MEDICINE CLINIC
2510 Webster Street
Berkeley, CA 94705

(415) 549-1228

Kenneth R. Pelletier, PhD, Director

A staff of medical doctors and other professional practitioners provide treatment through acupuncture, clinical biofeedback, cancer counseling and visualization therapy, orthomolecular and dietary medicine, relaxation and meditation methods, and psychotherapy.

6. INSTITUTE FOR RESEARCH INTO WHOLISTIC THERAPEUTIC ENERGIES
c/o University of the Trees
P.O. Box 644
Boulder Creek, CA 95006

(408) 338-3855

Steven Langer, MD, Director

Programs include the relationship between

color and personality, aura balancing, toning and chanting, specialized meditation for children and senior citizens, dream analysis, and "creative conflict": a growth process facilitating communication and emotional awareness.

7. BIOLOGY OF THE MIND/BODY
Department of Behavioral Biology,
School of Medicine
University of California
Davis, CA 95616

(916) 752-3259

Jim Polidora, PhD, Instructor
P.O. Box 709
Davis, CA 95616

An extensive course series offered to medical students which covers such areas as neurophysiology, nutrition, Eastern philosophy, yoga, transpersonal psychology, and bodywork.

8. NATIONAL ARTHRITIS MEDICAL CLINIC
13630 Mountain View Road
Desert Hot Springs, CA 92240

(714) 329-6422

Robert Bingham, MD, Medical Director

A nonprofit community clinic dedicated to the treatment of all forms of arthritis.

9. VITAL HEALTH CENTER
17200 Ventura Boulevard
Suite 305
Encino, CA 91316

(213) 990-9270

Gary R. Robb, DC, Director

Provides chiropractic treatment with dietary, herbal, and homeopathic supplementation.

10. MEDICINE HOLISTICS
364 South Clovis Avenue
Fresno, CA 93727

Dave Edwards, MD, Medical Director

A treatment facility which accepts referrals from health professionals and offers classes to the community.

11. WHOLISTIC MEDICINE AND PERSONAL GROWTH CENTER
11633 South Hawthorne
Boulevard, Suite 401
Hawthorne, CA 90250

(213) 973-7830

Richard L. Ferman, MD,
Medical Director

Provides a comprehensive program of outpatient counseling services and an adult voluntary admission inpatient mental health care unit.

12. ISLA VISTA OPEN DOOR MEDICAL CLINIC
970 Embarcadero del Mar
Isla Vista, CA 93017

(805) 968-1511

Wendy E. Assad, Administrator

Supplements traditional general medical practice with herbal medicines, iridology, nutritional counseling, and a general preventive approach.

13. COLLEGE OF NATURAL THERAPEUTICS
1434 Fremont Avenue
Los Altos, CA 94022

(415) 967-1232

Roy B. Oliver, ND, Dean

Nonaccredited, correspondence courses offered in homeopathy, naturopathy, nutrition, and magnetic healing.

14. BARAKA
11110 Ohio Avenue, Suite 204
Los Angeles, CA 90025

(213) 473-0881

Lee Baumel, MD

A holistic center for therapy and research.

15. FEMINIST WOMEN'S HEALTH CENTER
1112 South Crenshaw Boulevard
Los Angeles, CA 90005

(213) 936-7219

A nonprofit corporation dedicated to providing quality medical care to women at modest prices.

16. A HEALING PLACE
2476 South Overland Avenue
Suite 307
Los Angeles, CA 90064

(213) 204-0111

R. Frank Hoffman, MD.
Medical Director

Staffed by an MD, a rabbi, and a clinical psychologist, A Healing Place is dedicated to the "exploration of consciousness-expanding vehicles, our resistance to making full use of them, and their utilization in dealing with emotional, physical, and spiritual disease."

17. THE HOLISTIC HEALTH CENTER
8907 Wilshire Boulevard
Beverly Hills, CA 90069

(213) 652-5084

Griffith Page, MD, Medical Director

A treatment and education center for the whole person.

18. INSTITUTE OF REALITY AWARENESS
8217 Beverly Boulevard, Suite 7
Los Angeles, CA 90048

(213) 658-8600

Leslie J. Kent, DD, Director

A nonprofit, holistic healing arts organization.

19. KHALSA MEDICAL AND COUNSELING ASSOCIATES
8733 Beverly Boulevard
Suite 400
Los Angeles, CA 90048

(213) 652-2101

Jas Want Sing Khalsa, MD, MA,
Director

A nonprofit holistic healing center, balancing treatment and training in kundalini yoga with traditional Western medicine, homeopathy, kinesiology, anthroposophic medicine, acupuncture and acupressure, hypnotherapy, nutrition, and spinal manipulation.

20. WHITE CROSS SOCIETY
Punita
Box 576
Lucerne Valley, CA 92356

(714) 248-6163

Offers classes and experiential training in massage, herbology, nutrition, tissue salts, and homeopathy.

21. INSTITUTE FOR CREATIVE AGING
P.O. Box 142
Malibu, CA 90265

(213) 456-6297

Evelyn Mandel, Director

Seeks to enrich the lives of persons 65 years and older, and to establish this period of life as a time of richness and productivity.

22. McCORNACK CENTER FOR THE HEALING ARTS
499 Howard Street
Mendocino, CA 95460

(707) 937-5834

Peter H. Barg, MD, Director

A multidisciplinary holistic treatment facility.

23. WELLNESS RESOURCE CENTER
42 Miller Avenue
Mill Valley, CA 94941

(415) 383-3806

John Travis, MD, Director

Defining "wellness" as a state of health beyond the mere absence of illness, the Center assists people to take charge of their own lives and to experience greater levels of aliveness and satisfaction.

24. WHOLISTIC HEALTH AND NUTRITION INSTITUTE
150 Shoreline Highway
Mill Valley, CA 94941

(415) 332-2933

Richard Shames, MD, Medical Director

Provides medical care, herbal treatment, nutritional guidance, hypnosis, biofeedback, and somatic psychology for the wholistic care of the whole person.

25. AUTOGENIC HEALTH CENTER
6401 Broadway Terrace
Oakland, CA 94618

(415) 658-5913

Vera Fryling, MD, Director

Uses a holistic approach to personal growth and stress reduction using Autogenic Training, visual imagery, and "graduated hypnosis."

26. OAKLAND FEMINIST WOMEN'S HEALTH CENTER
2930 McClure Street
Oakland, CA 94609

(415) 444-5676

Provides a self-help clinic for women.

27. OPEN EDUCATION EXCHANGE
6526 Telegraph Avenue
Oakland, CA 94609

(415) 655-6791

Bart Brodsky, Coordinator

A nonprofit organization, making available noncredit adult education courses serving the Greater Bay Area.

28. SAN ANDREAS HEALTH CENTER
531 Cowper Street
Palo Alto, CA 94301

(415) 324-9350

Susan Harmon Stuart, President

A group of health professionals offering a variety of techniques for attaining and maintaining optimum health.

29. THE LIFE AND HEALTH MEDICAL GROUP
511 Brookside Avenue
Redlands, CA 92373

(714) 824-1750

Bruce W. Halstead, MD, Director

Concerned with treatment of chronic degenerative diseases, especially atherosclerosis, senility, cardiovascular diseases, and arthritis.

30. SACRAMENTO MEDICAL PREVENTICS CLINIC, INC.
2811 "L" Street, Suite 205
Sacramento, CA 95816

(916) 452-7011

Howard Greenspan, DO

A wholistic clinic, using computer diet evaluation, hair analysis, thermography, treadmill electrocardiograms, comprehensive blood analysis, and physical examinations.

31. AGE OF ENLIGHTENMENT CENTER FOR HOLISTIC HEALTH
3545 Revere Street
San Diego, CA 92109

(714) 270-4600

Harold H. Bloomfield, MD, Director

An integrative clinical facility centered around the Transcendental Meditation program as taught by Maharishi Mahesh Yogi.

32. BEACH AREA COMMUNITY CLINIC
3705 Mission Boulevard
San Diego, CA 92109

(714) 488-0644

Juanita Hollisey, RN,
Outreach Coordinator

Staffed by physicians, nurses, trained health workers, and volunteers.

33. THE NATIONAL CENTER FOR THE EXPLORATION OF HUMAN POTENTIAL
6731 Bamhurst Street
San Diego, CA 92117

(714) 278-8210

Herbert A. Otto, PhD,
Chairperson

A nonprofit educational organization conducting training programs in wholistic healing.

34. THE PHOENIX INSTITUTE
976 Chalcedony Street
San Diego, CA 92109

(714) 488-0626

Kathryn Breese-Whiting, DD,
Founder and President

Offers classes, workshops, and seminars in the inner creative action of science, art, and religion. The Institute is licensed by the State of California to give degrees.

35. SAN DIEGO NATURAL HEALTH CLINIC
4459 Morrell Street
San Diego, CA 92109

(714) 274-2482

John Caldwell Luly, DC, Director

A holistic natural clinic.

36. EAST-WEST ACADEMY OF HEALING ARTS
60 Ora Way
San Francisco, CA 94131

(415) 285-9400

Effie Poy Yew Chow, PhD, RN, President

Offers coursework for nurses and other health care professionals in acupressure, therapeutic touch, nutrition, herbology, iridology, and psychic healing.

37. HOLISTIC LIFE UNIVERSITY
Holistic Life Foundation
1627 Tenth Avenue
San Francisco, CA 94122

(415) 665-3200

William Staniger, President

Consists of four programs for the training of "life-support professionals," holistic health, holistic childbirth, yoga, and life-death transition.

38. NURSE CONSULTANTS AND HEALTH COUNSELORS: THE HEALING CENTER
465 Brussels
San Francisco, CA 94134

(415) 468-4680

Counselors and therapists provide services to individuals and groups in various modes of holistic healing.

39. SAN FRANCISCO WOMEN'S HEALTH CENTER
3789 24th Street
San Francisco, CA 94114

(415) 282-6999

Educational center dedicated to teaching women concepts and methods for self-health care.

40. ASSOCIATED PSYCHOLOGISTS OF SANTA CLARA
160 Saratoga Avenue, Suite 38
Santa Clara, CA 95050

(408) 296-5600

A group of eight holistically oriented psychologists dedicated to the client's psychological-structural-nutritional integration, and his or her realization of optimal well-being and satisfaction.

41. UNIVERSITY OF CALIFORNIA EXTENSION
Santa Cruz, CA 95064

(408) 429-2971

Carl Tjerandsen, PhD, Dean

Offers courses for both nurses and laypersons in acupressure and healing energies, laying on of hands, the healing power of sound (including both mantras and sounds of nature), and the role of stress in disease.

42. FAMILY PRACTICE CENTER
3325 Chanate Road
Santa Rosa, CA 95402

(707) 527-2826

Roger D. Snyder, PhD, Director

A staff of medical doctors and behavioral scientists provide an interdisciplinary family systems approach to medicine.

43. COMMUNITY FREE SCHOOL
Box 1724
Boulder, CO 80302

(303) 447-8734

Holds ongoing seminars and workshops in holistic healing modalities.

44. INTEGRAL HEALTH SERVICES, INC.
245 School Street
Putnam, CT 06260

(203) 928-7729

Sandra McLanahan, MD, Director

Associated with the Satchidananda Ashram which is under the direction of Sri Swami Satchidananda.

45. THE STAMFORD CENTER FOR THE HEALING ARTS
The First Congregational Church
Walton Place
Stamford, CT 06901

(203) 323-0200

Gabe Lewis Campbell, Minister

Provides training programs in prayer and meditation from a Judeo-Christian perspective, therapeutic touch, nutrition, herbs, reflexology, and cooking.

46. MANKIND RESEARCH FOUNDATION, INC.
1640 Kalmia Road, N.W.
Washington, DC 20012

(202) 982-4001

Carl Schleicher, PhD, Director

Provides information and educational programs in suggestology, biofeedback as a treatment for hypertension, Oriental medicine, moxibustion, yoga and meditation for alcohol and drug rehabilitation, and color and music therapy.

47. YES EDUCATIONAL SOCIETY
1035 31st Street, N.W.
Washington, DC 20007

(202) 338-7676

Lee Lewis, Coordinator

Offers a selection of 5- to 10-week courses at low cost with emphasis on holistic healing.

48. CORNUCOPIA CENTERS, INC.
5808 Northeast Fourth Court
Miami, FL 33137

(305) 758-9000

Gary Schwartz, MA, and
Deborah Schwartz

Educational programs and classes in such areas as T'ai Chi, acupressure, reflexology, nutrition, spiritual healing, vision training, and holistic health applications of altered states of consciousness.

49. HIMALAYAN INSTITUTE COMBINED THERAPY CENTER
1505 Greenwood Road
Glenview, IL 60025

(312) 724-2273

Richard M. Ballentine, MD,
Director of Therapy Programs

A branch of the Himalayan Institute founded by Swami Rama, the Center provides a quiet setting for patients who come for ten-day to three-week intensive treatment.

50. CENTERS FOR HEALTH AND LIFE, INC.
Des Moines Center
2600 Harding Road
Des Moines, IA 50310

(515) 277-6155

Kenneth G. Brockman, DC, and
Robert L. Burns, DDS, Directors

A wholistic treatment facility dedicated to educating, treating, and preventing disease, sickness, and illness through natural-biologic means.

51. MARTIN BUBER INSTITUTE
The Meeting House
5885 Robert Oliver Place
Columbia, MD 21045

(301) 730-6044

Rabbi Martin Siegal

Offers courses and workshops in New Age alternatives to Western medicine, such as massage, homeopathy, yoga, nutrition, meditation, gestalt, structural patterning, and rebirthing.

52. THE INSTITUTE FOR PSYCHOENERGETICS
126 Harvard Street
Brookline, MA 02146

(617) 738-4502

Buryl Payne, PhD, Director

Offers an integral program of mind-body balancing which includes bioenergetics, therapeutic massage, rolfing, yoga, biofeedback, dehypnosis, and meditation.

53. ACUPUNCTURE CENTER OF MASSACHUSETTS
93 Union Street
Newton, MA 02164

(617) 965-3306

James Doyle, DO, Director

Wholistic treatment center utilizing acupuncture, osteopathy, nutrition, and ancillary bioenergetic psychotherapy.

54. INTERFACE
63 Chapel Street
Newton, MA 02158

(617) 965-4491

Rick Ingrasci, MD, Co-Founder

". . .a freeform association supporting creative individuals and groups who reflect a holistic awareness of the evolutionary process."

55. NATURO-NUTRIC-BIONICS
Box 24
Mound, MN 55364

Kenneth Brockman, DC, and
Robert L. Burns, DDS

Offers a seminar in preventive health care focusing on the development of a Health Recommendation Plan.

56. THE FEATHERED PIPE RANCH
2409 Colorado Gulch
Helena, MT 59601

(406) 442-8196

A retreat, associated with the Holistic Life Foundation in San Francisco, offering programs on holistic health, yoga, and meditation.

57. DESERT LIGHT FOUNDATION, INC.
P.O. Box 40147
Albuquerque, NM 87106

(505) 268-2156

Harold Cohen, MD, President

Maintains a holistic health clinic (with one medical doctor and one chiropractor) with individual counseling services.

58. CHRISTOS SCHOOL OF NATURAL HEALING
P.O. Box 1503
Taos, NM 87571

William LeSassier, ND,
Founder and Director

Counseling in the areas of nutrition, natural birth, and body release therapies.

59. THE PEOPLE'S HEALTH CENTER
438 Claremont Parkway
Bronx, NY 10457

(212) 583-8010

John Lichtenstein, MD

A community-patient-health worker controlled nonprofit care facility.

60. INSTITUTE FOR SELF-DEVELOPMENT
50 Maple Place
Manhasset, NY 11030

(516) 627-0048

Makes available a course in self-development, including studies in yoga, meditation, T'ai Chi Kung, Chinese acupuncture, Korean massage, chirotherapy, nutrition, pulse diagnosis, and Chinese herbal medicine.

61. ARTHRITIS MEDICAL CENTER
320 West End Avenue
New York, NY 10023

(212) 595-1503

J. Sheridan Bell, MD,
Medical Director

Offers a three-fold treatment program for arthritis sufferers consisting of hormonal treatments, nutritional supplements and counseling, and special exercises.

62. HEALTH MAINTENANCE CENTER
1370 Avenue of the Americas
New York, NY 10019

(212) 489-0855

A preventive medicine clinic, with a computerized diagnostic system called "automated multiphasic testing."

63. ODYSSEY ASSOCIATION
333 East 49th Street
New York, NY 10017

(212) 751-5239

Jodi Desmond and Edna B. Kucher,
Founders

Sponsors teachers of spiritual, parapsychological, and esoteric systems which are supportive of the spiritual/psychic/physical growth of the whole person.

64. REILLY'S ON 34TH STREET
120 East 34th Street
New York, NY 10016

(212) 684-1472

Stanley Kestenbaum, PhT,
Director

Specializes in the application of colonic irrigations, therapeutic massage, exercises, paraffin baths, and other physical therapy treatments.

65. TREE OF LIFE
101 West 125th Street
New York, NY 10027

(212) 865-2000

Kanya Kekhumba, Founder

Offers workshops in such areas as astrology, herbology, psychic awareness, nutrition, yoga, and meditation.

66. THE ALTERNATIVE HEALTH EDUCATION CENTER
715 Monroe Avenue
Rochester, NY 14607

(716) 442-5480

Thaddeus Bukowski, Coordinator

Disseminates information to the community through workshops and lectures on such topics as nutrition, homeopathy, yoga, and fasting.

67. THE MOUNTAIN PEOPLE'S CLINIC
Eagle Street
Hayesville, NC 28904

(704) 389-6091

Jim Campbell, MD, Director

A clinic in a country farmhouse.

68. P.S.I. CENTER
(People Seeking Illumination of the Physical,
Spiritual and Intellectual)
Endicott Building, Room "M"
Cincinnati, OH 45218

(513) 742-2266

Robert J. Rothan, DDS

A clinical, educational, and research facility for the treatment of the whole person.

69. MERETA GROUP
Box 14191
Columbus, OH 43214

(614) 846-1187

William J. Strandwitz

A group of professional counselors, therapists, and teachers interested in the physical, mental, and spiritual aspects of healing.

70. THE INSTITUTE OF PREVENTIVE
MEDICINE
6171 Southwest Capitol Highway
Portland, OR 97201

(503) 246-7616

Mark J. Tager, MD, Director

Offers individual holistic medical and dental counseling.

71. CLYMER HEALTH CLINIC
R.D. 3, Clymer Road
Quakertown, PA 18951

(215) 536-8001

G. E. Posenecker, ND, DC, Director

A total natural treatment facility with inpatient accommodations if desired.

72. THE ESOTERIC PHILOSOPHY
CENTER, INC.
523 Lovett Boulevard
Houston, TX 77006

(713) 526-5998

William David, Executive Director

Provides a community educational program aimed at formal integration of personality as well as spiritual and self-awareness.

73. THE COMMUNITY HEALTH CENTER
260 North Street
Burlington, VT 05401

(802) 864-6309

A community-based health clinic offering services either free or at minimal cost.

74. ASSOCIATION FOR
BIOCOSMOLOGICAL RESEARCH, INC.
Box 9545
Rosslyn Station
Arlington, VA 22209

(703) 751-5776

Sponsors conferences and seminars in various natural healing modalities.

75. HOME CENTER
2100 Mediterranean Avenue
Virginia Beach, VA 23451

(804) 425-1170

Paul R. Thompson, DC, Director

A medical education center aimed at prevention.

76. PREVENTIVE MEDICINE CLINIC
800 156th Avenue, N.E.
Bellevue, WA 98008

(206) 746-4024

James C. Johnston, MD, Director

Holistic medicine practice founded on the belief that each individual is a unique being based on spiritual-emotional life with nutritional-biochemical and structural-anatomical expressions.

77. SUNSHINE MEDICAL SHOW
2316 Northeast 85th
Seattle, WA 98115

(206) 524-8083

Charles Thompson, MD

A holistic clinic comprised of a medical doctor, an acupuncturist, psychotherapist, and a Reichian breathing therapist.

78. THE PAIN AND HEALTH
REHABILITATION CENTER
Route 2, Welsh Coulee
LaCrosse, Wi 54601

(601) 786-0611

C. Norman Shealy, MD, Director

A holistic healing center emphasizing treatment of severe, chronic pain.

79. PINE FREE CLINIC
1985 West Fourth
Vancouver, British Columbia
Canada, V6J 1M7

(604) 736-2391

Follows a "whole-person" approach to medical (especially gynecological) problems.

80. SERENITY HEALTH EDUCATION CENTRE
P.O. Box 4886
Vancouver, British Columbia
Canada V6B 4A6

Provides classes and correspondence courses in nutrition, reflexology, color therapy, herbal remedies, yoga, spiritual healing, natural birth control, Oriental medicine, and related subjects.

index

Human development (*cont.*)
  holistic approaches, 115–22
  holistic philosophy, 100–101
  infant and early childhood,
    105–7
  interpersonal, 125–28
  intrapersonal assessment,
    122–25
  principles, 105
  research, 104–14
  stages, 104
  tasks, 104
  terminology, 99
  theories, 104–14
  youth and adolescence, 107–9
Humanistic caring, 19
  helping relationship, 74–76
Humanistic education, 381–88
Humanistic learning, 367–71
  principles of, 372–73
Humanistic medicine, 13, 14, 31
Humanistic movement, 74–76
Humanistic nursing:
  applying caring, 81
  description, 26
  humanistic nurse, 84
Human lifestyling elements, 20
Human needs theory, 362–63
Human potential, 100–101
Human relations training, 387, 405
Humility, 72–73
Hypertension, 147
Hypnosis, 14
Hypoglycemia, 200

I

I-Ching, 10–11
Identification, 91
Illich, Ivan:
  change, 413
  definition of health, 5
  medicalization of life, 63-64
Imagery, 39
Inclusion, 408
Independent learning, 315–16
Individual make-up, 142–43
  personality, 142
  Type A, 143
  Type B, 143
Induction, 315–17
Infant and early childhood
    development, 105–7
  community programs, 129
Institute for the Study of
    Humanistic Medicine, 8, 76,
    78

Intensive Journal, 177–78
Interpersonal lifespace, 23
Interpersonal system, 23
Intrapersonal lifespace, 23
Intrapersonal system, 23
Intuition, 315–17
Iridology, 15, 336–37
Iron, 198
Irrational ideas, 180-81

J

Jacobson's progressive relaxation,
    237–38
  shorteed version, 240–41
Jensen, Bernard, 336–37
Jin Shin Jyutsu, 15, 84
Journals:
  definition, 38
  Intensive Journal, 38
  topics, 39–40
Jung, Carl, 52, 92, 110–11
  archetypes, 110–11
  individuation, 110

K

Kennell, John K., 117–18
Kinesics, 284
Kinesiology, 16, 329 (*see also*
    Touch for Health)
Kinlein, Lucille, 63
Kirlian photography, 86
Klaus, Marshall H., 117–18
Knowing:
  direct, 71
  experimental, 71
  indirect, 71
  intuitive, 71
  professional, 71
Knowledge, absolute, 36
Koans, 36, 281–82, 286
Kohlberg, Lawrence:
  affective education, 384
  moral stages of development, 109
Kramer, Marlene, 424
Krieger, Dolores, 86, 88–90

L

Laying-on-of-hands healing,
    84–86, 90
Leadership, 403–9
  autocratic, 404
  group dynamics, 408–9

Leadership (*cont.*)
  interpersonal relationships,
    405–7
    concluding phase, 407
    orientation phase, 407
    working phase, 407
  laissez-faire, 404
  participative, 404
  terminology, 403
  theories, 403–5
Leadership and change, 396–435
  Committee for Integrated
    Health, 428–29
  East West Academy, 427
  holistic health movement,
    425–34
  holistic nursing, 425–26
  holistic paradigm, 21, 431, 433
  holistic politics, 427–28
  legal considerations, 429–31
  nursing and, 397–98
  preparation of nurses, 400–402
  role of nurses, 398–400
  role of women, 398–400
  self-determination, 427–28
  self-responsibility, 426–27
  Well-Being Centers, 429
Lean body mass, 210, 213
Learning, 100 (*see also*
    Teaching/learning):
  assessing own style, 374–75
  change, and, 410
  definition, 357
  independent, 375–76
  learning theories, 365–73
  meditation, and, 366
  philosophy of, 373
  principles of, 371–73
  self-learning modules, 376–77
LeBoyer, Frederick, 15, 116–17
Lecithin, 204
Levinson, Daniel, 99
Lewin, Kurt, 411
Life change index, 16
Life course, 99
Life cycle, 99
Life Events and Illness Index,
    157–59
Life processes, 22, 23
  caring, 26, 69–96
  communication, 28, 279–309
  human development, 26–27,
    97–132
  leadership and change, 30,
    396–435
  lifestyling, 27–28, 171–278

Nutrition, Health, and Activity
Profile, 16, 156, 450–71